The medical enlightenment of the eighteenth century

The medical enlightenment of the eighteenth century

Edited by
ANDREW CUNNINGHAM
and
ROGER FRENCH
Wellcome Unit for the History of Medicine,
University of Cambridge

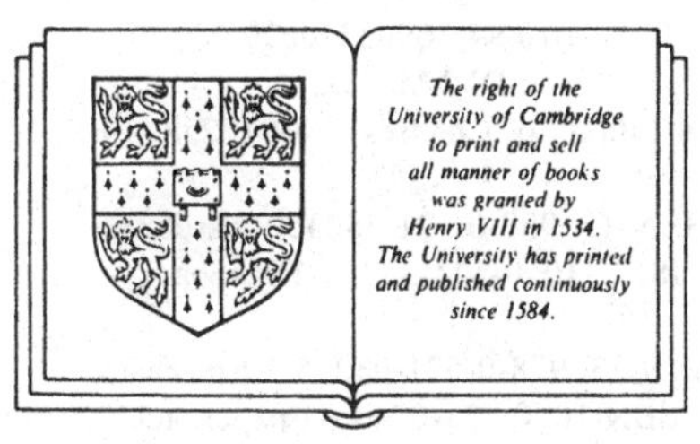

CAMBRIDGE UNIVERSITY PRESS
Cambridge
New York Port Chester
Melbourne Sydney

CAMBRIDGE UNIVERSITY PRESS
Cambridge, New York, Melbourne, Madrid, Cape Town, Singapore, São Paulo

Cambridge University Press
The Edinburgh Building, Cambridge CB2 2RU, UK

Published in the United States of America by Cambridge University Press, New York

www.cambridge.org
Information on this title: www.cambridge.org/9780521382359

First published 1990
This digitally printed first paperback version 2006

A catalogue record for this publication is available from the British Library

Library of Congress Cataloguing in Publication data

The medical enlightenment of the eighteenth century / edited by Andrew
Cunningham and Roger French.
p. cm. – (History of medicine)
Includes index.
ISBN 0-521-38235-1
1. Medicine – Europe – History – 18th century. 2. Medicine – Great
Britain – History – 18th century. I. Cunningham. Andrew.
II. French. R.K. (Roger Kenneth) III. Series: History of medicine
(Cambridge. England)
[DNLM 1. History of Medicine. 18th century. 2. History of
Medicine. 18th century – Great Britain. WZ 70 FA1 M33]
R148.M36 1990
610 94-109033–dc20
DNLM/DLC
For Library of Congress 89-17258 CIP

ISBN-13 978-0-521-38235-9 hardback
ISBN-10 0-521-38235-1 hardback

ISBN-13 978-0-521-03095-3 paperback
ISBN-10 0-521-03095-1 paperback

Contents

List of illustrations *page* vii
List of tables ix
Preface xi

Introduction 1
1 The politics of medical improvement in early Hanoverian London 4
ADRIAN WILSON
2 Medicine to calm the mind: Boerhaave's medical system, and why it was adopted in Edinburgh 40
ANDREW CUNNINGHAM
3 Georg Ernst Stahl's radical Pietist medicine and its influence on the German Enlightenment 67
JOHANNA GEYER-KORDESCH
4 Sickness and the soul: Stahl, Hoffman and Sauvages on pathology 88
ROGER FRENCH
5 Sauvages's nosology: medical enlightenment in Montpellier 111
JULIAN MARTIN
6 Honour and property: the structure of professional disputes in eighteenth-century English medicine 138
DAVID HARLEY
7 Medicine, morality and the politics of Berkeley's tar-water 165
MARINA BENJAMIN

8 North America, a western outpost of European medicine 194
HELEN BROCK

9 John Haygarth, smallpox and religious Dissent in eighteenth-century England 217
FRANCIS M. LOBO

10 'Living in the light': dispensaries, philanthropy and medical reform in late-eighteenth-century London 254
ROBERT KILPATRICK

11 Measuring virtue: eudiometry, enlightenment and pneumatic medicine 281
SIMON SCHAFFER

Index 319

Illustrations

PLATES *page*

1 Title-page of Herman Boerhaave, *De Comparando Certo in Physicis* (Leyden, 1715); Wellcome Institute Library, London, reproduced by permission 52

2 Title-page of Herman Boerhaave, *Sermo Academicus de Chemia Suos Errores Expurgante* (Leyden, 1718); reproduced by permission of the Syndics of Cambridge University Library 53

3 The Rt. Revd George Berkeley, Bishop of Cloyne, from a painting by Vanderbank, *c.* 1735, known only from an engraving by W. Skelton, 1800; reproduced by permission of the Governors and Guardians of Marsh's Library, Dublin 193

4 Title-page of John Haygarth, *A Sketch of a Plan to Exterminate the Casual Small-pox from Great Britain* (London, 1793); reproduced by permission of the Syndics of Cambridge University Library 246

5 Title-page of the second edition of John Haygarth, *An Inquiry How to Prevent the Small-pox* (London, 1801); reproduced by permission of the Cambridge Philosophical Society 250

6 Table from the second edition of John Haygarth, *An Inquiry How to Prevent the Small-pox* (London, 1801); reproduced by permission of the Cambridge Philosophical Society 251

7 Title-page of M. Landriani, *Ricerche fisiche intorno alla salubrità dell'aria* (Milan, 1775), Wellcome Institute Library, London, reproduced by permission 297

8 First page of M. Landriani, *Ricerche fisiche intorno alla salubrità dell'aria* (Milan, 1775); Wellcome Institute Library, London, reproduced by permission 298

9 Table 2 from M. Landriani, *Ricerche fisiche intorno alla salubrità dell'aria* (Milan, 1775); Wellcome Institute Library, London, reproduced by permission 299

10 Table 4 from Felice Fontana, *Descrizione e usi di alcuni stromenti* (Florence, 1775); reproduced by permission of the Royal Society, London 303

FIGURE

General structure of voluntary hospitals 12

Tables

page
1 Westminster Infirmary: select early chronology 17
2 Founders of the Westminster Charitable Society, 1716 and 1719 22
3 The promotion of smallpox inoculation by public experiments, 1721–2 28
4 Politico-religious allegiance and attitudes to inoculation, 1721–46 30
5 Morbi evacuatoria 126
6 Classificatory changes within a class of diseases 128

Preface

The title of this volume should serve to link it with two other volumes in an informal series on the history of medicine published by Cambridge University Press: *The Medical Renaissance of the Sixteenth Century*, edited by A. Wear, R. K. French and I. M. Lonie (1985), and *The Medical Revolution of the Seventeenth Century*, edited by Roger French and Andrew Wear (1989).

With the exception of David Harley from Oxford, all the contributors are, or were, members of the Wellcome Unit for the History of Medicine at Cambridge University, or of the Department of the History and Philosophy of Science at Cambridge.

We would like to thank the Wellcome Trust for their generous support of the conference from which this volume arose.

We dedicate the volume to the memory of a former colleague and outstanding scholar, Iain Lonie.

Introduction

The eighteenth century has been relatively neglected by English-speaking historians of medicine. This is perhaps understandable, given its position between the twin peaks of the so-called 'Scientific Revolution' of the seventeenth century on the one hand, and the triumphs of 'scientific medicine' – the clinic and the laboratory – of the nineteenth century on the other. French and German historians of medicine, by contrast, have long seen the eighteenth century as a period of great change in medicine: as part of that great intellectual blossoming known as the Enlightenment. This volume is an attempt to help redress the balance, and renew interest in the far-reaching changes in medicine which occurred during the century of the Enlightenment.

The term 'Enlightenment' corresponds to terms coined and used at the time, particularly by Voltaire (*siècle des lumières*) and Kant (*Aufklärung*), and is a valuable concept to convey the radical intellectual switch which happened during the eighteenth century: from a world where Revelation was still the highest form of truth, to one where Reason had dethroned Revelation. A secular world, with secular values, replaced a religious world with religious values. People came to believe that Superstition had been replaced by Reason. Authority, the new Rationalists claimed, was no longer to be venerated simply because it was old. Enlightenment thinkers, such as Voltaire, Diderot and Condillac, based their thinking largely on the natural-philosophical and philosophical work of Isaac Newton and John Locke, and claimed that society could only be happy and stable if it was structured and operated in accordance with the operations of Natural Law, and that – happily – Natural Law was accessible to man in a way that divine law was not. Even rulers, such as Frederick the Great and Catherine the Great, became enlightened by Reason, 'enlightened despots', seeking to run their states according to rational principles and Natural Law.

Such radical changes in attitudes were reflected in and affected the medicine of the period; in medicine too there was an 'Enlightenment'. There was a renunciation of authorities: Galen, venerated as the prime medical authority since antiquity, now ceased to be held in esteem. Instead, every man became his own authority, and there was a proliferation of people offering new medical 'systems'. The religious dimension of traditional medical theory came to be downplayed. The soul became less a subject of central concern when dealing with the body, and the body came to be seen less as the 'instrument' of the soul and more in mechanistic terms, simply as a machine operating according to natural laws and with all its operations open to being numbered, weighed and measured. 'Psychology', a term whose old meaning was to do with the operations of the soul (*psyche*), came to be about the operations (and loss) of *reason*, and hence madness became a new subject of medical fascination and intervention. The *anima* (the Latin equivalent of *psyche*), which had been held responsible for 'animating' animal and human bodies and producing their gross actions, all but vanished from the discussions of medical men. Its place was taken by 'mechanism': the necessary transfer of motion through a set of physical structures. *Pneuma*, the self-mobile, quasi-material 'spirit' of earlier centuries, gave its name to a new university discipline of 'pneumatology', which occupied the space of the old soul and spirits, and which was welded to a deistic metaphysics and a necessitarian Natural Law. The God whose justice had visited disease upon the wicked became the 'Author' of a regulated and rational world. In this world the doctor could now expand his activities into new areas. The rational doctor, pursuing also his new interest as a 'professional', increasingly came to offer an interventionalist medicine and to medicalise normal life. Hospitals for the very first time in history became commonplace, filled with the poor on whom the physician and surgeon could demonstrate, practise and teach in the name of 'philanthropy', dispassionate love of mankind. Childbirth, and this too was for the very first time in history, came to be treated as a primarily medical rather than a natural event, whose dangers could only be circumvented by the skills of a male practitioner.

The causes of all the intellectual changes in this period lie of course outside categories of 'Enlightenment', 'Progress' and 'Reason'. They lie instead in certain great dynamic changes in the economic and political structure of eighteenth-century Europe, which culminated in the downfall of the absolute governments which had failed to meet the expectations of their people or of their burgeoning bourgeoisies. It all exploded in the French Revolution, itself fuelled by Enlightenment ideas and ideals which even 'enlightened despots' could not meet. Ultimately the bourgeoisie were to replace the aristocrats in power. In this light, the improvements in medicine that we are here embracing under the title of 'the medical Enlightenment' may be seen as some of the first effects of the new, professionalising, middle class bringing their more secular values and interests to bear on the traditional domain of medicine.

Almost half of the chapters in the present book deal with the most free country of eighteenth-century Europe, Britain, the country whose bourgeoisie least needed to displace their political ambitions into purely intellectual endeavours, and which thus (it is sometimes claimed) hardly qualifies as having had an 'Enlightenment' at all. But Britain was certainly the model to which many continental Enlightenment thinkers looked and to which they aspired. The active, participatory political arena was one place in Britain where issues of health and medicine were fought over publicly. And in Britain, it was the non-enfranchised part of the bourgeoisie who played the most active role in innovations: those Protestants who 'dissented' from the doctrines and disciplines of the Church of England, and who thus disqualified themselves from state employ. They busied themselves with philanthropy, industry and medical improvements.

The chronological arrangement of the chapters in the present volume enables one to follow in the case of medicine some of the changes typical of the 'Enlightenment': the change from the religious to the secular world; the change from a real concern with the soul as medically active, to the mathematical measurement of 'virtue'; and the change from the closed world of the doctor–patient relationship, to ambitious schemes of rational social planning to eliminate diseases once and for all. We hope that the studies in this book will contribute to awareness and appreciation of the importance of the great changes in medicine in the century of Enlightenment.

1

The politics of medical improvement in early Hanoverian London

ADRIAN WILSON

EIGHTEENTH-CENTURY 'IMPROVEMENT' AND MEDICINE

How does medical history fit into history at large – into 'general' or 'political' or 'social' history? The history disciplines themselves both imply and construct an answer: the relationship is the non-relationship of parallel stories, linked only by the fact that they inhabit the dimension of time. We have a sub-discipline called medical history, with its own sources, methods, topics, problems and concerns; this is more or less walled off from that series of other sub-disciplines which together comprise mainstream academic history – political, social and economic history. These in turn are to some extent sealed off from each other; so too a similar hermetic quality is to be found in all the sub-disciplines, such as ecclesiastical history, history of art, history of science. Worst of all, perhaps, is the fate of the study of what is deemed literature: hived off into an entirely separate discipline. What historians have sundered, let no woman or man put together again: there are

Editors' note. The term 'whig' and its derivatives are used in this chapter in two senses. One (whig, whiggery), to refer to the Whig political party and its values; this is to be contrasted with 'Tory'. Two (whig, whiggish), to refer to a certain kind of history-writing in which the criteria for deciding what counts as 'interesting' and what constituted 'success' or 'progress' in the past, are drawn from the criteria of what counts as 'interesting', 'success' or 'progress' *in the present*; on this usage see Herbert Butterfield, *The Whig Interpretation of History* (London, 1931).

Acknowledgements: The research for this paper was supported by the generosity of the Wellcome Trust. Manuscript and printed sources were consulted in the Greater London Record Office; the British Library; the Wellcome Institute Library; and Cambridge University Library. I am grateful to the staffs of all these institutions for their help. From 1983 to 1986 I was fortunate to have the opportunity to teach on these topics in the Wellcome Unit for the History of Medicine, Cambridge. Participants in the discussion at the 1987 conference, especially David Harley, offered valuable comments. For detailed advice I wish to thank Jonathan Clark, Mark Goldie, Gill Hudson, Robert Kilpatrick and Julian Martin. Craig Rose and Simon Schaffer have given me extended help in the course of many valuable discussions. Finally, I am particularly grateful to Andrew Cunningham for several years of generous encouragement, stimulation and advice in the exploration of the themes treated in this paper.

many individual examples of the transcending of these barriers, yet these remain isolated examples which have little or no effect on the structure of the discipline. Thus even when eighteenth-century English history is hotted up by recent fierce debate, the battle has been conducted largely on the traditional high-ground of political history, with only occasional side-glances elsewhere.[1]

Most of my own research concerns early-eighteenth-century England. One of the striking characteristics of that society was the vast and profound influence exercised by its capital, the metropolis of London, a concentration of population which when set against its hinterland had no parallel or precedent in European history. (Paris had more inhabitants, but could not compare with London's astonishing share of its nation's population – something approaching 10 per cent.) The complex threads of trade, migration, politics and propaganda tied even the remotest parts of the kingdom to London. The social history of London in the eighteenth century, then, must comprise a very important part of English, indeed British, history at large.

Historiographically, one work has now towered over this field for over sixty years: Dorothy George's *London Life in the Eighteenth Century*.[2] Published in 1925, that book was to prove the most enduring and successful monument to the labours of the remarkable 'first wave' of English women historians – the circle including Eileen Power and Alice Clark, and centring around the influence of the redoubtable Olive Schreiner.[3] George's study was an extraordinary *tour de force*, a commanding survey of many aspects of eighteenth-century London life (from the family to the economy) and, no less so, of the vast pamphlet literature of the period. To this day no challenge has been mounted to George's synthesis, and it is not difficult to see why: the terrain she covered remains dauntingly vast. I doubt whether any historian since has read a tenth of the materials she covered: the Old Bailey Sessions Papers (almost her sole manuscript source); the Bills of Mortality; the writings of Hanway, Fielding, Place, Colquhoun, and a host of less eminent reformers, projectors and improvers; and dozens

[1] I refer to the debate opened up by J. C. D. Clark, *English Society 1688–1832: Ideology, Social Structure and Political Practice during the Ancien Régime* (Cambridge, 1985). For a discussion of the implications of what has been called 'tunnel history' see T. G. Ashplant and Adrian Wilson, 'Present-Centred History and the Problem of Historical Knowledge', *The Historical Journal* 31 (1988), pp. 253–74.

[2] M. Dorothy George, *London Life in the Eighteenth Century* (London, 1925; Harmondsworth, 1966).

[3] See the discussion by Jane Lewis in Miranda Chaytor and Jane Lewis, 'Introduction' to Alice Clark, *Working Life of Women in the Seventeenth Century* (London, 1982, reprint of 1919 first edition).

of tracts concerning the regulation of wages, the administration of the Poor Law, the constructing of hospitals, the managing of police – and even medicine. In its breadth and intensity, her study is reminiscent of the writings of her equally daunting predecessors, Sydney and Beatrice Webb. These days, few historians even consider tackling topics of this scale.

What place did medicine find in this remarkable synthesis? The answer can be given in a single word: *improvement*. In this respect medicine simply exemplified George's wider themes: the story she told was precisely one of 'improvement' across a vast social terrain: improvements in housing, in lighting, in hygiene, in the care of children, in policing, in prisons, in diet. Down to roughly the mid-century, conditions were squalid and crowded and probably worsening; thereafter, a series of schemes for improvement brought about a gradual, but eventually massive, amelioration. In some spheres of life there would be a temporary decline – for instance, an 'epidemic of gin-drinking' in the 1720s and 1730s, or the massive abandonment of children when the Foundling Hospital's doors were temporarily thrown open between 1756 and 1760. But each such instance brought about the appropriate response: the Gin Act of 1736 and the restriction of Foundling Hospital admissions in 1760. In some contexts there were schemes for improvement at an unusually early date – as, for instance, in the parish of St James Westminster, with its workhouse, infirmary and provision for lying-in women, all evident by 1732; other parishes lagged far behind, yet a variety of supra-parochial initiatives eventually spread such benefits across the capital. Thus the story of improvement was by no means simultaneous or geographically homogeneous. Yet that story was indeed the general pattern; and in broad terms, the mid-century marked a watershed. Most of George's central improving characters – Hanway, Fielding, Colquhoun and Howard – were active after 1750.

It would be going far beyond my present brief to offer that general critique of George's work which remains wanting from the historical profession as a whole. Not until we have become able to mount such a critique, I suggest, will we be able to move beyond George's achievement and thus to build constructively on the foundations she laid: as long as we remain mesmerised by her achievement, our horizons will remain defined by her problematic. Thus the task of appraising George's study cannot properly be attempted here. Nevertheless, if we are to move forward at all, we must make some attempt to characterise the boundaries of her approach, the limits of her problematic; and in this spirit three observations are in order. First, it is striking that for George, the process of 'improvement' she chronicled in such detail never posed an *explanatory* problem. The need for improvement, in her eyes, was self-evident: squalor itself begat the schemes for its abolition; the Hanways and the Fieldings emerged, so to speak, by spontaneous generation from the filth and disorder, the crime and the uncertainty, of London. Given Gin Lane, we have Hogarth, and given Hogarth, we have the Gin Act; a logical necessity generated amelioration. Second, the towering absence in George's book is the sphere of *politics*. One would never have guessed from her study that eighteenth-century London was riven by political faction; that Jacobites plotted in coffee-houses; that the charity schools were the arena not only of education but also of faction; that this was the city where the cry 'Wilkes and Liberty' brought tens of thousands onto the streets in the 1760s; that here, a generation later, the first Corresponding Society came into being. This should begin to trouble us when we notice that some of these phenomena impinged directly on George's own themes. We see this at the beginning of the century with the charity schools, and at the end with the fact that Francis Place – George's most favoured observer – was heavily involved in the London Corresponding Society and in later schemes for electoral reform, culminating of course in Chartism. Strangely enough, George's idea of social history turns out to conform remarkably well to the definition offered by her near-contemporary G. M. Trevelyan: 'history with the politics left out'.[4] Is it not curious that we now remember Trevelyan's description only with amusement, yet we continue to be held in thrall by George's study, which in fact embodies that very definition at work?

A third observation concerns George's source materials. I am not suggesting that the historian is the passive prisoner of her or his sources: on the contrary, the historian constitutes the sources, above all by selecting them. And George's selection, as we have already noticed in passing, was overwhelmingly concentrated upon printed materials. Now these materials – the pamphlets and accounts which George used on such a massive scale – have this in common: they were *appeals* for public support. The printed pamphlet was an intervention in a market-place: what was at stake was support, both political and financial, for the given scheme of improvement, whether it be the raising of a tax on spirituous liquors, or the marshalling of a more effective police force, or the preservation of the lives of parish children.

[4] G. M. Trevelyan, *English Social History* (London, 1944), p. vii.

Any such scheme for improvement began as the plan or dream of a small and select group – sometimes, indeed, of a single individual – and then had to mobilise wider support. The pamphlet literature was precisely the means by which that mobilisation was brought about. Now in order to achieve this, the pamphleteer was subject to one cardinal rule: he or she (it was usually he) had to present the given scheme as having universal benefits or, to be more precise, benefits universal amongst the intended audience, that is, the politically and financially active class. And this had two general effects. First, there was a rigorous suppression of any *particular* interest which lay behind the given scheme. The key to success was precisely presenting interests as general: thus, for instance, in propounding a Tory scheme for a workhouse, the pamphleteer would carefully conceal the party provenance of the initiative. Secondly, and relatedly, there was developed a specific rhetoric for such appeals: the rhetoric of 'improvement'. It was the concept of improvement which permitted the eighteenth-century projector or reformer to couch his (or, rarely, her) scheme in a language of potentially universal appeal. 'Improvement' seized the moral high ground: opponents could appear as the obstructors of progress. Thus the medium of print and the market-place for support inexorably pulled the language of the pamphlets in the direction of 'improvement'.

These three aspects of George's work were inextricably bound together. The vocabulary of improvement gave her an instant rapport with a certain set of source materials – for that vocabulary, taken up and developed by nineteenth-century progressives, remained in force for George's own generation and precisely for her own intellectual circle. George's own indifference to party-political themes found ample confirmation in the pamphlets' concealment of the particular interests which had given rise to their various schemes. And this happy collusion between the historian and her materials was what excluded explanatory questions from the historiographic agenda: identification, such as George's identification with Hanway or Fielding, does not breed the curiosity which alone can provoke the search for a causal explanation. George's eighteenth-century London became an early-twentieth-century England writ onto an earlier canvas: a struggle for social improvements, not so much against the forces of reaction as against the forces of poverty. Amelioration was neither a class cause nor a party cause, but the cause of humanity itself; if there was a central enemy, this comprised not a specific political force or set of forces but rather a set of living conditions with their associated products of poverty, overcrowding, dirt and disease. Hence perhaps George's particular vision: a massive humanity deployed without a political cutting-edge.

The corollary of this analysis is that if we wish to discover the social causes of the process of 'improvement', we must dissolve the boundary between political and social history; and we must either turn to different sources from those George used, or else find a different way of reading such public appeals. The key, I suggest, is the identification of *interests*. Projects for 'improvement' may appear to the twentieth-century historian – of George's day or our own – to look forward to the future; yet their genesis lay in the past, in the specific constellations of interests which brought such projects into being. To specify the particular interests at work in any given case is to reinsert the scheme in question back into its original context. In this chapter I shall be attempting a series of exercises in this spirit.

As we have seen, medicine was one of the spheres of George's 'improvement': her first specific theme in fact was 'life and death in London', and the improvement in this sphere (evidenced from the Bills of Mortality) could be attributed not only to changes in living conditions but also to advances in medicine. Those advances, like most other aspects of improvement, were most marked after the mid-century; the early decades of the eighteenth century represented the more or less stagnant ground-level against which the post-1750 takeoff could be favourably compared. In this respect George's picture of eighteenth-century medicine anticipated a much later minor classic of whiggish medical history: Le Fanu's 1972 paper bearing the revealing title, 'The Lost Half-Century in English medicine, 1700–1750'.[5] If we were to take either George or, especially, Le Fanu as our guide, we would come to the conclusion that early-eighteenth-century English medicine was a vast lacuna between the heroic ages which preceded and succeeded the calm, not to say the tedium, of this so-called 'Augustan age'. Le Fanu's account is an edifice of negatives: Arbuthnot 'contributed no new knowledge'; he and Radcliffe were 'unprogressive physicians' who 'made almost no advance towards deeper understanding of disease and its treatment'; it was a 'quiescent period', a 'pause' in history; medical men 'made little effort to devise new techniques'; 'advanced medical teaching . . . was sadly wanting'; there was 'no interest in experimentation', and 'a similar neglect of instruments'; it was a 'barren age' marked by a general 'lack of urgency'. By the end of his paper Le Fanu's

[5] William R. Le Fanu, 'The Lost Half-Century in English Medicine, 1700–1750', *Bulletin of the History of Medicine* 46 (1972), pp. 319–48. I quote below from pp. 321, 322, 323, 330, 334, 335, 340, 343, 345 and 348.

rhetoric became even stronger: from 'almost no advance' it had shifted to 'no real advance'. Physicians, he concluded, like divines, 'wrote pietistic, tranquilising books'. In sum, this was 'an empty age'.

It is strange to reflect that it took Le Fanu some thousands of words merely to summarise the many non-events, as he saw them, of this 'lost half-century'. Stranger still is the fact that many of the post-1750 improvements which he (like George) recognised and celebrated, actually had well-known roots in pre-1750 developments. This chapter is devoted to three of these medical themes: the creation of voluntary hospitals; the adoption of inoculation for smallpox; and the rise of man-midwifery. In each of these cases, it is beyond dispute that crucial advances took place well before 1750. In each case, again, it is widely accepted that the given 'improvement' had major long-term consequences. Those consequences have attracted considerable historiographic interest; but to the best of my knowledge, no historian has ever seriously asked what were the *causes* of these three advances. It is precisely as we turn from effects to causes that we will begin to explore – that is, to *find* – the 'lost half-century' from 1700 to 1750. One of my purposes here will be to demonstrate that this period was not barren, but creative; not dull, but exciting; not an ocean of consensus but rather a whirlpool of conflict. In short, this will be an invitation to historians to investigate further what is probably the most neglected period in English medicine after 1600. The interest of that period is by no means confined to those spheres where we can demonstrate, by whiggish criteria, a permanent 'advance', a piece of 'improvement'. But against the historiographic background I have been outlining, it is surely best to start by putting this period on the map of what is whiggishly interesting. Hence the choice of the three particular case-studies to which I shall now turn.

VOLUNTARY HOSPITALS: THE ORIGINS OF THE WESTMINSTER INFIRMARY

The voluntary hospitals were amongst the most important permanent institutions produced by Hanoverian England. They comprised a new kind of philanthropy, financed by voluntary subscriptions (hence the term 'voluntary' to describe them); they constructed a new political space for the practice of medicine; and as a result they produced and fostered many new medical initiatives in the eighteenth century and afterwards. Through their impact on the French hospital reformer Jacques Tenon they may have contributed indirectly to the Paris 'birth of the clinic'; and they were certainly the site of an independent London medical revolution along similar lines.[6] Their founding is usually described as a 'movement', and it was certainly a large-scale development: by 1750 there were seventeen of them in England, when in 1718 there had been none. We can distinguish three types of voluntary hospital: London general hospitals (the first to be founded); provincial general hospitals (beginning with the Winchester County Hospital in 1736); and London specialist hospitals (such as the Lock Hospital for venereal disease and the Smallpox Inoculation Hospital, both founded in 1746).

In order to grasp the way these institutions operated, it is easiest to proceed from a particular example. The figure sets out the organisation of the Lying-in Hospital in Brownlow Street (established in 1749), some six or seven years after its foundation.[7] First, it is no accident that the people at the centre of the diagram are neither doctors nor patients, but rather the subscribers. It was these men and women – mostly men – who usually started the institution and who always maintained it by their annual donations, typically of a guinea or more. The subscribers appointed the medical staff; a committee of the subscribers supervised the running of the hospital; and last, but not least, the subscribers had the role of recommending prospective patients for admission. For a poor man or woman, the month or two spent in a voluntary hospital was a massive subsidy from his or her social superiors, and thus there was never any shortage of would-be patients. But in order to get admitted, the prospective patient had to be recommended by an individual subscriber; and thus this form of charity reinforced the power of the elite by enabling them to dispense

[6] For Tenon see C. C. Gillispie, *Science and Polity in France at the End of the Old Regime* (Princeton, 1980), pp. 254–7. On the transformation of the Paris hospitals and its effects, see Michel Foucault, *The Birth of the Clinic*, trans. A. M. Sheridan (London, 1973). London developments are discussed in Robert Kilpatrick's 1989 Cambridge Ph.D. thesis, entitled 'Nature's Schools: The Hunterian Revolution in London Hospital Medicine, 1780–1825'. The voluntary hospital movement as a whole has been reviewed by John Woodward, *To Do the Sick No Harm* (London, 1974); David E. Owen, *English Philanthropy 1660–1960* (Cambridge, MA, 1965), pp. 36–57; and A. Delbert Evans and L. G. Redmond Howard, *The Romance of the British Voluntary Hospital Movement* (London, n.d.). For brief but very perceptive comments see Charles Webster, 'The Crisis of the Hospitals During the Industrial Revolution' in E. G. Forbes (ed.), *Human Implications of Scientific Advance* (Edinburgh, 1978), pp. 214–23; and Roger French, 'Disease, Theory and Practice in a Voluntary Hospital' in F. M. Ricci (ed.), *A Social History of the Biomedical Sciences* (Milan, in press).

[7] The diagram is based on *An Account of the Rise, Progress and State of the British Lying-in Hospital for Married Women, Situated in Brownlow-Street, Long-Acre, from its Institution in November, 1749 to Lady-Day, 1756* (London, 1756). It was from this date that the hospital took the name 'British'. Details varied: thus this hospital's perpetual Presidency seems not to have been typical.

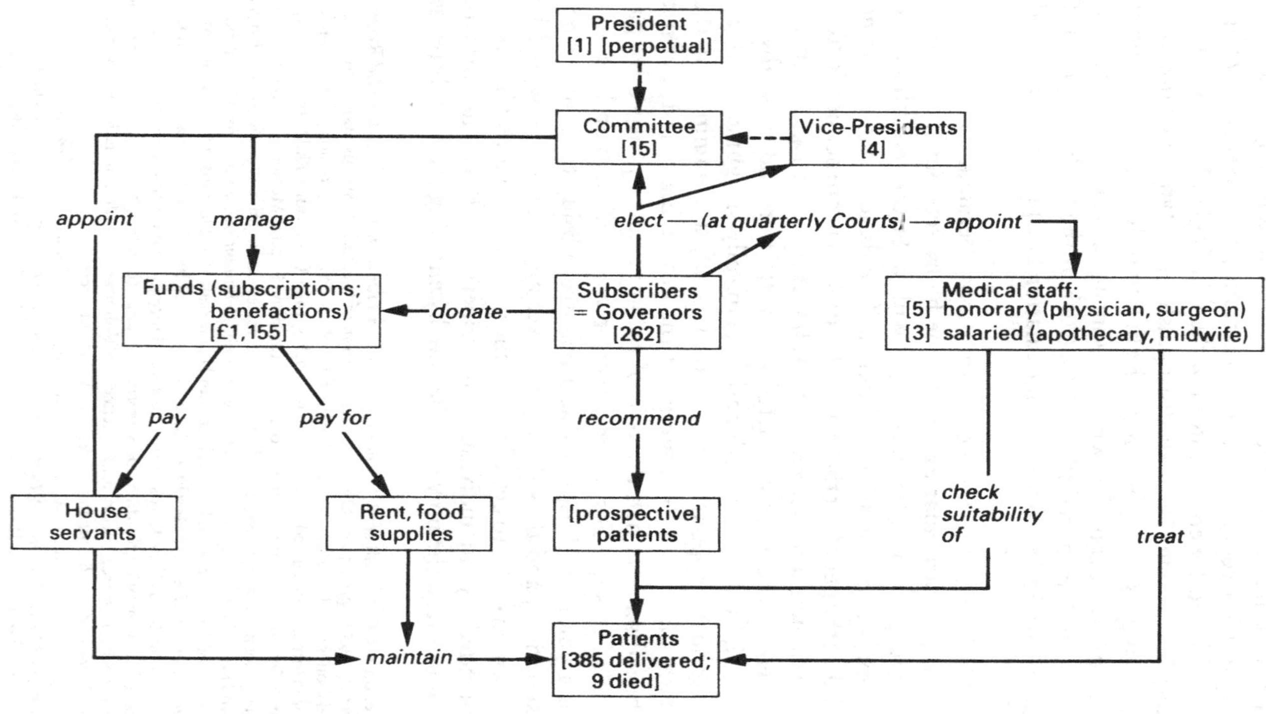

General structure of voluntary hospitals, illustrated by the particular case of the Lying-in Hospital, Brownlow Street, with [numbers] as for 1755–6

selectively a new form of largesse. The subscribers, then, were at the hub of the whole institution. The second important point which emerges from the figure is how *small* these institutions were. The Brownlow Street lying-in hospital was thriving, yet it had an annual budget of barely £1,000; it delivered fewer than 400 patients; and there were only 262 subscribers. Against this we have to remember that the potential number of subscribers in London at this time would have been comfortably of the order of 10,000.[8] This in turn has two important corollaries. For one thing, would-be founders did not need to convert a vast mass of people to their point of view; all that was required was to recruit a few hundred supporters. For another, despite the apparent popularity of the voluntary-hospital 'movement', the fact is that this was a *minority* activity amongst the London elite at this period. This becomes still more true if we focus not on the mass of subscribers but on the much smaller core of key activists who ran any given voluntary hospital, and who probably recruited many of their more passive fellow-subscribers. Each voluntary hospital was in practice the result of dedicated activity by a small and probably close-knit group of philanthropic individuals.

Against this background we can begin to open up the explanatory question as to why these institutions were founded. The voluntary hospitals resulted, not from the general interest of the elite, but rather from the particular interests of specific groups within that elite. The way forward in our understanding of these institutions must begin by identifying the interests involved. For the mass of subscribers this is no easy matter; but the leading individuals are often relatively easy to identify in standard sources, which enables each given institution to be located on the complex politico-religious map of interests in this period. Here is an attractive and important field for research; so far as I am aware, every one of these London voluntary hospitals still awaits study in these terms.

I have suggested that it was the subscribers who were the founders, as well as the managers, of these institutions. In fact the voluntary hospitals came into being in three distinct ways. Most usual was for a group of lay subscribers to get together and set up such an institution: such was the case with the very first of the voluntary hospitals, the Westminster Infirmary, as we shall see in a moment. But secondly,

[8] A guesstimate, based on a London population of over 500,000; assuming a household size of about 5, i.e., 100,000 families; allowing 10 per cent of these families to have the wealth required to subscribe to a voluntary hospital; and assuming only one subscriber per household. The latter two assumptions are almost certainly very conservative; relaxing these, we might estimate a pool of potential subscribers of the order of 20,000 or even more.

some such institutions arose by a process of splitting: a group of subscribers would secede from a hospital through some disagreement within the ranks. Such a process is illustrated by St George's, the second of the London voluntary hospitals, which split off from the Westminster in 1733. Thirdly, it sometimes happened that a medical man was the first initiator, such as John Harrison who set up the third such institution in London, the London Hospital, in 1740. He would of course have to mobilise a group of subscribers in order to achieve this, which reinforces the key role of subscribers; nevertheless this comprised a distinct style of foundation. The third route was subsequently responsible for two of the four London lying-in hospitals: the General (founded in 1752 by Felix Macdonogh) and the Westminster New Lying-in Hospital (set up by John Leake in 1767).[9]

Finally, in considering the character of these institutions, we must attend to the complex and specific *relations of power* which obtained within them. Here, although the role of the hospital's paid servants is also important, the key issue concerns the triangular relationship between subscribers, medical practitioners and patients. The medical practitioners served in two very different capacities. On the one hand, the physician (and in most cases the surgeon) gave his advice gratis; on the other hand, most hospitals had a salaried apothecary (rarely, a surgeon) who of course was part of the staff of servants. For the physician the rewards of the honorary post were considerable: not only would his name be printed in the published appeals of the hospital, thus instantly advertising his good charitable name to a prospective clientele of elite patients, but also the hospitals served increasingly as a site for teaching. Moreover, and this applied to the salaried apothecary as well, the hospital made it possible to experiment on the patients. Experimentation and teaching were both rooted in the same crucial fact, that voluntary hospitals created a new and distinctive political environment for medical practice. In the patronage-dominated world of eighteenth-century England, where one success or failure with an aristocratic patient had more implications than a dozen countervailing experiences with less affluent patients, the medical man was necessar-

[9] See, for St George's, G. C. Peachey, *The History of St. George's Hospital* (London, 1910–14); for the London, A. E. Clark-Kennedy, *The London: A Study in the Voluntary Hospital System* (London, 1962); for the General Lying-in Hospital, *An Account of the Rise, Progress, and State of the General Lying-in Hospital, the Corner of Quebec-Street, Oxford-Road* (London, 1768) and Jean Donnison, 'Note on the Foundation of Queen Charlotte's Hospital' *Medical History* 15 (1971), pp. 398–400 ('Queen Charlotte's' was the name later given to the General Lying-in Hospital). The Westminster New Lying-in Hospital is the subject of Philip Rhodes, *Doctor John Leake's Hospital* (London, 1977); confusingly, this became known as the 'General Lying-in Hospital'.

ily deferential towards his patients.[10] But in the voluntary hospitals the possibility was opened of far greater medical authority over the patient: hence the use of patients as raw material for experimentation and teaching. Nevertheless the subscribers could intervene to prohibit or to limit such practices; the medical man was not wholly free from the dictates of patronage. The voluntary hospital was not simply a medical space, nor merely a charitable space; rather, it comprised a *medico-charitable* space, whose interior practices and events were governed *both* by the lay subscribers *and* by medical men. The corollary is that throughout the history of the voluntary hospitals there ran a recurrent, though intermittent, theme of tension between medical men and lay subscribers. Each group wanted power; conflict between the two groups thus inevitably flared up from time to time. A simple instance of this is the fact that when a *minority* of the subscribers of the Westminster seceded in 1733 to form St George's, *all* the medical staff (both honorary and salaried) went off to the new institution, leaving the Westminster in the position of having to recruit an entirely new medical staff. Nor did this end the conflict: only a few years later, a struggle arose within St George's itself over the wish of some of the medical men to perform experiments on their patients.[11]

By now it should be clear that the founding of the Westminster Infirmary in 1719 was crucially important. Not only was this the first of the voluntary hospitals; it was also the parent of the second, since St George's was created in 1733 as a split-off from the Westminster. Thus in terms of London general hospitals, the voluntary-hospital 'movement' in its first two decades – from 1718 to 1739 – in fact consisted of the history of this single institution and, after 1733, its offspring. Thus the origins of the Westminster Infirmary command attention, not just as one case-study amongst the many that need to be carried out, but as the birth of the voluntary-hospital movement as a whole.

The origins of the Westminster Infirmary lay in the meetings of just four men, calling themselves 'the Charitable Society', between January and May 1716. The meetings lapsed thereafter for over three years, whereupon they suddenly resumed – with an enlarged and somewhat different personnel – in December 1719. From the latter date the

[10] See N. D. Jewson, 'Medical Knowledge and the Patronage System in Eighteenth-century England', *Sociology* 8 (1974), pp. 369–85. Recently Jewson's neglected argument has been taken up and developed in a highly fruitful way by Malcolm Nicolson, 'The Metastatic theory of Pathogenesis and the Professional Interests of the Eighteenth-Century Physician', *Medical History* 32 (1988), pp. 277–300.

[11] See Peachey, *History of St George's Hospital* and *HMC Egmont Diary*, vol. 2, *passim*.

society had a permanent existence, and it was at this stage that the actual Infirmary was created. But in order to grasp the origins of the institution, we must attend to both these two phases of founding. Table 1 tabulates the dates of all the 1716 meetings, and goes on to specify some highlights of the post-1719 phase, down to the 1735 move into premises which were to be kept for almost a century.[12]

The Charitable Society of 1716 was intended to be both the seed for wider developments, and the umbrella organisation which would oversee those developments. It was intended:

> to establish particular societies in distant parts of this City . . . who may be mutually helpful and assistant to one another . . . all under the general direction of the Society.

There was no intention of setting up an infirmary. The purpose of the charity was to relieve the sick and needy *in their own homes*, both to supplement and to reinvigorate the Poor Law:

> Notwithstanding the provision settled by our laws and the [assistance of voluntary collections] for the relief of the poor, it is obvious to anyone who walks the streets that [this] is [insufficient], to the great grief of all good men, and the no small reproach of our religion and country . . . How deplorable [then] must the condition be of such persons whose poverty is accompanied with sickness . . . it seems above the power of humane laws to remedy this evil. Nothing but the revival of the true Christian spirit of justice and charity in the persons employed to take care of the poor and the voluntary assistance of others acted by the same spirit . . . can effectually redress the grievances they [the poor] suffer and make their deplorable condition more tolerable and easy to them.

The aim, then, was to infuse a Christian and charitable spirit into the operation of the Poor Law, mainly by force of example. The means proposed for doing this were several, but did not include any mention of an infirmary or hospital. Five activities were put forward: (1) free medical advice for the sick; (2) lodging and nursing for lying-in women; (3) visitation and relief of sick prisoners; (4) the repatriation of sick and destitute foreigners; and lastly (5) 'to take care of the souls of those who are sick and needy as well as of their bodies'.

Conspicuous by its absence amongst these aims and methods is any mention of the 'improvement of physic'. Thus the usual claim, that this group was responding to the recent suggestions of John Bellers (1714),

[12] The following account is based on Greater London Record Office, Westminster Charitable Society/Infirmary, Minutes, vol. 1, *passim*. (The roll of early subscribers to the Society is held in the Westminster City Libraries; this document, which I have not examined systematically, suggests that Whig as well as Tory subscribers and benefactors were recruited in the course of the 1720s. I am grateful to Colin Brooks for drawing my attention to this source.)

Table 1. *Westminster Infirmary: select early chronology*

1716	January 14 February 1, 26 March 5, 12, 20, 26 April 3, 7, 14, 21, 28 May 5	Charitable Society meetings – St Dunstan's Coffee-House, the Strand (except April 7, at Revd Cockburn's house)
	January 14	Cockburn 'desired to draw up a scheme of this design'; a messenger to be found; repositories for gifts-for-sick-poor to be sought.
	February 26	'In order to collect subscriptions some of the Proposals were ordered to be bound . . .'
	March 5	500 copies have been printed by Mr Downing (Hoare)
	20	Hoare declines to be Treasurer; Wogan 'was prevailed upon to accept the same for the first year . . .'
	April 3	Cash crisis; 'resolved to admit no more patients till the contributions come in; and that our principal care be confined to the sick and needy . . . of St Margarets Westminster until it shall please God that our stock increase.' Letter from Dr John Colbatch (to Mrs Frowde, here via Wogan): has seen the proposal, wishes to help, and notes that the City of London has 'several noble foundations to relieve the needy sick', but Westminster has none, 'which is a great reproach to it'.
	April 14	Mr Saville (apparently employed as apothecary) to buy drugs, utensils, a still; Society trying to get hold of Colbatch.
	April 28	Colbatch attends, 'and offered his service . . . gratis'.
	May 5	. . . routine meeting, no hint of discontinuing . . .
1719	December 2	refounding 'after long intermission'
1720	March 23 to April 20	Petty-France house taken (in-patients from 1 May)
1724	March to June 10	Chapel Street house taken instead
1733	June	. . . first moves towards 3rd infirmary . . .
1733	October to	
1734	January	. . . St George's Hospital splits off . . .
1734	January 8 to	
1735	February 24	St James's Street house taken (kept till 1834)

is refuted.[13] Whatever the stimulus for setting up the Charitable Society, this did not come from the Quaker Bellers.

Why did the Society lapse in 1716? One historian has suggested that there was strife between the four original founders, observing that two of them were no longer members when the Society was refounded in 1719.[14] Another possibility, not incompatible with this, is that conflict arose over the suggestion received in April from Dr John Colbatch (mentioned in table 1), which implied that a residential hospital should be set up, that is, a departure from the original aims. Thirdly, there may have been too little response to the public plea for subscriptions: this would certainly have discouraged the original founders. Some subscriptions came in – one of twenty guineas – but neither the number nor the total sums were very great. We shall return to this question later, after considering the political provenance of the Society.

In 1719 it 'pleased Almighty God to stir up the hearts of some persons to revive the charitable design of relieving the sick and needy'. Accordingly they met – at the same venue, St Dunstan's Coffee-House in the Strand – 'to consider of the most proper and effectual methods for putting the same in execution'. Now there were twelve founders – two out of the original group of four, and ten new ones. At this very first meeting of the new group, the Society resolved to set up an infirmary as the means to its charitable ends. Proposals were again published, and this time there was an immediate and sustained response. In the first year, subscriptions to the value of about £200 were received; after four years, income from this source stood at £400 per year. This was mostly made up of small subscriptions – one or two guineas per year – and, as this implies, there were over 100 subscribers by 1723. Meanwhile, the plan of founding an Infirmary had rapidly come to fruition: a house was leased in March 1720 (that is, within four months of the re-founding), and patients were admitted in May of that year. From this point on, the history of the Charitable Society becomes the history of the Westminster Infirmary.

Nevertheless some of the earlier themes persisted; three aspects of the group's activities should particularly be mentioned in this regard.

[13] Woodward, *To Do the Sick No Harm*, pp. 9–11, citing the anonymous study, 'The Origin and Evolution of the Eighteenth-Century Hospital Movement', *The Hospital* 55 (1913–14), pp. 290, 428, 485, 538, 596, 649 and 706. Bellers's idea resembled William Petty's much earlier concept of a 'nosocomium': see Charles Webster, *The Great Instauration: Science, Medicine and Reform in England, 1626–1660* (London, 1975), pp. 293–5.

[14] John Langdon-Davies, *Westminster Hospital: Two Centuries of Voluntary Service* (London, 1949), chapter 1. See also W. G. Spencer, *Westminster Hospital* (London, 1924) and J. G. Humble and Peter Hansell, *Westminster Hospital 1719–1966* (London, 1966).

(1) The Society continued to visit the sick and to give medical advice to non-resident sick and needy people. These were now described as 'out-patients', to distinguish them from those actually admitted to the Infirmary; and they were now expected to turn up at the Infirmary each week. Nonetheless this represents a continuation of what the Society had been doing before an Infirmary was ever mentioned. (2) The Society continued to operate at two levels, the parochial and the supra-parochial. Before the first house was taken, it was made clear (by a special order relating to persons from other parishes) that the infirmary was primarily designed to meet the needs of St Margaret's Westminster – the parish in which it was situated, and the same parish to which the Society had decided to confine its efforts in 1716 (see table 1). At the same time, the Infirmary did receive sick poor from other parishes, as both in- and out-patients. In such cases, the recommender of the patient was obliged 'to take care of the said person upon his recovery and return to his [own] parish'. It seems likely, in fact, that the Society's aim was to stimulate the creation of an entire network of parochial infirmaries, or of charitable societies, emulating its example across the metropolis. This, however, signally failed to occur. (3) The Society continued to be very much a *participatory* enterprise. It did not use committees: instead, all the subscribers were free to attend the weekly meetings, held on Wednesday nights, and it was at these meetings that all the important business took place, including the admission and discharge of patients. Thus all the subscribers could involve themselves fully, if they wished, in the running of the Society. This was a direct continuation of the initial aim, the 'revival of the true Christian spirit of justice and charity'.

All this was based on a specific model, namely *the charity-school movement* and its leading organisation, the SPCK (Society for the Promotion of Christian Knowledge).[15] The SPCK had begun in 1698 with just four founders – the same number as initiated the Charitable Society some eighteen years later. The SPCK had acted as an umbrella organisation, and had set up individual schools in dozens of parishes; again this was mirrored in the aims of the Charitable Society. Further, when the Charitable Society retreated from its wider goals and decided, in April 1716, 'that our principal care be confined to the sick and needy . . . of St Margaret's Westminster', it was now modelling itself on the individual charity school. These schools were parish-based; and they had always manifested the participatory methods which we have

[15] See M. G. Jones, *The Charity-School Movement: A Study of Eighteenth Century Puritanism in Action* (London, 1964).

seen were a conspicuous feature of the work of the Charitable Society. Of course the charity school had its salaried professional – the teacher – and so too did the Charitable Society, in the form of its apothecary. In each case, the status of the professional person involved neither professional autonomy, nor mere subservience. He was paid, but paid to exercise a trust; in the conduct of charitable affairs he and the trustees met as complementary equals. Finally, there were many direct links between the SPCK and the Charitable Society, links which appear at three levels. Two of the members of the Society, Henry Hoare (a member in both 1716 and 1719) and Samuel Wesley (1719 only), were members of the SPCK itself. Further, Hoare was for many years the chairman of the complementary umbrella organisation, the Grand Committee of London Charity Schools. Thirdly, there were tangible links with one specific charity school, namely the Grey Coat School (so named from the uniforms of its pupils), the largest, the most successful and the most famous of all the charity schools.[16] It had been founded in 1698, as the charity school of St Margaret's Westminster – that is, the same parish as the Charitable Society's later focus. Hoare and Wesley were both on its board, so was another 1719 Charitable Society member (Thomas Wisdom), and there were other individuals who were subscribers or benefactors of both the school and the Society. And in 1720, it was in the Grey Coat School that the Society held its weekly meetings – after their re-founding meeting at St Dunstan's Coffee-House, and until the first Infirmary building was fitted out.

To sum up: the Charitable Society, which created the Westminster Infirmary, was designed to extend into the care of the sick poor a form of charitable provision which had already worked effectively for the education of the children of the poor. It drew on the same personnel, the same methods and the same religious motive: the care of the sick was linked with their eternal salvation, just as the education of children was designed to this end. The trustees of the Charitable Society were not trying to lower the death-rate, any more than the trustees of the charity school were trying to raise the literacy-rate. *They were instead seeking actively to Christianise the society in which they lived.* They saw themselves as active instruments of a beneficent Providence; every new subscription was proof of God's approval of the design, and every patient was required, after receiving the help of the Society, to render thanks 'to God and to the Society'.

Why then was this initiative taken at this time? The SPCK dated

[16] For the Grey Coat School, see Elsie S. Day, *An Old Westminster Endowment* (London, 1902).

from 1698; it had flourished for eighteen years without any move into this new sphere of charitable activity. What led to this sudden extension of participatory philanthropy in 1716 and 1719? We can approach this question by considering who the founding fathers were; when they founded it; and, first of all, the changing political complexion of the SPCK. As the researches of Craig Rose demonstrate, the SPCK was created as a specifically Anglican missionary society, an attempt to revitalise the Christianity of the Church of England in the wake of the new flourishing of Dissent – and particularly of Dissenting education – resulting from the Toleration Act of 1689.[17] The Established Church was threatened by toleration with becoming merely one amongst many sects; the SPCK sought to strengthen the Church by catechising and educating the young. (The simplest way to grasp this objective is by analogy with the more familiar case of Methodism, a generation or so later. It is perhaps no accident that Samuel Wesley was prominent in the SPCK and that his sons were leaders of the Methodist movement for spiritual revival within the Anglican church.) In the political climate of the reign of Anne, this aim made for an inexorable drift of the SPCK away from its initial, rather eirenic Anglicanism towards a High-Church, Tory and even Jacobite orientation. Thus by the time the Charitable Society was founded – early in 1716 – the SPCK was firmly placed at the Tory end of the political spectrum.

We would therefore expect that the founding fathers of the Charitable Society were specifically Tories and High Churchmen. And in fact, wherever information as to their allegiance can be found, this does indeed turn out to have been the case. Table 2 sets out the names of the fourteen men involved; I have identified the allegiance of just six of these men, but the pattern is so clear for these six that we can be confident it extended to the whole group.[18] To mention only the four

[17] Craig Rose, personal communication, 1988, drawing on his forthcoming Cambridge Ph.D. dissertation on charities in London, *c.*1680–1720.

[18] For Cockburn, Hutton and Wesley, see the *Dictionary of National Biography*. Hoare belonged to the Goldsmiths' Company, Witham to the Vintners' Company, and these were two of 'the three great tory London guilds' (the other being the Grocers' Company): Linda Colley, *In Defiance of Oligarchy: The Tory Party, 1714–60* (Cambridge, 1982), p. 87. Both men voted Tory in 1713: see W. A. Speck and W. A. Gray (eds.), 'London Pollbooks 1713', in H. Horwitz (ed.), *London Politics 1713–1717* (London Record Society, vol. xvii, 1981), pp. 94 and 128. Finally Trebeck must have been at least a Tory and possibly a non-juror in June 1715, since a sermon of his was strongly approved by Thomas Hearne at that time: see D. W. Rannie (ed.), *Remarks and Collections of Thomas Hearne*, vol. 5 (Oxford, 1901), p. 67. (Trebeck, however, went over to the Court in the middle of the 1720s.) Note in addition that Wogan is probably to be identified with the man of that name in the DNB, whose precise allegiance at this time is unclear to me. Wesley's wider circle is discussed by Thomas E. Brigden, 'Samuel Wesley Junior, and His Circle, 1690–1739', *Proceedings of the Wesley Historical Society* 11 (1918), pp. 25–38, 97–102, 121–9 and 145–53.

Table 2. *Founders of the Westminster Charitable Society, 1716 and 1719*

1716 only	1716 and 1719	1719 only
Revd Patrick Cockburn	Henry Hoare	Revd Mr Fitzgerald
Robert Witham	William Wogan	Revd Pengrey Hayward
		Revd John Hutton
		Revd Dr. Alexander Innes
		Revd Richard Russell
		John Russell
		John Thornton
		Revd Andrew Trebeck
		Revd Samuel Wesley
		Thomas Wisdom

most prominent cases: *Henry Hoare* was a member of the Tory family of bankers and goldsmiths. *John Hutton* was a non-juring clergyman, who had lost his living and had supported himself by taking in boarders from Westminster School, itself a centre of high-flying Toryism. *Patrick Cockburn* was at this period technically a Jacobite, since he had been removed as curate of St Dunstan's, Fleet Street, for refusing to take the oath of abjuration on the accession of George I. (Later, in 1726, he became reconciled to the Hanoverian succession, took the oath and duly obtained a living.) *Samuel Wesley* was closely associated with Atterbury, was head usher at Westminster School and belonged to a substantial circle all of whose members were High Churchmen. Thus these four men were so far to the Tory end of the spectrum that it is difficult to imagine their working with colleagues who did not share their basic principles; we may safely infer that the whole group, both in 1716 and 1719, was of deeply Tory allegiance. The same conclusion is suggested by the simpler fact that so many of these founding fathers were clergymen; seven of the 1719 group of twelve were in holy orders. At this period almost all the lower clergy were of Tory persuasion, believing that under the Whigs the Church of England was 'in danger'.

In this context we can begin to grasp the significance of the date of founding. By January 1716, when the Charitable Society was set up, the Tories had witnessed in turn the accession of George I and the associated flight of Bolingbroke to France and the creation of a Whig ministry; a crushing defeat in the General Election which followed; and the abortive Jacobite uprising of 1715, which was now in the process of being mopped up. They well knew that they were about to be consigned to the political wilderness; the only question was for how long. The Whigs were already setting about purging Tories from a variety of local offices, tightening their own grip on all levels of government and creating a one-party State. As one instance amongst many, the Commission for Building Fifty New Churches, set up under Anne in 1711 as a High Church initiative, was purged of Tories and filled with Whigs; the date at which this took effect was 5 January 1716, that is, nine days before the first meeting of the Charitable Society, and one of the Commissioners purged was Henry Hoare.[19] A further move in the same direction was the Close Vestries Bill, which came before Parliament at about this time; this was designed to wrest control of parish vestries in London from Tories and to replace them with Whigs.[20] No wonder that Henry Hoare and his colleagues began to feel that the Poor Law was insufficient: it was now likely to be administered by their political enemies, men whom they probably regarded as infidels.

The subsequent disbanding of the Society in May 1716, and its refounding in December 1719, may also be intelligible in this light. The Close Vestries Bill was a key issue for the Tories, who put a major effort into lobbying against it. Given their strong emphasis on the parish as the unit of activity, Hoare and his associates may well have diverted their efforts in this direction once the Bill came before the House of Commons in April 1716. In the Commons such efforts were unsuccessful; but the Tories won a famous victory in the Lords, where the Bill was thrown out on 1 June. It is just conceivable that with this success they lost the impetus which had fuelled the Charitable Society. But why then did it 'please Almighty God to stir up the hearts of some persons to revive this charitable design' in December 1719? All these questions deserve to be explored through a study of vestry affairs in St Margaret's Westminster; but it can be suggested that it was now electoral politics which provided the crucial stimulus. The City of Westminster, which sent two MPs to the House of Commons, was one of the largest, the most democratic and the most keenly fought of all electorates in the country. By reviving the Charitable Society in 1719, Hoare and his associates may have been preparing for the General Election of 1722. Charity was a means of securing respect, affection and political leverage: this is amply shown by Rose's work on the City

[19] See M. H. Port (ed.), *The Commissions for Building Fifty New Churches: The Minute Books, 1717–27, a Calendar* (London, 1986), pp. xvi, xvii and 45.

[20] See John Oldmixon, *The History of England*, vol. 2 (London, 1735), p. 633; *House of Lords Journal* 20 (1716), pp. 365–8 and 372.

hospitals, St Thomas's and St Bartholomew's, where the struggle for political control had been intense throughout the reigns of James II and William III.[21] If the underlying aim of the 1719 re-founding was indeed political, then this succeeded – for the Tories won both seats in the Westminster electorate in the 1722 election.

The two motives I have suggested – religious and political – were not at odds, nor was the one altruistic and the other interested. Politics and religion were different facets of the same set of issues: it had been over a religious question (the succession of a Catholic monarch) that the Whig/Tory split within the elite had developed in 1679, and while that split had evolved into new shapes after 1688, chiefly through the impact of war and the resulting problem of the National Debt, it nevertheless retained a fundamentally religious orientation. Thus, for the founders of the Charitable Society, to promote the Tory cause in politics and to work for a Christian revival in daily life were the same thing.

This case-study amply bears out the earlier contention, that behind the founding of any given voluntary hospital there lay not the general interests of the leisured classes but rather some particular set of interests within those classes. The chief sphere in which such interests were demarcated was, throughout our period, politico-religious. In the case of the Westminster Charitable Society, it was specifically the Tory interest which was at work. What prompted the founders to involve themselves in the care of the sick, and thus eventually to found the first voluntary hospital, was the new political conjuncture arising from the accession of George I and the creation of a Whig one-party State.

INOCULATION OF SMALLPOX

Smallpox inoculation is one of those forgotten medical practices which, while playing an immensely important historical role, must be distinguished from the later techniques which succeeded it.[22] The term 'inoculation' simply meant *engrafting*, and indeed it was this word which was first used to describe it: the language, then, was taken from horticultural botany. Purulous matter was taken from one of the many pustules on the body of a sufferer from smallpox. This matter was then

[21] Craig Rose, forthcoming Ph.D. and his paper on St Thomas's and St Bartholomew's in Lindsay Granshaw and Roy Porter (eds.), *Hospitals in History* (London, 1989).

[22] See Genevieve Miller, *The Adoption of Inoculation for Smallpox in England and France* (Philadelphia, 1957); Peter Razzell, *The Conquest of Smallpox* (Firle, 1977); Derrick Baxby, *Jenner's Smallpox Vaccine* (London, 1981); J. R. Smith, *The Speckled Monster: Smallpox in England, 1670–1970, With Particular Reference to Essex* (Chelmsford, 1987).

'prepared' in some way – for instance, by drying. Meanwhile the recipient individual, someone who had never had the disease, was also 'prepared' by manipulation of regimen. Finally the noxious matter was inserted into or under the skin of the recipient, again by any of a variety of techniques, chiefly through an incision (sometimes deep, sometimes shallow). The recipient then, within a few days, would develop a very mild form of smallpox – marked above all by the presence of far fewer pustules than were usually observed with the natural disease. In another week or so the pustules would fade away and the recipient would recover. The result, it was alleged by promoters of inoculation, was permanent immunity from the natural disease, an immunity just as effective as that acquired from a natural attack. The advantage of inoculation-conferred immunity was that the inoculated disease was far less lethal than the natural smallpox: not only did it produce far fewer pustules on the individual, but it also produced far fewer deaths amongst the mass. (The typical mortality seems to have been about one in seventy or eighty from inoculations, as against one in six or seven from smallpox itself.)

The long-term history, viewed in whiggish perspective, was to vindicate dramatically the claims of the inoculators. Inoculation was promoted by the Royal Society through the 1720s, and gradually came to prevail against a stubborn resistance mounted by various critics. From the middle decades of the eighteenth century it was more and more widely adopted, chiefly through the remarkable activities of the Suttons, who developed a cheaper and simpler technique. In a rural village there would be a 'mass inoculation' of the whole population as soon as an epidemic of smallpox threatened. Large towns, on the other hand, were more reluctant to adopt the practice, since here a universal inoculation was a practical and political impossibility, and it was widely feared that an *inoculated* person could transmit the *natural* and lethal disease to someone who had not been inoculated, thus starting an epidemic. It was to combat this fear and to promote inoculation in the towns that John Haygarth and his colleagues at Chester Infirmary created their new practice of inoculation-with-isolation, together with the accompanying rationale that infection obeyed an inverse-square law of diminishing effects with diminishing distance. Their success – much promoted by the Howard-Percival network of social reformers in the late eighteenth century – led by the 1790s to a campaign for the actual eradication of the disease in Britain.[23] It seems to have been this

[23] Francis M. Lobo, 'John Haygarth, Smallpox, and Religious Dissent in Eighteenth-Century England', this volume, pp. 217–53.

rival stimulus which prompted Edward Jenner to intensify his researches on the immunity to smallpox conferred by the diseases of cowpox in cows and 'grease' in horses. Hence Jenner's 1798 experiments and publication on what was soon to be called *vaccination* – the inoculation of cowpox (so called from the Latin *vacca*, a cow). Vaccination rapidly triumphed over inoculation (despite the sustained opposition of Burdett, Cobbett and other radicals), swiftly receiving military use and State backing.[24] In the nineteenth century a series of moves towards *compulsory* vaccination led to political campaigns against the practice; one of the monuments of this struggle was Creighton's massive *History of Epidemics*, animated by his opposition to vaccination.[25] Meanwhile Pasteur and Koch were extending the basic technique to other diseases; the word 'vaccination' lost its connection with cowpox and was used by Pasteur for the creation of artificial immunity in general. Thanks to all this and to the involvement of the laboratory in these researches and experiments, we have the scientific field of immunology and a vast range of 'vaccines' against specific diseases. It is in the promotion of inoculation for smallpox in the 1720s that this heroic story finds its real roots. Consequently, it is difficult to resist the basic assumption that the inoculators were 'right' and their opponents were 'wrong'.

Yet from the perspective of around 1720, the question appears in a very different light. Not only could the long-term results not be anticipated, but also the success of inoculation itself lay in the future. And inoculation was extraordinary, for it consisted in deliberately *giving a disease* to someone in health – the very inversion of the notional role of the physician. It is thus hardly surprising that inoculation was resisted; what requires explanation is not so much this resistance, as the very fact that the practice was promoted at all. We are fortunate to have the excellent study of Genevieve Miller – an important classic of medical history – on *how* inoculation was promoted. But Miller, proceeding from the modern perspective I have already outlined, was not concerned with the question as to *why* an important cadre of physicians set about promoting it.[26] As we shall see, an exploration of this question takes us again into the realm of early Hanoverian politics and religion.

We may approach the question of the 'why' by looking in some detail at the mechanics of the 'how'. The practice of inoculation arose chiefly in the Middle East, where it appears to have been a popular or

[24] See Paul Saunders, *Edward Jenner: The Cheltenham Years 1795–1823* (Hanover, New England and London, 1982).

[25] Dorothy Porter and Roy Porter, 'The Politics of Prevention: Anti-Vaccinationism and Public Health in Nineteenth-Century England', *Medical History* 32 (1988), pp. 231–52.

[26] Unless otherwise stated, my account here follows Miller, *Adoption of Inoculation*.

folk practice. (Thus here, just as with Jenner's later vaccination and much earlier with cinchona for malaria, Western medicine is indebted to popular or indigenous traditions for some of its most heroic achievements.) Reports of its success reached the Royal Society, chiefly through John Woodward, in 1714. But it was not until Lady Mary Wortley Montagu returned from her stint as wife of the ambassador to Constantinople that any campaign for inoculation was mounted. Lady Mary persuaded the apothecary Charles Maitland to inoculate her three-year-old daughter; since Maitland had been with the Montagues in Constantinople, he was familiar with the practice, yet it required some pressure from Lady Mary to convince him to perform the act. With remarkable speed the idea was taken up by Hans Sloane, who used the Royal Society to promote an investigation into the efficacy of inoculation. This may appear as an open-minded study, but all the evidence suggests that Sloane and his backers were convinced in advance that inoculation would work. The crucial moves were a series of experiments, carried out in the nine months from June 1721 to March 1722. Table 3 summarises their chronology and content. All these experiments deserve detailed study as pieces of public theatre, but I shall focus simply on the first of them, 'Experiment I' in my own terminology. Sloane and some of his colleagues – including opponents as well as supporters of inoculation – went down to Newgate prison and selected six prisoners, all condemned to death, all in good health, and offered them repeal from execution if they would submit to an experiment in inoculation. It was not difficult to get the prisoners to agree to this: certain death was exchanged for the uncertain. The six prisoners were duly inoculated: significantly, the inoculator was Charles Maitland, so that here as with other experimental innovations we see the necessity for physical and personal transfer of techniques from one context (Constantinople) into another (London). The inoculated prisoners were carefully observed, over the next few weeks, by the interested physicians of both the pro- and the anti-inoculation camps. In due course they developed pustules and other symptoms and then recovered. None of them died; the experiment had succeeded. On 6 September 1721 they were given a public pardon and release. For these six prisoners, then, inoculation certainly worked: it saved their lives.

The whiggish perspective, then, is that inoculation worked; and this, from a different point of view, was also the conclusion of the pro-inoculators. But the anti-inoculators interpreted the experiment quite differently. In the publications of William Wagstaffe on the one hand, and Charles Maitland on the other, we have two quite different

Table 3. *The promotion of smallpox inoculation by public experiments, 1721–2*

1721 April:	Lady Mary Wortley Montagu prevails on Charles Maitland to inoculate her 3-year-old daughter
June:	[Experiment I] already under way, probably at the initiative of Sir Hans Sloane
Aug 9:	[Experiment I]: Six condemned prisoners in Newgate prison inoculated in exchange for their lives. Inoculator: Chas Maitland In charge: Sloane and Dr John George Steigerthal
Sept 6:	Public pardon and release. [Expt I] complete.
Oct:	[Experiment II]: Performed by Maitland under direction of Sloane and Steigerthal, on a 19-year-old woman, one of the subjects of [Expt I). She is exposed, in 2 different ways, to natural smallpox; survives.
[Oct]:	[Experiment III]: Performed by Maitland, at Hertford: inoculated children pass the disease on.
1722 Feb to March	[Experiment IV]: Performed by Maitland, in London: six 'persons' inoculated, then displayed to the public. Announcement in the newspapers, etc.
March	[Experiment V]: Maitland inoculates a child with pus from a person with the inoculated disease.
March	[Experiment VI]: Five pauper children from the parish of St James's, Westminster inoculated and displayed to the public. (This expt had been publicly initiated, the previous November, by the Princess of Wales.)

accounts of the 'same' experiment. For Maitland, what had happened was that the prisoners had received a mild form of smallpox and had duly recovered: this was what a pro-inoculation person *saw* in the experiment. But an anti-inoculation physician, Wagstaffe, saw something quite different: some odd-looking pustules, not the same as the smallpox pustules; an inflammation surrounding the pustules, different from what was observed with smallpox; and a constellation of other, febrile symptoms, once again quite different from smallpox. Here we have an elegant example of the structuring of perception by the preconceptions of the observer. The result, of course, was that Wagstaffe was totally unconvinced of the alleged results of the experiment, whereas Maitland was confident that the inoculation had worked.[27]

[27] William Wagstaffe, *A Letter to Dr Freind; Showing the Danger and Uncertainty of Inoculating the Small Pox* (London, 1722); Charles Maitland, *An Account of Inoculating the Small-pox* (London, 1722; second edition, enlarged, 1723); *Mr Maitland's Account of Inoculating the Smallpox Vindicated from Dr Wagstaffe's Misrepresentations* (London, 1722). I owe the latter reference to the kindness of Robert Kilpatrick.

This pivotal experiment thus illustrates some basic principles of the historical sociology of science. But what should also command our attention is the political precondition of the experiment. In order for the experiment to be performed, Sloane and his allies had to be given the power of life and death over the six prisoners. *The State handed over to the Royal Society its control over six human lives.* Without this fundamental resource, the experiment could not have been carried out; and the availability of that resource was an extraordinary political fact, a quite remarkable donation from the State to a select group of its citizens. This can only mean that inoculation had prior support from the Crown and the ministry. And this was indeed the case. Inoculation was specifically a project of the Court Whigs; opposition to the practice came exclusively from Tories. This fundamental cleavage of attitudes to inoculation was to persist until at least the 1740s.

Table 4 sets out the association between political allegiance and attitudes to inoculation, between 1721 and the late 1740s, for those individuals who can be allocated a position in both spheres. There is a powerful connection between Whig allegiance and support for inoculation, and between Toryism and opposition to the practice; the odds against this being a chance association are 77 to 1.[28] Only two out of sixteen individuals go against the stream, and in each of these cases their departure from the main pattern is at least partly intelligible. *John Arbuthnot* was the only Tory supporter of the operation so far identified; and it is striking that he alone, of all the authors under discussion, published anonymously. What lay behind his support was apparently his interest in statistical questions, and perhaps also his involvement in the recent discussions leading up to the Quarantine Act for control of plague (discussed below).[29] *Sir Richard Blackmore* was the only known Whig opponent of inoculation, and in fact his opposition fits with other aspects of his eccentric career. He was a much older Whig than most of the supporters, having been knighted by William III. From about 1720 he was apparently moving rapidly away

[28] Using the Fisher exact-probability test, for which see Sidney Siegel, *Nonparametric Statistics for the Behavioural Sciences* (Tokyo, 1956), pp. 96–104. At least another twenty individuals with known attitudes to inoculation can be identified from Miller's study, split approximately evenly between supporters and opponents. This table includes only those of known politico-religious allegiance; the latter has been identified from standard sources, chiefly the *DNB*.

[29] For Arbuthnot, see Larry Stewart, 'The Edge of Utility: Slaves and Smallpox in the Early Eighteenth Century', *Medical History* 29 (1985), pp. 54–70, at pp. 55 and 65; Ian Hacking, *The Emergence of Probability* (Cambridge, 1975), pp. 166–71; and the entry for him in the *Dictionary of Scientific Biography*. Arbuthnot's approach is particularly intriguing in view of the otherwise Whig associations of the statistical approach to inoculation, discussed below. On the later ramifications of this statistical theme, see Leslie Bradley, *Smallpox Inoculation: An Eighteenth-Century Mathematical Controversy* (Nottingham, 1971).

Table 4. *Politico-religious allegiance and attitudes to inoculation, 1721–46*

Whigs/Dissenters/members of Royal household	Tories/Non-jurors
Supporters of inoculation	
Claude Amyand	
Dr Samuel Brady	
Ephraim Chambers	
Dr James Jurin	
Dr Richard Mead	
Lady Mary Wortley Montagu	
Rev Daniel Neal	
Dr Thomas Nettleton	
Sir Hans Sloane	
Dr John George Steigerthal	Dr John Arbuthnot
Opponents of inoculation	
Sir Richard Blackmore	Dr John Byrom
	Dr Peirce Dod
	Revd Edmund Massey
	Dr William Wagstaffe

from the Court; this was signalled by his various published attacks on 'modern Arians', that is, on the religious tendencies manifested by the new Court divines Samuel Clarke and William Whiston. He retired to the country in about 1722, and then began to publish medical works which argued against the monopolistic practices and pretensions of the Collegiate physicians. After his death in 1729 he was mentioned with affection and respect by two Tory medical writers. Blackmore, then, was fast becoming a 'Country' Whig at the time of the inoculation campaign.[30] The exceptions (Arbuthnot, Blackmore) are thus intelligible; and the main pattern has further evidence for its support. For one thing, the most sustained opposition to inoculation in the newspapers of the day came from *Applebee's Original Weekly Journal*, which was a Tory paper. For another, consider the following passage from Edmund Massey's *Letter to Mr Maitland* of 1722. Here, towards the end of his counter-attack against Maitland, Massey referred also to the the pro-inoculation (and anti-Massey) text of Samuel Brady of Portsmouth:

[30] For Blackmore, see his entry in the *DNB* and the various works of his cited there. The later respectful Tories were Edmund Chapman, *A Treatise on the Improvement of Midwifery, Chiefly With Regard to the Operation* (London, 1735), p. 101, and Henry Bracken, *The Midwife's Companion* (London, 1737), p. 186.

I had almost forgot to take notice, that amongst all the advantageous symptoms of inoculation, I do not remember any that are so squeamish as the following, viz., that it is a diagnostic of a man's affection or disaffection to the government; for, says your brother Brady, I wish the happy conduct of the Royal Family in this particular has not, out of an abundant respect, occasioned some people's zeal against the practice. I assure the Doctor, that I neither have, nor expect, place or pension under the government; and yet I . . . am certain, that I am as good a subject as some who have . . .

Thus Brady had insinuated that opponents of inoculation were Jacobites; and Massey, who was a Hanoverian Tory, found this smear deeply offensive ('squeamish').[31] Here we have a rare occasion on which the political connections of the contending medical interests actually become explicit.

It is not difficult to see why Tories were opposed to inoculation. As David Harley observes, the Tory doctrine of passive obedience to the monarch was naturally transferred into the realm of the supernatural as this impinged on the affairs of man.[32] Diseases were judgements of God; resistance to such judgements was impious. We can find something like this position elegantly articulated by John Byrom, in a poem he wrote against inoculation (emphasis added):

I heard two neighbours talk, the other night,
About this new distemper-giving plan,
Which some so wrong, and others think so right.
Short was the dialogue, and thus it ran:
– 'If I had twenty children of my own,
  I would inoculate them every one.'
– 'Aye, but should any of them die, what moan
  Would then be made for venturing thereupon!'
– 'No; I should think that I had done the best,
  And be resigned, whatever should befall.'
– 'But could you really be so quite at rest?'
– 'I could'. – '*Then why inoculate at all*?'
– 'Since, to resign a child to God, Who gave,
  Is full as easy, and as just a part,
  When sick and led by Nature to the grave,
  As when in health, and driv'n to it by Art'.

The very *possibility* of a fatality from inoculation, Byrom was arguing, refuted the practice. To inflict disease, and thus the possibility of death, was to usurp the role of God.[33]

[31] Edmund Massey, *A Letter to Mr Maitland, in Vindication of the Sermon Against Inoculation* (London, 1722), p. 22. (Brady was also mentioned at the beginning of the text, p. 2.)

[32] David Harley, comments in conference discussion, September, 1987. This interpretation is amply borne out by Massey's writings. See Edmund Massey, *A Sermon Against the Dangerous and Sinful Practice of Inoculation* (London, 1722), and his subsequent *Letter to Mr Maitland*, cited in the previous note. The *Sermon* must have been popular, for it ran to at least three editions in 1722.

[33] *Remains Historical and Literary Connected with the Palatine Counties of Lancaster and Chester*, new series, vol. 29 (Manchester, Chetham Society, 1894), pp. 204–5.

But what of the reasons for the Whig support for the 'new distemper-giving plan'? Part of the reason may lie in the fact that smallpox, already a subject of bitter contention amongst physicians as to the right method of treatment, was likely to become a concern of the State.[34] At the time when the first experiment was carried out (it started in June 1721), the ministry was recovering from the ravages of the South Sea Bubble, which had burst in 1720, and was dealing with the threat of the plague epidemic, raging in France and widely feared as imminent in England. The Bubble had brought to power the 'screen-master general', Walpole; the government response to the plague scare was the Quarantine Act of February 1721. (What with these upheavals, Atterbury's Jacobite plot of 1721–2, and the Black Act of 1722, the 'political stability' allegedly achieved by 1725 appears as a rather delicate equilibrium.)[35] Plague posed a passive threat not only to human life but also to trade and to public order; hence the draconian measures of the Quarantine Act. Since smallpox had recently assumed a new and more virulent form, there was reason to fear that another, different but scarcely less fatal plague was already developing – one which quarantine would be quite powerless to prevent. Against smallpox, what was needed was a pre-emptive strike; it can be seen as a blow struck, not just against the disease, but also against the *fear* of the disease. If smallpox could be depicted as preventable, the public could be massaged into a grateful tranquility. Hence its political importance.

On this reading, inoculation was backed by the Whigs simply because the Whigs were in power: it was they who held the reins of State, and thus they who had most to gain and to lose from the success or failure of the management of disease. Yet there are grounds for suspecting that a deeper predisposition was at work. The arguments deployed in favour of inoculation rested upon a distinctive morality, one which ran precisely counter to Byrom's views already described. For James Jurin, the most publicly active supporter of inoculation in the Royal Society, the question of the merits of inoculation was statistical. What was the death-rate from natural smallpox? What was the death-rate from inoculation? If the latter was lower than the former, then inoculation was justified. (This rested implicitly on the

[34] On the controversy of *c.*1718 over the treatment of smallpox, in which Freind and Mead were ranged against Woodward, see Miller, *Adoption of Inoculation*, p. 36; R. J. J. Martin, 'Explaining John Freind's *History of Physick*', *Studies in History and Philosophy of Science* 19 (1988), pp. 399–418; Joseph M. Levin, *Dr Woodward's Shield* (Berkeley, 1977), pp. 9–17. For the connection with plague, quarantine and the Bubble, see Stewart, 'Edge of Utility', *passim*.

[35] Compare J. H. Plumb, *The Growth of Political Stability in England, 1675–1725* (London, 1967), and E. P. Thompson, *Whigs and Hunters: The Origins of the Black Act* (London, 1975).

premise, which was probably false, that everyone caught smallpox at some stage in his or her life.) Here we see a concept of *utility*, a weighing of this good against that evil, in which individual life is an atomic entity to be viewed *de haut en bas*. Such a morality – some would see it as an anti-morality – had powerful Whig and Latitudinarian roots.[36] The corollory was that man did indeed have a God-like role: against disease there was a right of resistance. (Meanwhile the traditional Whig doctrine of a right of *political* resistance was fast becoming a forgotten shibboleth: by labelling Tories as Jacobites, by repealing Habeas Corpus and by passing the Septennial Act, Walpole and his colleagues rapidly constructed a new Whig compound of loyalty to the ministry and to the Hanoverian succession, with resistance consigned to the single moment of 1688.) It is tempting to see inoculation for smallpox as the Whig and Hanoverian equivalent of the Stuart practice of touching for scrofula, for the 'king's evil'.[37] In each case we have State action against a familiar and disfiguring disease. In each case this action was deployed with massive publicity in an orchestrated campaign. But whereas the Royal Touch mobilised divine powers, based on hereditary right, inoculation deployed natural powers harnessed by man, with the monarch as the benevolent onlooker rather than indispensable participant. This role for the sovereign – involved yet marginal – precisely fitted the Walpolian Whig political role assigned to George I, just as the thaumaturgical power of the Stuart monarchs corresponded to the Tory conception of the relationship between Crown and subject. The strongly theatrical character of the early inoculation experiments, together with the fact that relatively few actual inoculations were carried out in the 1720s, similarly suggests that inoculation was political massage as well as medical intervention.

These are only speculations as to the underlying motivations behind the inoculation campaign. Here, just as with the voluntary-hospital movement, we have a large and open field which invites further exploration. Inoculation remained controversial until at least the 1750s, and generated a variety of new initiatives, from the creation of

[36] The emerging concept of utility can be traced in different ways within Margaret Jacob, *The Newtonians and the English Revolution* (Ithaca, New York, 1976), and Lorraine C. Daston, 'Probabilistic Expectation and Rationality in Classical Probability Theory', *Historia Mathematica* 7 (1980), pp. 234–60.

[37] See Mark Bloch, *The Royal Touch: Sacred Monarchy and Scrofula in England and France*, trans. J. E. Anderson (London, 1973); Keith Thomas, *Religion and the Decline of Magic: Studies in Popular Beliefs in Sixteenth- and Seventeenth-Century England* (first published 1971; Harmondsworth, 1978), pp. 227–41; French, 'Disease, Theory and Practice'; W. E. Tate, *The Parish Chest* (Cambridge, 1946; third edition, 1969), pp. 157–61.

the London Smallpox-inoculation Hospital in 1746 to Haygarth's remarkable work at Chester in later decades. Larry Stewart has shown how inoculation was swiftly taken up by the slave-traders of the Africa Company, with the heavy involvement of Sloane, the Royal Society, and the Duke of Chandos;[38] similarly the subject can and should be pursued further in many local contexts. Once such research is carried out, it will no doubt become possible to develop a more nuanced and concrete account than I have been able to offer here. But it is already certain that this theme, like that of the voluntary-hospital movement, opens directly into the terrain of political and religious conflict and allegiance in early Hanoverian England.

CONCLUSION

My third case-study – on the rise of man-midwifery – will be considered only briefly; it has been discussed in detail elsewhere, and space permits only a summary here.[39] After outlining this third theme I shall reflect on the significance of the overall pattern.

The emergence of man-midwifery, which took place in London between about 1720 and 1750, was one of the most remarkable and consequential changes in English medicine at any point in the past. Down to the early eighteenth century, male involvement in childbirth was almost entirely restricted to difficult births: the typical form of male practice was the emergency call. A transition period, which we will examine in a moment, can be observed in the next few decades. Then, from about 1750, we find male practitioners acting *in lieu of a midwife*, delivering normal births – setting up a competition between the midwife and the man-midwife which was to continue, in a complex and unfolding struggle, until the beginning of the present century. The 1750 shift in the nature of male practice had effects on the scope of technical knowledge: thus William Hunter, the most successful exponent of the new form of male practice, brought the womb itself within the domain of male knowledge with his *Anatomy of the Gravid Uterus*, published in 1773 but based on researches started around 1750. The

[38] Stewart, 'Edge of Utility'.

[39] For a more detailed treatment, and for supporting references at greater length, see Adrian Wilson, *A Safe Deliverance: Ritual and Conflict in English Childbirth, 1600–1760* (Cambridge, in press), chapters 6–10. See also Herbert R. Spencer, *The History of British Midwifery from 1650 to 1800* (London, 1927); Jean Donnison, *Midwives and Medical Men: A History of Inter-Professional and Women's Rights* (London, 1977); and Margaret Connor Versluysen, 'Midwives, Medical Men and "Poor Women Labouring of Child": Lying-in Hospitals in Eighteenth-Century London' in Helen Roberts (ed.), *Women, Health and Reproduction* (London, 1981), pp. 18–49.

watershed of practice simultaneously generated a series of (largely ineffective) counter-attacks, starting in the 1750s, which criticised the new man-midwifery as immodest and interventionist and sought to raise the status and skills of midwives so that they could reverse the new trend. The transformation was most marked in the wealthier classes, that is, in the more lucrative sphere of practice. It has been variously seen as a heroic 'revolution in obstetrics' and as a tragic 'decline of the midwife', according to the viewpoint of the observer.[40] It embodied a new form of practice, not only by specialist *accoucheurs* such as Hunter, Smellie and Denman, but also amongst humbler surgeon-apothecaries, who now found that the management of normal birth was one of the standard tasks of their 'general practice'.[41] Its causes are baffling: it has usually been attributed to the dual influences of fashion and the midwifery forceps; yet the first of these explanations begs the question as to how the new 'fashion' got started, while the forceps was explicitly restricted to the small minority of difficult births.

It is on the phase of transition, from about 1720 to 1750, that I shall focus here. This was the period in which the midwifery forceps – one of the alleged causes of the 'revolution in obstetrics' – came into wider use (it had previously been a family secret amongst its inventors, the Chamberlen family), was published (in 1733–5), and was systematically taught to a new generation of male practitioners (by William Smellie in the 1740s).[42] With whiggish hindsight, the forceps seems to have played a critical role; and thus we have a story of a single, uncomplicated, unidirectional transition in this period. Yet, in fact, the forceps were *contested* from the outset. The crucial resource deployed against it was the suite of obstetric theories and techniques of the Dutch surgeon Hendrik van Deventer. Deventer's works, first published in 1701, were translated into English by Robert Samber in 1716; thereafter, a protracted struggle ensued between forceps practitioners on the one hand and the followers of Deventer on the other. The many and unprecedented public initiatives in midwifery in this period – the publication of treatises, systematic teaching, the creation of lying-in hospitals – were blows struck in a battle. That battle was not, as it appears with hindsight, between the old (midwives) and the new (men-

[40] J. H. Aveling, *English Midwives: Their History and Prospects* (London, 1872). p. 86; Donnison, *Midwives and Medical Men*, chapter 2.

[41] Irvine Loudon, *Medical Care and the General Practitioner* (Oxford, 1986), pp. 85–93.

[42] J. H. Aveling, *The Chamberlens and the Midwifery Forceps: Memorials of the Family and an Essay on the Invention of the Instrument* (London, 1882); Wilson, *A Safe Deliverance*, chapters 2, 8 and 9.

midwives); rather, it was between two parties of men-midwives, struggling for hegemony over practice and theory. Nor was the aim of this generation of men-midwives to replace the female midwife. Rather, their purpose was to gain much earlier access to difficult births; the midwife's role was intended to be circumscribed and defined, limited to managing easy natural labours, but there was no intention of displacing her. Earlier male access to difficult births meant the delivery of a living child, rather than a dead child; it meant a different social 'path' to the delivery-room;[43] and it made for substantially higher fees for the male practitioner. This was the domain of practice being contested between forceps practitioners and Deventerians. The struggle between the two groups has been obscured from historical vision by the fact that the forceps party eventually triumphed and Deventer's methods were forgotten. But this outcome was by no means inevitable; the struggle was keenly contested throughout this 'period of transition'.

The two parties of men-midwives were distinguished not just by obstetric allegiance but also in other ways. And amongst the *differentiae* between them was party-political allegiance. The early forceps practitioners, so far as their allegiance can be identified, were Tories; the followers of Deventer, by contrast, were Court Whigs. A shift took place in the 1740s, when the leading teacher of the forceps, William Smellie, was a Whig; but his was a Country rather than Court allegiance (signalled by his close association with Smollett), and meanwhile the Court Whig men-midwives continued to follow Deventer. The same battle still generated new initiatives: thus in 1746, when Smellie got one of his pupils to translate into English the earlier midwifery treatise of La Motte, this was a blow struck against Deventer's methods, while the Court Whig men-midwives who ran the lying-in wards of the Middlesex Hospital (1747) and who created the Brownlow Street Lying-in Hospital (1749) deployed Deventerian arguments and eschewed the forceps. Thus the teaching activities of Smellie and the creation of lying-in hospitals, which were seen by Dorothy George as a single movement, were in fact the visible effects of an underlying struggle and rivalry.[44]

The domain of man-midwifery thus illustrates yet again the role of party-political allegiance in the medical initiatives of the early Han-

[43] See Adrian Wilson, 'William Hunter and the Varieties of Man-Midwifery' in W. F. Bynum and Roy Porter (eds.), *William Hunter and the Eighteenth-Century Medical World* (Cambridge, 1985), pp. 343–69. In the terminology developed there, it was *onset calls with a midwife* which were now being sought.

[44] George, *London Life in the Eighteenth Century*, pp. 60–1.

overian period. The contest appears as a battle between Whig and Tory in the 1720s and '30s, and between Court and Country in the 1740s, with the Deventerians consistently on the Court Whig side, and forceps practitioners in the oppositional role. Whether this association between obstetric and party-political allegiances was a matter of accidents of patronage, or whether by contrast it reflected some deeper affinity between the two spheres, is a question for further research. But it is clear that there was such an association; that this helped to fuel the conflicts over technical obstetrics; and that each party of men-midwives had its lay supporters. The rise of man-midwifery can no more be grasped in isolation from the political history of the period than can the emergence of the first voluntary hospital or the campaign for smallpox inoculation.

We have examined three central instances of medical 'improvement' in early-eighteenth-century London: the creation of the first voluntary hospital; the campaign for smallpox inoculation; and the rise of man-midwifery in place of traditional obstetric surgery. Each of these developments turns out to have strong associations with political allegiance: the first was Tory, the second was Whig, and the third was a site of contest between the two parties. The concrete nature of the connections between medicine and politics remains to be explored, but at least we have established the existence of such connections in all three cases. It would be interesting to pursue a corresponding investigation for the other main site of practical medico-surgical innovation in this period, namely the treatment (both surgical and medical) of the excruciating and widespread complaint of stone in the bladder. Moreover the vast terrain of medical *theory* in this period awaits exploration along these lines. With the new resource of a listing of *Eighteenth Century Medics* – their book-subscriptions, education, apprenticeships – it is now becoming possible to locate medical practitioners within the complex and shifting networks of eighteenth-century patronage, thus vastly facilitating further explorations of the kind attempted here.[45] (If only the correspondence of Hans Sloane could be published, or at least calendared and indexed, the rich possibilities for further research would be still more handsomely demonstrated.) My aim has been both substantive and historiographic: not only to suggest some interpretations, but also to invite other scholars to engage in

[45] Peter J. V. Wallis, Ruth Wallis, Juanita Burnby and T. D. Wittet, *Eighteenth Century Medics (Subscriptions, Licences, Apprenticeships)* (Newcastle, 1985), and the associated lists of books published by subscription. New editions of these works, incorporating still more details, are now in press.

further exploration along these lines. As has repeatedly emerged, there is no shortage either of interesting topics or of source materials for investigation.

The central result of the findings outlined here is to insert medical history firmly within the matrix of the political history of the period. We began by observing the disciplinary phenomenon of 'tunnel history': the division of the past into separate zones such as political history, social history, ecclesiastical history, history of science. By now it should be clear that these divisions, applied to our period, have robbed the past of much of its meaning and interest. No doubt political historians who read *Applebee's* noticed its attacks on inoculation, but so far as I am aware, none of them thought this interesting or relevant to their own concerns. Similarly, historians of medicine have been well aware of party-political conflict in our period, without apparently noticing that this had medical implications. Similar arguments can be advanced against *all* the walls which modern sub-disciplines have erected within the past. Literature emerged from a social matrix; demographic phenomena were intertwined with economic matters and thus with politics; natural philosophy was a sphere of active contests which connected, for instance, with the critique of the stage.[46] It is precisely in their interconnectedness that the events and phenomena of the period can be understood and explained. Total history is the only viable approach, difficult though this may be to construct. What is required in the first instance is active collaboration between historians of different competences. Alas, institutional divisions make such collaboration very difficult to sustain.

If there is a single dramatic question which arises from the present findings, this concerns the *chronology* of the processes explored above. Strikingly, in all three spheres we have investigated, the crucial moment of conflict and initiative turns out to be the first five years or even less of the reign of George I. It was in 1714 that the first reports of smallpox inoculation were transmitted to the Royal Society; in 1716 that the Westminster Charitable Society was first set up; and in 1716, again, that Deventer's treatises were first translated into English. Yet party-political conflict – the explanatory resource I have deployed here – did not begin in 1714; on the contrary, it had begun, in the form of a Whig/Tory contest (though over different issues), well over a genera-

[46] See Simon Schaffer, 'Electricity, the People, and the Wrath of God: The Martin–Freke Debate', *Isis*, forthcoming; and compare Rosemary Bechler, '"Triall by what is Contrary": Samuel Richardson and Christian Dialectic' in Valerie Grosvenor Myer (ed.), *Samuel Richardson: Passion and Prudence* (London, 1986), pp. 93–113, at pp. 94–8.

tion before. Were the battles of the Exclusion Crisis (1679–81) and subsequent developments translated into medical initiatives? If so, what were those initiatives? If not, why not? It is precisely for the exploration of questions such as these that collaborative research is required.

The general claim that medical initiatives had politico-religious roots, while novel for the period, is of course highly familiar for the seventeenth century. Let us remind ourselves how Charles Webster summed up the findings of his *Great Instauration*:[47]

> Each group . . . tended to develop an attitude towards nature consistent with its social, political and religious position . . . strongly contrasting styles of science were being evolved in response to differing intellectual standpoints . . . The borderlines between the various groups were never defined rigidly; certain individuals gradually reoriented themselves . . . nevertheless, at any one point in time it is possible to discern a mosaic of competing groups wedded to different value systems. The various groups identify themselves both by the type of phenomenon chosen for investigation and by their method of approach . . .

Adding medicine to science, and incorporating practical innovations as well as theoretical investigations, this can serve as an apt description of the picture I have tried to paint of some key developments in early Hanoverian London.

[47] Webster *Great Instauration*, pp. 497–8.

2

Medicine to calm the mind Boerhaave's medical system, and why it was adopted in Edinburgh

ANDREW CUNNINGHAM

PEACE OF MIND

Herman Boerhaave (1669–1738) was by far the most famous medical man in Europe in the first half of the eighteenth century. He ran at Leyden what was for over thirty years the world's most celebrated medical school, to which thousands flocked from abroad. His enthusiastic students rushed back to their homes to found new medical schools on the model of his. We shall be investigating the one at Edinburgh later, but there were others in Vienna and Göttingen too. His lectures he turned into little books, and these became the new medical textbooks of Europe; they were then piously elaborated into exhaustive works by other ex-pupils such as Van Swieten and Haller. He was at the centre of an international network of correspondence, offering postal diagnoses and prognoses of their patients to other physicians on request, discussing chemical problems, and exchanging botanical specimens and plants. His fame stretched to Constantinople and Russia and beyond: it is said of him that a letter from China, addressed simply 'Boerhaave, Physician, Europe', immediately found its addressee.[1] Yet Boerhaave, who played such a large role on the stage of eighteenth-century medicine, is a mystery to us. Despite the excellent work of a number of Dutch historians,[2] we still know virtually nothing

Acknowledgements: my special thanks to Adrian Wilson, as the theme of the first part originated in discussions with him when we were teaching together. Dr Ole Grell kindly advised me on Dutch religious matters.

[1] G. A. Lindeboom, *Herman Boerhaave, the Man and his Work* (London, 1968), p. 3.

[2] Professor Lindeboom has been chief amongst them, with his biography, *Herman Boerhaave*, and his editing of *Analecta Boerhaaviana*, which includes the bibliography, iconography and correspondence of Boerhaave. My account is deeply indebted to these works. More recently has appeared *Boerhaave's Orations*, translated with introductions and notes by E. Kegel-Brinkgreve and A. M. Luyendijk-Elshout (Leyden, 1983).

of his motivations and concerns; we know nothing of why he produced so many writings, dealt with such a wide range of subjects, or attracted so many pupils. And if we know nothing of the man, I would claim, we know nothing of the medicine. Equally, until we know the medicine, we will know nothing of the man. My aim here is to explore this issue, and thus to see what it was about Boerhaave's medicine which so excited his pupils – especially those from Scotland, such that they organised a new medical school at Edinburgh on the basis of it.

One of the reasons why Boerhaave is so unknown today, seems to lie with the fact that he is not associated with any particular major discovery or innovation or invention (except for a greenhouse heater) – and historians of science and medicine have been obsessed with originality. It is not that time has passed Boerhaave by, with the historians using a different criterion of achievement than did Boerhaave's own contemporaries. For his lack of effective innovation was well known in his own day too. Here is an account of his time with Boerhaave in about 1710 by James Houston, which illustrates this. Houston was a typical young Scot of his day, of the kind whose eye for the main chance shocked the English and prompted J. M. Barrie's much later remark that there are few more impressive sights than a Scotsman on the make.

> I can no more judge of the *Genius* and Temper of the *Dutch*, than if I had never lived amongst them, for I knew no Dutchman, but my Professors; but, if I am allowed to take Dr *Boerhaave* for a Sample of the whole, I do say, that he was the most extraordinary Man of his Age, perhaps in the whole World; a clear Understanding, sound Judgement, with Strength of Memory that nothing could exceed, and indefatigably laborious [i.e. painstaking]: It is true, he had not that Brightness of Invention, that some Authors may have; but with these his Talents he has done more Service to the World in the Knowledge of *Physick*, than all his Predecessors in the whole World put together; by digesting a huge Heap of Jargon and indigested Stuff into an intelligible, regular, and rational System.[3]

Happy was it for Medicine, Houston concludes, when this great man was advised to turn his attention from Divinity to Medicine. This is praise indeed from anyone; from a Houston it is the highest conceivable praise. What an astonishing impression Boerhaave must have made on his pupils!

Boerhaave's service to the world, according to Houston, was in 'digesting a huge Heap of Jargon and indigested Stuff into an intelligible, regular, and rational System'. It is beginning to sound as though Boerhaave was a *systematiser* (and probably an *eclectic* one at that). And this indeed has been the common judgement of historians. If so,

[3] J. Houston, *Dr Houston's Memoirs of his own Life-Time*, ed. Jacob Bickerstaff (London, 1747), pp. 56–7.

Boerhaave may be said to have started a fashion, for the eighteenth century has been characterised as the age of 'systems' – the period when every physician had to produce his own 'system' in order to drum up business for himself.[4] But to ascribe Boerhaave's success to his 'systematising' does not *account* for that success, it merely redescribes it. For why should any medical students at this time have wanted or needed a medical 'system'? Why (if they did) did they find Boerhaave's so attractive? Would just any old system do, or did there have to be something special about it? If so, what was it that was special about Boerhaave's 'system'? In other words, we are back where we started: trying, in the absence of any sign of innovation or invention on his part, to discover what made Boerhaave's medicine special, what was unique and so highly attractive about it.

To answer this conundrum, let us first glance at where Boerhaave achieved his triumphs: the Leyden medical school. During the sixteenth and seventeenth centuries, the centre of economic power and productivity in Europe had moved from the Mediterranean to the north (where it still resides today). Amsterdam, a canal city built on water-borne commerce, came to supplant Venice, another canal city built on water-borne commerce, as the commercial entrepôt of the world. To put it in terms appropriate to the history of medicine: the pre-eminence of Padua (university town of Venice), came to be supplanted by that of Leyden. As had been the case with Venice, with prosperity went a very large measure of toleration: indeed the toleration may have been an enabling cause of the prosperity. Business was too important to be held up by confessional differences. Back in 1619 James Howell had recorded on a visit, 'I believe in this Street where I lodge, there be well near as many Religions as there be Houses; for one Neighbour knows not, nor cares not much what Religion the other is of',[5] and the case was still the same a century later. The official church, the Dutch Reformed Church, was Calvinist in doctrine and Presbyterian in organisation, but it was perfectly possible for Catholics and for refugee Jews to practise their religions. As a republic, there was also room for the intellectually and politically disaffected from England and Scotland to take refuge from the difficulties of James II and VII's

[4] On which see N. D. Jewson, 'Medical Knowledge and the Patronage System in Eighteenth-Century England', *Sociology* 8 (1974), pp. 369–85; Malcolm Nicolson, 'The Metastatic Theory of Pathogenesis and the Professional Interests of the Eighteenth-Century Physician', *Medical History* 32 (1988), pp. 277–300.

[5] *Epistolae Ho-Elianae: The Familiar Letters of James Howell, Historiographer Royal to Charles II*, ed. Joseph Jacobs, 2 vols. (London, 1890–92), vol. 1, p. 29, writing from Amsterdam.

rule at home. Intellectually too, the United Provinces were open, tolerant and flourishing. As Boerhaave's first biographer remarked (revealing his own prejudices thereby), 'From history it appears that ever since the rise of the Athenian commonwealth, the sciences have flourished most in states free from despotic sway, especially in republics.'[6] Leyden University had been flourishing, but in the last years of the seventeenth century was undergoing something of a dip in its fortunes. It was controlled by three Curators chosen by the states of Holland and by four Burgomasters of the city. They ran it as a business, and were determined that it should flourish again, and were seeking the best professors wherever they could be found. The medical faculty had five professors, who received a small salary and were dependent for the rest of their income on fees from the students they could attract. The hour called forth the man and, as is so often the case in such circumstances, it turned out that he was a local lad.

In the Leyden medical school Boerhaave had a startling rise to fame and position. He had been intending to enter the ministry, but changed his mind as he was (falsely) under suspicion of having Spinozist leanings. In 1701, aged thirty-two, he was appointed Lector on the Institutes of Medicine. He was not considered experienced enough to be appointed a Professor. The 'Institutes of Medicine' was the Theory of Medicine. The lectures Boerhaave gave here were published by him in 1707. To give some idea of the topics covered in the Institutes, we can note the main sections of the *Institutiones*: (1) The oeconomy (or workings) of the animal, (2) On diseases, (3) On signs, (4) On preserving health and (5) On the cure of diseases. It was not a comprehensive medical course, but the theoretical side of such a course. In this position he also chose to lecture on practical medicine in the form of a series of 'Aphorisms on recognising and curing diseases',[7] and these he published in 1708. Then in 1709 he was appointed also to the chair of Medicine and Botany, which he held for twenty years. With this chair came the charge of the large and flourishing University Botanic Garden. In 1714 Boerhaave was also given the chair of practical medicine ('clinical'), with the care of a twelve-bed hospital, where he took pupils to show them patients suffering under various diseases. Then in 1718 Boerhaave was also made Professor of Chemistry, a post he held until 1729. Thus, at the maximum, that is between the years 1718 and 1729, Boerhaave held four major teaching positions simultaneously out of

[6] William Burton, *An Account of the Life and Writings of Herman Boerhaave* (London, 1743; second edition, 1746), p. 2.
[7] Lindeboom, *Herman Boerhaave*, p. 61.

the six in the faculty: three professorships and a lectorship. It was not a chair of medicine that he held, but a whole sofa!

Some of these positions Boerhaave got through internal politics of the university; for example he had since 1703 been promised the first vacant chair, which turned out to be that in Medicine and Botany (of which he knew nothing at the date of his appointment). But the most important fact about these appointments is that it was effectively the Town Council who did the appointing. Anywhere else at this period (at Cambridge, for instance) if one person had held several chairs at once, it would be evidence of corruption and nepotism. At Leyden, however, it was a sign of the efficiency and effectiveness of the holder of these positions, i.e. of Boerhaave, for Boerhaave drew the students in, to the profit of the whole of Leyden – a fact that he well recognised himself.[8] Success bred success, and thus Boerhaave dominated the teaching of all branches of medicine at Leyden and, through the huge number of students who attended his teaching, he dominated medical teaching throughout the north of Europe for decades, in a way that no-one has done before or since.

On the principle that Boerhaave is likely to be a good authority on Boerhaave, in order to discover the man behind the medicine I want to take as the central document the *Commentariolus*, the autobiographical fragments written in 1738 and found amongst his papers after his death.[9] In this we shall find the key to Boerhaave's success. For here we can trace Boerhaave's education and his attitude to life and medicine. Boerhaave refers to himself in the third person. At first Boerhaave was taught by his father, a minister in the Dutch Reformed Church:

> The father of Herman was versed in Latin, Greek and Hebrew; he was very accomplished in history and knowledge of peoples (I) . . . Boerhaave's father himself undertook to instil into him, when he was very young, the principles of Latin and Greek, using the grammar of Vossius, and to explain the dialogues of Erasmus and the comedies of Terence. To the reading and explaining of the New Testament he added a survey of universal history, as expounded in the *Theatre*[10] of Christian Matthias (III).

[8] Lindeboom, *Herman Boerhaave*, p. 83, and *Orations*, pp. 143–4: Boerhaave's oration of 1709, inaugurating his professorship of Medicine and Botany.

[9] These are printed in Latin in Burton, *Life and Writings of Boerhaave*, who offers English versions in his text; and in his Appendix by Lindeboom, *Herman Boerhaave*, with translations. The roman numerals refer to the paragraphs as numbered by Lindeboom. I have used Lindeboom's translation with modifications.

[10] This is Christian Matthias, *Theatrum Historicum Theoretico-Practicum, in quo Quatuor Monarchiae . . . Nova et Artificiosa Methodo Describuntur, Omniaque ad Usum Oeconomicum, Politicum et Ecclesiasticum Accomodantur* (first edition 1648; third edition Amsterdam, 1668). The list of Roman monarchs is taken up to date in the person of the Holy Roman Emperor. The work is full of moral lessons.

The 'three languages' of the Renaissance are there: Latin, Greek and Hebrew, together with the writings of the greatest advocate of these languages, Erasmus. There is also much history, together with familiarity with the diversity of peoples in the world. Then Boerhaave went to the university at Leyden in 1684. Here he learnt dialectic, metaphysics, natural philosophy, the use of globes, and politics. But more than this:

> Perceiving the use and necessity of mathematics, Boerhaave gave some attention to that subject in the year 1687, and soon, enchanted by its elegance, advancing speedily through geometry and trigonometry and their applications, he came to algebra. This was wonderfully agreeable to his talents. He admired especially the geometrical synthesis of the ancients, cultivating it in order to exercise his intelligence, and the geometrical analysis of the moderns, for the purpose of discovering new things (VII).

Thus it was in the very year of Newton's great work, the *Philosophiae Naturalis Principia Mathematica*, that Boerhaave became an enthusiast for mathematics. At some time Boerhaave 'taught mathematics to the most choice young men' (x). And while still a student, he kept reading history: Trigland (the Leyden Professor of Divinity) on Hebrew antiquities, and Spanheim (another Leyden professor) on ecclesiastical history (VIII).

Boerhaave was studying both theology and medicine, intending to graduate in medicine and then enter the ministry in the usual way (XV) and practise both. His system of learning theology was as follows:

> a daily reading of the Church Fathers, in their chronological order, beginning with Clement of Rome and proceeding through the centuries, in order that he might understand the teaching of Jesus Christ, as handed down in the New Testament, through the interpretation of the early Fathers of the Church. In them he admired the simplicity of their pure doctrine, the sanctity of their discipline, and the blamelessness of a life devoted to God. He regretted that the subtleties of the Schools had later corrupted theology. He greatly regretted that the interpretation of Holy Scripture was sought for among the sects of the Sophists; and that the metaphysical reflections of Plato, of Aristotle, of Thomas Aquinas, of [Duns] Scotus, and – in his own time – of Descartes, were considered as laws according to which sentiments of the Holy Scriptures about God should be amended (IX).

The effect of his reading of history is becoming evident: Boerhaave reads the Fathers in chronological order. But in addition to this, Boerhaave takes it as given that the earlier the Father, the purer the doctrine. For, he believed, subsequent ages had corrupted the original simple doctrine: the Schools had brought in the philosophers and metaphysicians to explain the Holy Scriptures, and had made *their* opinions the test and guide of the Scriptures! He continues, recalling his time at Leyden:

He experienced bitter differences of opinion, and that from these are born and fostered the most passionate disputes, and the hatreds and ambitions, of the most acute minds, so much in contrast to peace with God and man. Nothing was more repugnant to him, than that all asserted that the Holy Scriptures speak in a human way, but that they should be explained in a divine sense, and that they each define the divine sense according to the tenets of their own metaphysics. Therefore he deplored that the prevailing opinion of the dominant sect prescribed the path and the rules of orthodoxy only according to the dictates of the Metaphysicians and not of the Sacred Writings – whence such varied opinions concerning the most simple doctrine (IX).

The Scriptures speak in a simple way; their message has become obscured by interpreting them through the teachings of one or other school of metaphysics; this has resulted in differences of opinion and hence – worst of all – 'the most passionate disputes, and hatreds and ambitions . . . so much in contrast to peace with God and man'.

This peace Boerhaave desperately wanted:

The doctrine, handed down in Holy Writ in Hebrew and Greek, he recognised and felt as the only one that was salutary to the soul. On every occasion he professed that the teaching expressed by Jesus Christ, by His words and His life, alone gives peace of mind (*tranquillitatem menti*). To his friends he always declared that peace of mind (*pacem animi*) is scarcely to be found save only in the great precept of Moses concerning a sincere love of God and man, if well observed; and that nowhere outside the Holy Scriptures is to be found anything which calms the mind (*quod mentem serenet*) (XVIII).

Hebrew and Greek are the means to reach that simple message in the Scriptures, and that simple message brings *peace of mind.*

PEACE IN MEDICINE

It may sound as though this has little to do with Boerhaave's medicine. Until, that is, we notice that Boerhaave adopted exactly the same technique in learning medicine – because he had exactly the same attitudes there. It is perhaps incredible, he wrote in retrospect, that when he was a student of medicine he did not attend lectures by any professor of medicine, except for a few by the celebrated Drélincourt shortly before Drélincourt's death (XI). He did not need to, because he was following a programme of self-education identical to the one he employed for theology: 'He began his reading of the ancient medical writers in chronological order, starting with Hippocrates' (XII). Hippocrates, then, was the equivalent for Boerhaave of the Bible, and just as pristine: 'he quickly realised that the later authors owed to Hippocrates everything that was good in their work; therefore to Hippocrates alone he devoted a long time, reading him, summarizing and analysing him' (XII). Had Boerhaave been attending the university lectures on medicine, this long time he was spending mastering Hippocrates would, of course, have been spent imbibing more up-to-date opinions and writers. But Boerhaave, when he turned to reading through the other medical writers after Hippocrates, found most of them defective: 'Running through the more recent writers he paused at Sydenham, whom he worked through several times, each time more eagerly' (XII). And that is the only other medical writer he mentions in these autobiographical fragments. Thomas Sydenham, who was still alive when Boerhaave was a young man (Sydenham died in 1689), seems to be the only medical writer after Hippocrates who was worth studying!

Boerhaave did indeed, according to these fragments, study other writers on subjects related to medicine. On anatomy he studied Vesalius, Fallopius and Bartholin, and conducted numerous animal dissections, and followed the anatomical demonstrations of Nuck (XI); in botany he used the Flora of Hermann – though he did not attend his lectures – but mostly he learnt botany in the university physic garden. Chemistry too, he recalled, he studied day and night, but does not mention having read any particular author (XII). But on the theory and practice of medicine, the two core subjects in the medical curriculum, the only authorities he speaks of are Hippocrates and Sydenham.

Boerhaave was very happy in Leyden, and turned down repeated offers to transfer to The Hague. For in Leyden he could be free:

> He was satisfied with a free life, far from the crowd, a life altogether devoted to the continuation of his studies, where he would not be forced to say some things that he did not feel, and to feel some things that he had to conceal; to be snatched from the devotion of his loved ones; to be ruled by others. Such at this time was his life: visiting the sick, and directly thereafter devoting himself to the Muse in his home; stoking the furnace of Vulcan, and studying attentively all branches of medicine; also teaching mathematics to others; reading Holy Scripture and those authors who profess to teach a sure way to love God (XVII).[11]

Freedom of thought, aversion to the crowd, peace of mind: these Boerhaave wanted in both theology and medicine, simultaneously. Boerhaave's medicine was his theology – itself built round a desperate desire for peace of mind – in another domain.

If the desire for peace of mind is the key to understanding Boerhaave's attitude to medicine, and hence to the kind of medicine he taught (and hence, in turn, to why it had such a strong appeal to others), then it deserves a little further consideration here. This atti-

[11] Lindeboom, *Herman Boerhaave*, p. 48, takes this as referring to a very early period in Boerhaave's career, i.e., 1693–1701; I see no reason why it may not be referring equally to later periods.

tude of Boerhaave's is readily recognisable. Scholars refer to it as 'eirenic', a term which had come to be quite extensively used in the seventeenth century. 'Irenical Theology . . . presents the points of agreement among Christians, with a view to the ultimate unity . . . of Christendom.'[12] As its Greek root reveals, it is the pursuit of *peace* in religion, and hence in society. Peace of mind had, of course, been the traditional goal of the philosopher, especially of the Stoic; here it is made the goal of religion. This is an attitude which allows one to stay a member of one's own church – it is most definitely not a sectarian position or a new sect – and in this (though only in this) it is akin to ecumenicism today. The eirenic position had many prominent adherents in England in the middle and late seventeenth century, of whom the most important for our purposes was Robert Boyle. According to J. R. Jacob, Boyle wanted a broad church which would not divide men by emphasising the doctrinal differences which separated them, but rather would unite them by appealing to the Christian tenets they held in common; Jacob quotes a letter from Boyle of 1647: 'It is strange, that men should rather be quarreling for a few trifling opinions, wherein they dissent, than to embrace one another for those many fundamental truths, wherein they agree.'[13] The individual should strive for a certain inner calm or imperturbability of spirit,[14] and express his love of God through applying himself wholeheartedly to *work*.[15] Boyle's adherence to this position was a model to Boerhaave, for Boyle was one of his heroes.[16]

In Boerhaave's application of these same principles to both religion and medicine, we can see that he thought there was a basic core set of truths which, if discovered, are indisputable. How is one to find them? By looking at the authors/authorities that all men hold in common, and limiting oneself to these. In religion it is the Bible (as interpreted by the early Fathers), in medicine it is Hippocrates. So: one should go back to the beginning. Then, sedulously avoiding the adoption of any misleading metaphysical system, read your way forwards: where subsequent authors develop or build on this core set of truths, then they can be followed; where they do not, they are to be avoided. So *history* is

[12] P. Schaff, *Encyclopaedia of Religious Knowledge*, vol. 2 (1882–3,), p. 1,118, as quoted in the Oxford English Dictionary.

[13] J. R. Jacob, *Robert Boyle and the English Revolution* (New York, 1977), p. 23.

[14] *Ibid.*, p. 59. [15] *Ibid.*, p. 87.

[16] The references to Boyle are legion, but see especially the oration 'On Chemistry Purging Itself of its Own Errors', translated in Kegel-Brinkgreve and Luyendijk-Elshout, *Boerhaave's Orations*. Burton, *Account of Life and Writings*, claimed that Boerhaave liked to read Boyle's *Seraphic Love* (Burton, p. 23n.); on this work, see Jacob, *Robert Boyle*. On Boyle see also the most important study, Steven Shapin and Simon Schaffer, *Leviathan and the Air-Pump: Hobbes, Boyle and the Experimental Life* (Princeton, 1985).

the key: it is the key to the core doctrines, and hence to the promotion of peace! Always one should try to reconcile apparently competing doctrines, to play down the differences, and to promote what they have in common. And always avoid conflict: 'the sparks of calumny will be presently extinct of themselves unless you blow them', as Boerhaave said.[17] This is what Boerhaave's medical approach, his apparent 'systematising', is about. It is aimed at promoting peace in medicine and amongst medical men. And of course it worked spectacularly, if we may take Boerhaave's astonishing success as a teacher and inspirer as evidence.

Such an approach looks very innocent, and this is (presumably) how Boerhaave experienced it. He probably found no trouble in identifying which were the purest and most ancient doctrines, whether he was looking at Hippocrates or at some more recent writer of whom he approved. But while it may, in that sense, be innocent, this approach is hardly value-free. For what Boerhaave inevitably did was to *take to* Hippocrates, and other writers, certain attitudes from his own day. As a result he makes of both ancients and moderns some quite new persons: it is highly doubtful whether Boerhaave's Hippocrates or even his Sydenham would have recognised themselves in his characterisations of them. Boerhaave's success in creating these new images for the dead was so great that we today tend to hold Boerhaavian views of all the ancients and moderns of whom Boerhaave approved.

Boerhaave's enemies were Descartes, above all, and chemists in the tradition of Paracelsus and Van Helmont. His heroes were an odd bunch. The main ones were: Hippocrates, and then other Greek physicians almost as ancient, such as Aretaeus of Cappadocia (he produced an edition of his work) and Nicander. Then no-one for a millenium and a half. Then Francis Bacon, William Harvey, Robert Boyle, Thomas Sydenham and Isaac Newton, all from seventeenth-century England – of whom the greatest for him was Sydenham, the 'English Hippocrates'. We know that Boyle and Sydenham were friends, but we also know that Harvey despised Bacon, and that Newton had little time for the doctrines of Bacon. We also know that the followers of these great men were often at each others' throats – as were, for instance, the medical followers of Newton and Sydenham.[18] But what Boerhaave maintained, and firmly believed, was that all of

17 As quoted by Burton, *Life and Writings of Boerhaave*, p. 54.

18 See my 'Sydenham Versus Newton: The Edinburgh Fever Dispute of the 1690s Between Andrew Brown and Archibald Pitcairne' in W. F. Bynum and V. Nutton, *Theories of Fever from Antiquity to the Enlightenment*, (London, 1981), pp. 71–98.

them taught doctrines which were in harmony, and that Hippocrates had taught all these doctrines first! Thus, he could claim that Hippocrates 'was versed in the Philosophy of *Democritus*, which was the purest of any System, being founded on three Principles: Atoms, Gravity and a Vacuum; which have been in our Age again restored by the most solid Reasonings of Sir *Isaac Newton*.'[19] He could find, again quite innocently, that Hippocrates 'had under him a Class of young Physicians, who were employ'd in making Experiments' and passing on the results to Hippocrates,[20] which are thus incorporated in the Hippocratic writings! Boerhaave could instinctively portray Sydenham as a latter-day Hippocrates:

> *Sydenham*, whom no one ought to mention but with Honour. This Author laying aside all the Pomp of Learning and Systems, did nothing else but observe by the *Clinica Methodus* of the Ancients what happen'd in Distempers. He was excellent in this, that one may so know the Nature of Distempers as to admit no deductory Conclusions, to use no Authors, nor take up any Prejudice; but he tells what pre-existed in the Body and Life of the Patient . . . I know no one like him, his Method is most excellent . . .[21]

Eirenic themes – of how desirable it is to avoid sectarianism, of the need to clear away the debris of later metaphysical accretions from the ancient truths – pervade the great public orations that Boerhaave gave, and which were frequently reprinted.[22] The very first of these was given by Boerhaave before he ever entered medicine, and was 'On Cicero's judgement – properly understood – of Epicurus on man's highest good'. Epicurus had claimed that man's highest goal was giving himself over to self-indulgent pleasure; in modern times Gassendi had defended Epicurus. Boerhaave defends Cicero's ancient condemnation of Epicurus, on the ground that pandering to the senses fails to promote the proper goal of philosophy, tranquillity of mind.[23] The first of the specifically medical orations that Boerhaave gave (1701) was 'On Commending the Study of Hippocrates':

> who will be able to follow Nature as his sole guide when investigating things? Who will never go astray? Who will always avoid uncertainties? Only he, in my opinion, who is free from all sectarianism, unfettered by any preconceived ideas, devoid of all leanings towards prejudice; he who merely learns, accepts, and relates what he actually sees.[24]

[19] *Dr Boerhaave's Academical Lectures on the Theory of Physick. Being a Genuine Translation of his Institutes and Explanatory Comment, Collated and Adjusted to Each Other, as They Were Dictated to his Students at the University of Leyden*, 6 vols. (London, 1742), vol. 1, p. 27.

[20] *Ibid.*, p. 28.

[21] Quoted from the *Method of Studying Physic* (London, 1719), pp. 316–7, by G. A. Lindeboom, 'Boerhaave's Debt to British Science and British Medicine's Debt to Boerhaave' in his *Boerhaave and Great Britain* (Leiden, 1974), p. 13n.38. On Sydenham see my 'Thomas Sydenham: Epidemics, Experiment and the "Good Old Cause"' in R. K. French and A. Wear, *The Medical Revolution of the Seventeenth Century*, (Cambridge, 1988), pp. 164–190.

[22] For a translation of them see Kegel-Brinkgreve and Luyendijk-Elshout, *Boerhaave's Orations*; I have generally followed these translations.

[23] *Ibid.*, pp. 27–8, 36.

[24] *Ibid.*, p. 69.

Who did this? Hippocrates alone. We must follow him. In 1709, Boerhaave's address was 'on the Simplicity of Purified Medicine'. The true and certain tenets of medicine are few, but currently medicine is inflated with errors and deceit:

> And such deceit will certainly never be avoided more successfully than by rejecting everything sectarian. Truth will be discerned most easily when only that to which all experts unanimously agree is accepted as being sound. If medicine – currently inflated by a mass of alien elements – is corrected according to this rule, it will return to its proper condition and soon shrink to its own limited size.[25]

His oration in 1715 was 'On Achieving Certainty in *Physica*', the realm of natural philosophy (see plate 1). Its theme is that the postulating of first principles and then deducing truths from them, is barren and futile; it is the Cartesians primarily who are here condemned. In fact, Boerhaave claimed, 'only from the observations of our senses' can the knowledge of the properties of things be gained, and these 'either become known in the experimental manner, or can be deduced from this first category (as previously explored by that one and only way of *experience*) via foolproof mathematical reasoning'.[26] When he became Professor of Chemistry in 1718, Boerhaave orated 'On Chemistry Purging Itself of its Own Errors' (see plate 2): the history of chemistry shows that its earlier errors, associated with ancient superstitions, have been purged – especially by Robert Boyle!

> It is but fair, then, that we should greatly rejoice at the present most excellent state of chemistry throughout the whole of Europe, which is fostered by the united efforts of its votaries. For they are eager to set up experiments, yet full of cautious reserve about drawing conclusions from them, taking everything into account, warned by the hazards incurred by others; and they take no less pride in the correcting of errors than in substantiating their own theses. And the results envisaged really come up to their wishes and merits. We now have a purified, useful and trustworthy chemical discipline – so much so, that anybody who now trains his mind to follow the precepts of this discipline ends up by having a refined insight into the secrets of Nature and Medicine. He will avoid the snares set up by the wayward cleverness of rhetorical tricksters; he will not swear himself bondsman to the words of any master (*nullius in verba Magistri addictus jurare*), and will never be an inept supporter of any particular sect.[27]

Even the 1703 Oration 'On the Usefulness of Mechanical Reasoning in Medicine', though we might not expect so from its title, is on these same eirenic themes. We have already seen how, for Boerhaave, Hippocrates was an adherent of Democritean atomism (equivalent, for Boerhaave, to Newtonian natural philosophy). Recent investigators,

[25] *Ibid.*, pp. 124 and 129. [26] *Ibid.*, p. 155.

[27] *Ibid.*, p. 211. 'Nullius in verba' was of course the motto of the Royal Society of London, the Society of Boyle and Newton. On the adoption of the motto (it comes from Horace) by the Royal Society, see Dorothy Stimson, *Scientists and Amateurs: A History of the Royal Society* (London, 1949), p. 64.

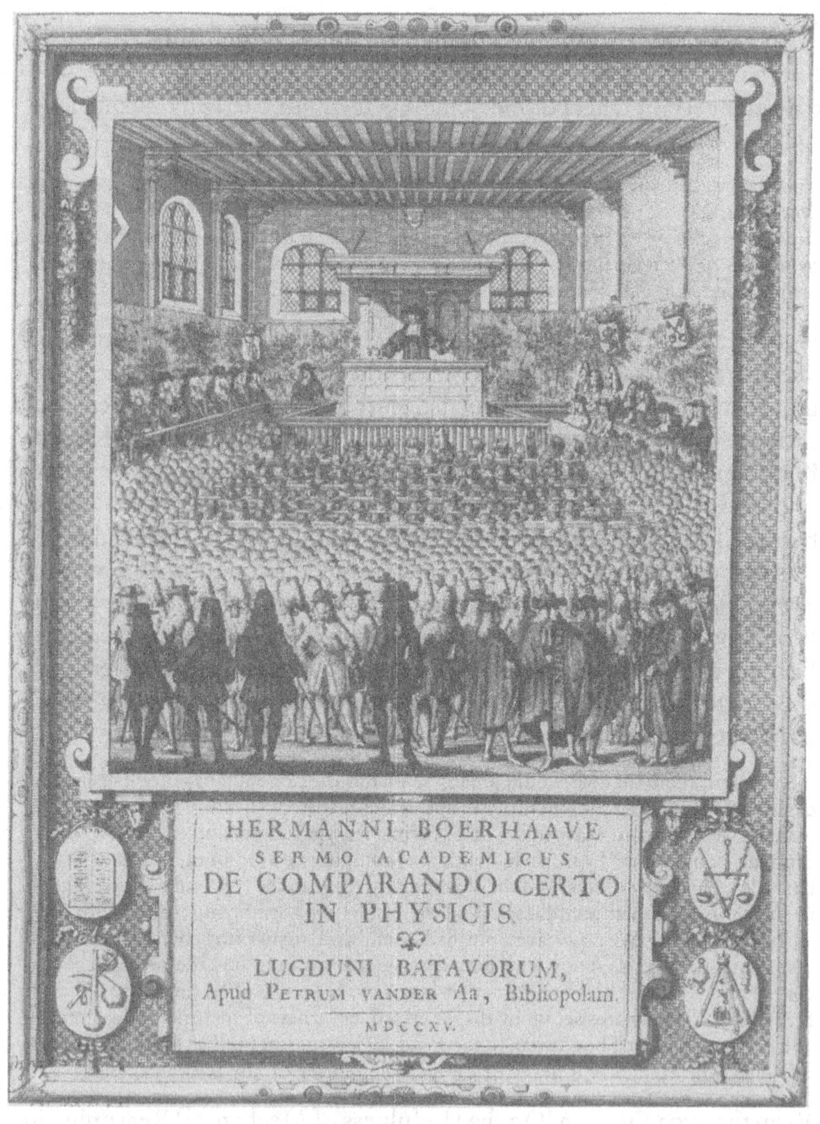

HERMANNI BOERHAAVE
SERMO ACADEMICUS
DE COMPARANDO CERTO
IN PHYSICIS
LUGDUNI BATAVORUM,
Apud PETRUM VANDER AA, Bibliopolam.
MDCCXV.

1 Title-page of Herman Boerhaave, *De Comparando Certo in Physicis* (Leyden, 1715)

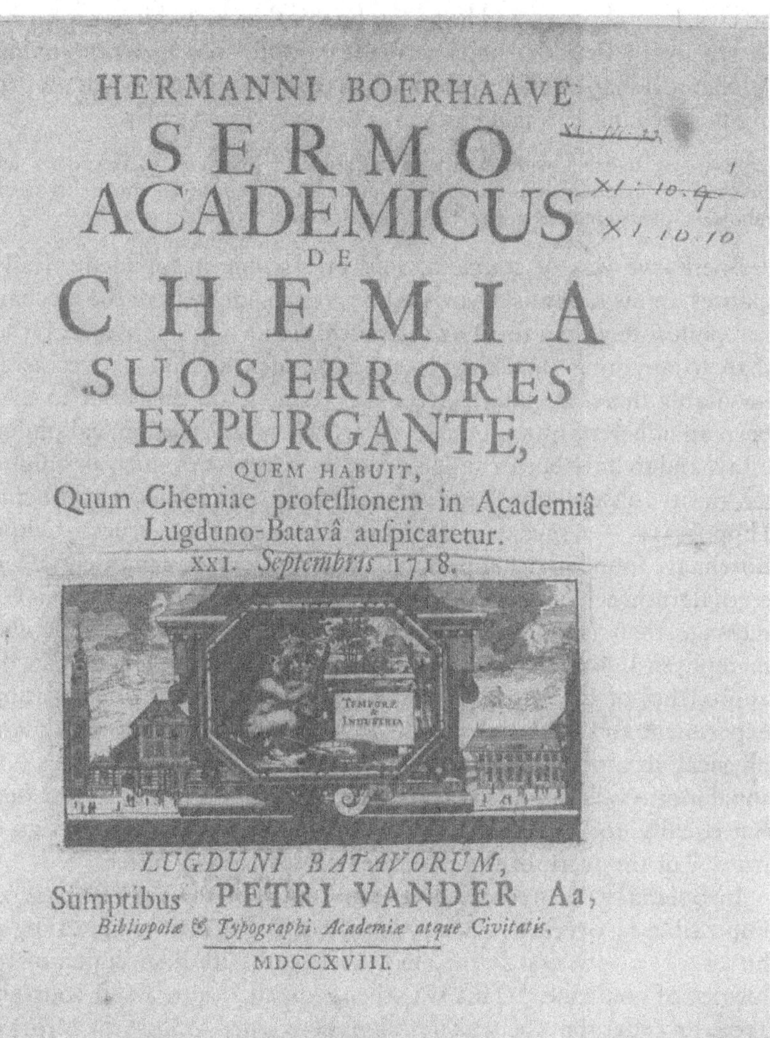

HERMANNI BOERHAAVE

SERMO

ACADEMICUS

DE

CHEMIA

SUOS ERRORES

EXPURGANTE,

QUEM HABUIT,

Quum Chemiae profeſſionem in Academiâ Lugduno-Batavâ auſpicaretur.

XXI. *Septembris* 1718.

TEMPORE & INDUSTRIA

LUGDUNI BATAVORUM,

Sumptibus PETRI VANDER Aa,

Bibliopolæ & Typographi Academiæ atque Civitatis.

MDCCXVIII.

2 Title-page of Herman Boerhaave, *Sermo Academicus de Chemia Suos Errores Expurgante* (Leyden, 1718)

he says, have shown – and he means by this that such things are visible to the eye – that the body is made of *solid* parts, arranged into mechanical shapes, and of *fluids* which pass through the solids according to mechanical principles and laws. Surprise, surprise,

> Hippocrates, together with the whole multitude of Babylonians, Egyptians, and Greeks in whose footsteps he walked, and with the entire school of his Greek followers, discovered only these two categories (*duo haec*).[28]

Boerhaave was of course a child of his time in his medical allegiances. In his case this meant that he was an adherent of the mechanical philosophy, in a form owing much to Newton and Boyle, rather than to anything smacking of atheism, such as that of Descartes. Inevitably therefore Boerhaave's Hippocrates too turns out to have been an adherent of the best seventeenth-century mechanical philosophy, and to have been a supporter of its watch-cries, such as simplicity, purity, observation[29] and the need to avoid speculation. It is *this* Hippocrates – a seventeenth/eighteenth-century construct – whom Boerhaave found in the Hippocratic writings, expressing essential and eternal truths which the proper physician ought to follow. Boerhaave's message, then, is: out with the sects; out with disagreement; out with metaphysical speculations; out with the godlessness inherent in the approaches of Epicurus, Descartes or Spinoza. In with observation, experiment and mathematics; in with sciences purged of their metaphysical accretions. In, above all, with simplicity. Boerhaave's personal motto was 'simplicity is the sign of truth', *simplex veri sigillum*. But equally, for Boerhaave, peace among medical men is the sign of truth – of the truth of the doctrines on which they agree.

In Boerhaave's approach, the importance of the use of history is impossible to overstate. Always, always, Boerhaave is appealing to history. His very first lecture in 1701 began with a specimen of the history of medicine.[30] This was then expanded into a full course in 1704, 'in order that the student might be warned against the errors of the past'.[31] The story was always the same: originally there were pure doctrines, subsequently they were perverted by followers of the metaphysical sects, and then they were rescued from the clutches of the sectaries by heroic moderns. The *Institutiones*, for instance, starts with an account of the Origin, Progress and Fate of Medicine. This shows the birth of medicine in antiquity, its development by experience,

[28] Kegel-Brinkgreve and Luyendijk-Elshout, *Boerhaave's Orations*, p. 102.
[29] On how Boerhaave based the teaching of clinical medicine on the senses, see Lindeboom, *Herman Boerhaave*, p. 106. [30] *Ibid*., p. 58. [31] *Ibid*., p. 68.

observation and experiment, its culmination in Hippocrates, follower of Democritus. Medicine thus cultivated (and as then organised by Aretaeus of Cappodocia) eventually reached Galen. And here was where medicine went astray, being shaped to the theories of a sect:

> Galen, making a collection of their various writings, digesting what was confused, and explaining everything from the dogmas of the Peripatetics, right to the point of the disgrace of slavery, brought great profit yet no less damnation to the good Art: he was responsible for Medicine having to be explicated, more subtly than truthfully, according to the elements, the so-called cardinal qualities, their gradations, and the four humours.[32]

Ultimately the immortal Harvey, having by his demonstrations overthrown every theory of his predecessors, laid a new, and certain, foundation for this science. And Boerhaave's message is also always the same: if pursued in an open-minded and disinterested way, the truths of medicine are everywhere accessible; but if one brings in *preconceptions*, if one tries to make nature and medicine fit the dreamt-up principles of some sect or other, then one perverts the truth and stops the progress of the sciences. The sects as Boerhaave presents and condemns them, both in religion and in medicine, are always concerned with metaphysics, but we need to remember that in this period every religious position – including Boerhaave's own – was also a political position. Boerhaave's message here is of course reminiscent of that nowadays often preached about science and medicine (especially by historians of these subjects): that disinterested open-mindedness is the only way to pursue them, and that 'interests' of any kind (whether philosophical, political, social, economic) have to be excluded lest the truth become polluted. That we agree with Boerhaave here does not however, in itself, show that he was right: only that he has had an enormous influence on the later development of attitudes toward the proper pursuit of medicine and the natural sciences.

It is not very easy to discover what it was in the circumstances of late-seventeenth-century Dutch life which had first elicited from Boerhaave the eirenic attitude which thereafter organised all his thinking. For Boyle, in mid-seventeenth-century England, it had been the discord of

[32] 'Ille sparsa colligens, digerens confusa, cunctaque ex Peripateticis dogmatibus, ad servitutis infamiam usque, explicans, emolumenti plurimum, neque minus tamen damni, bonae Arti attulit: dum auctor fuit, ut ex elementis, qualitatibus vulgo dictis cardinalibus, harum gradibus, et humoribus quatuor, subtilius, quam verius, explicaretur Medicina', *Institutiones Medicae in Usus Annuae Exercitationibus Domesticos Digestae ab Hermanno Boerhaave*, 6th edition (Paris, 1735), paragraph 15, my translation.

the civil war which prompted him to see the eirenic route as the only way forward. But in Boerhaave's case the spur is unknown, though it may perhaps have had something to do with the expulsion of the Huguenots from France in 1685 and their arrival in the Netherlands.[33]

The eirenic message that Boerhaave preached did get through to his pupils as they imbibed the easily assimilable medicine that he taught. But the message was of course reinterpreted in the light of each student's own views. Here, for instance, is the way in which his biographer, Burton, paraphrased Boerhaave's oration 'On Commending the Study of Hippocrates'; Burton thought the story was about

> the original conjunction of theory with practice, the abuse of the former by making speculation supersede, rather than build up observation and experience; the necessity of collecting naked and indisputable facts, and delivering them untainted by partiality or hypotheses, and the pre-eminence of this author [Hippocrates] on that account above the rest of the ancients.[34]

But the Boerhaavian message could also be used as a weapon against one's enemies, as it was in 1735 by the anonymous translator of the *Aphorisms* into English, here attacking the members of the Royal College of Physicians:

> Those Gentlemen, for whom I chiefly design'd this Translation, will here . . . be enabled to judge of the true Merit of Physicians and to distinguish . . . those, who are forced to hide their Ignorance, and confused unsettled Thoughts under the Cloak of a Jargon, which they themselves do not understand, or who have no other Merit than the noisy Clamour of *Oxford*, *Oxford*!, their Equipages, and the cunning sly Way of engaging Nurses or some ignorant Women in their Interest . . .[35]

So much for the peace that Boerhaave wished to inculcate! On the other hand, this particular instance may have happened because it was England. In what may have been a joke, Boerhaave warned a friend about the English just before the friend went to visit England: 'you will soon become acquainted with the customs of a most fierce race, and with its riches and wisdom, and you will praise the plain simplicity of the Dutch, who work untiringly'.[36] The Scots, however, were a different race, and we must now turn to see how Boerhaave's medicine brought peace to the medical warfare of Edinburgh.

[33] There is not much clue in F. L. R. Sassen, 'The Intellectual Climate in Leiden in Boerhaave's Time', in G. A. Lindeboom (ed.), *Boerhaave and his Time* (Leiden, 1970), pp. 1–16.

[34] Burton, *Life and Writings of Boerhaave*, p. 24.

[35] The anonymous 1735 English translation, printed in London by Bettersworth and others; Preface.

[36] Letter to Bassand, 21 October 1731, printed and translated in G. A. Lindeboom (ed.), *Boerhaave's Correspondence*, 3 vols. (Leiden, 1962–79), vol. 2, pp. 292–5.

PEACE IN SCOTLAND

The founding of the famous Edinburgh medical school can justifiably be looked on as the first public act of the Scottish Enlightenment.[37] It was formally founded in 1726 when, by decision of the Town Council, there were appointed (1) Dr Andrew St-Clair (Sinclair) and (2) Dr John Rutherford, to jointly be Professors of the Theory and Practice of Medicine; and (3) Dr Andrew Plummer and (4) Dr John Innes, to jointly be Professors of Medicine and Chemistry.[38] They had all been pupils of Boerhaave in Leyden in the years 1718–22, and had been teaching privately in Edinburgh for a while. It will be noticed that what they undertook to teach was virtually the same range of topics (though divided between four teachers) that Boerhaave taught in all his chairs. They taught these subjects out of Boerhaave's own books. Like Boerhaave himself they were to teach for fees (they were offered no salary), and hence what they were getting in 1726 was a grant of title and the use of certain facilities belonging to the town. Together with Alexander Monro, already appointed (1725) as Professor of Anatomy, they were to constitute the Faculty of Medicine of Edinburgh University. The whole thing turned out to be a vast success, and Edinburgh became the premier medical school for English-speaking students of medicine for more than a century. The teaching attracted many students to Edinburgh from England, Ireland and America, and hence brought very significant wealth to the town.

So popular was Boerhaave in Edinburgh in the early 1720s that there had been two other young Boerhaave pupils teaching there privately, Dr William Graeme and Dr George Martin. The Provost later said that the Town Council had had difficulty in choosing between their petitions to be granted title as Professors:

> At that time, we [the Town Council] were only making a trial, and were somewhat uncertain about its success; and yet they [the four teachers] thought themselves favoured by the Town-Council in giving them a preference in our choice to another set who petitioned us to appoint them. At that time I should have cheerfully come in to the Town's accomodating them with a laboratory, if our finances would have admitted of it.[39]

[37] See the prominent role ascribed to the beginnings of the medical school in R. A. Campbell and Andrew S. Skinner (eds.), *The Origins and Nature of the Scottish Enlightenment* (Edinburgh, 1982), esp. the essays by Ronald C. Cant, 'Origins of the Enlightenment in Scotland: The Universities' and Anand C. Chitnis, 'Provost Drummond and the Origins of Edinburgh Medicine'.

[38] The Town Council minute is reprinted in Jane Rendall, *The Origins of the Scottish Enlightenment 1707–1776* (London, 1978), pp. 52–3.

[39] Letter from George Drummond to William Cullen, February 1756, printed in John Thomson, *An Account of the Life, Lectures and Writings of William Cullen, M.D.*, 2 vols. (London, 1832–59), vol. 1, p. 95.

The Boerhaave formula worked for Edinburgh, and hence for Scotland. Why should this have been the case? Other historians[40] have pointed out the parallels between Leyden and Edinburgh, which facilitated this adoption of Dutch practices: the Town Council was in charge of the university; the university was run deliberately to attract students and hence make money for the town; both Scotland and the United Provinces were Calvinist Protestant. Such common features, however, can at best only count as necessary causes, not sufficient ones. Our characterisation of Boerhaave's teaching has been of an approach which was deliberately eirenic (and hence non-controversial), non-sectarian (and hence tolerant) and one which *as a consequence* was 'synthetic'. It was medicine to calm the mind; and it was (or its audience felt it was) comprehensive and exhaustive. In order to find some more compelling reasons for the successful grafting of this particular Dutch medicine on to Scottish stock, let us look at the state of Scotland and of medicine within Edinburgh and see how they needed the balm which only Boerhaave's medicine could bring.

Politically Scotland was in turmoil. But certain Scots were promoting what I shall call a 'Scottish mission to civilise Scotland' in order to quell the disquiet. I shall be claiming that the founding of a Boerhaave-type medical school was part of this political campaign. To understand this we need to go back to the arrival in Britain of the Prince of Orange, the Stadtholder of Holland, Prince William.

When in late 1688 James II fled the throne of England, in the so-called 'Glorious Revolution', many Scots considered that, as James VII of Scotland, he had abandoned the Scottish throne at the same time. Certain Englishmen of a 'Whig' persuasion (meaning that they were in favour of a limited, constitutional monarchy) had already turned to William and Mary, and invited them to the throne of England – under certain 'constitutional' conditions. Some Scottish nobles went down to London, and invited William and Mary to take the throne of Scotland too. In all the excitement of installing a new – an invited – monarchy, the Scottish Parliament suddenly found its own strength. *Party* strategies suddenly appeared, and the dominant faction was very like that dominant in the English Parliament: it was Whig. So not only did William have to acquiesce to constitutional concessions in Scotland, as he had had to do in England, before he formally got the throne, but the terms were as stringent as they had been in England. There was one

[40] For instance J. B. Morrell in his essay 'The Edinburgh Town Council and its University, 1717–1766' in R. G. W. Anderson and A. D. C. Simpson (eds.), *The Early Years of the Edinburgh Medical School* (Edinburgh, 1976). This work contains several valuable essays.

major difference: the established religion of Scotland was to be Presbyterianism. And this meant that the Covenanters – the clergy who had been forced to become outlaws in the reign of James – suddenly came to be in charge of the whole apparatus of the church, from the General Assembly down through the Synods and the Presbyteries, to the Kirk Sessions in the parishes. Scotland was their oyster, to make as God-fearingly Calvinist as they wished, and to make its monarch as subject to the Kirk as their traditions demanded. It looked as though Scotland was about to become highly intolerant.

The Scottish Parliament, in the 1690s and the first years of the new century, experienced a quite unprecedented degree of activity, and became a centre of national life. Parliament took on itself the role of planning for Scotland's future. In particular it actively sought to rival the Dutch in fishing and the English in cloth-making. Unfortunately, the proximity to England meant that all its well-meaning projects were doomed: Scotland was trying to compete with industries already flourishing in England; its attempt to create colonies on the English pattern was ruthlessly destroyed by England. England, both advertently and inadvertently, just would not let Scotland develop economically. All that the Scots could do to protest, and to protect their own interests, was to refuse to settle the succession to the Scottish throne on the Hanoverians as the English had done. In order to defuse the instability that this threatened to themselves, the English bought off the Scots with Union in 1707.

Only a handful of Scots were in favour of the Union at the time: and, by a strange chance, almost all of them seemed to have been in Parliament, brought round to favour Union either by financial persuasion, or by the genuine belief that Union would bring to Scotland all the economic advantages that England possessed. At all events, the consequence of Union was that Scotland no longer had a Parliament; it no longer had a centre for political life. Certainly, under the terms of the Union treaty, there was representation for Scottish nobles and MPs in the new Parliament of Great Britain; but they were swamped in that great institution, and Scotland's voice could not be heard in London. Instead it suffered neglect: England's interests were paramount in Parliament, Scotland's forgotten. But the Scots still had a weapon: when sufficiently disenchanted, many of them were prepared to turn to the hope that a restoration of the Stuart monarchy in Scotland – the restoration of Scotland to the status of independent kingdom – could solve all their problems. And this hope was the basis of *Jacobitism*: some Jacobites being principled and loyal supporters of the House of

Stuart, others temporarily seeing in it their salvation from the most recent indignities of neglect heaped upon them by the English. So, although Scotland was something that English government ministers ignored as long as they could, it was a lion that might stir at any time. Luckily for the English government, they had voluntary allies amongst the Scots. It was these allies who ran what I am calling the mission to civilise Scotland.

They were the supporters of the 1689 Revolution, determined to preserve it and to unite the nation behind the new monarchy. Some of these people, who tended to be 'sober' Presbyterians (which is a technical term of the period) as well as sober Whigs (which is not), had brought from their exiles in Holland – enforced on them during the reign of James – ideals of a moderate kind. They quickly inserted themselves into the Kirk and into educational establishments. Their early leader was William Carstares, chaplain to William in Scotland, who in time became Moderator of the Church of Scotland, and Principal of Edinburgh University.[41] He proceeded to modify both institutions. He calmed the fanaticism of the General Assembly, and counselled it to abstain from challenging the power of the monarchy and State. This was an amazing achievement, and was carried out with consummate skill. With respect to Edinburgh University, both as *éminence grise* behind Gilbert Rule, and then as Principal himself, he inherited charge of an institution which was still pursuing its original role as an instrument of Edinburgh Presbyterianism; and he turned it into an institution worthy of the name of university, and one designed to produce tolerant graduates. To this end he introduced a professoriate on the Dutch principle, incorporated new studies such as law, and studies calculated to introduce an attitude of tolerance toward the other churches, such as the Regius Professorship of Ecclesiastical History. He also tried to create a professorship of medicine and chemistry in the university in 1713, when Dr James Crawford suggested his own eligibility, as a Leyden graduate, to hold such a post.[42] Crawford was given rooms in the university, where he certainly taught chemistry, but an attempt by Carstares to get him a salary from royal funds did not succeed, and Crawford does not seem to have taught much medicine.

It was people of Carstares's persuasion who were quick to import

[41] On Carstares see A. Ian Dunlop, *William Carstares and the Kirk by Law Established* (Edinburgh, 1967); Sir Alexander Grant, *The Story of the University of Edinburgh*, 2 vols. (London, 1884).

[42] Edinburgh University MSS La II 676, and Da 4; Helen Armet, *Extracts from the Records of the Burgh of Edinburgh, 1701–18* (Edinburgh), p. 258.

into Scotland those novel English institutions, 'societies'; in 1691 was established a Scottish version of the Society for the Reformation of Manners; and 1699 saw the first, informal, appearance of the Scottish Society for the Propagation of Christian Knowledge.[43] This latter organisation was Presbyterian in Scotland, and it took as its primary target the nation within the nation, the Highlanders. Here was a prime instance of the need to civilise Scotland. The Highlanders outraged the sensibilities of the Lowland Whiggish Scots on many counts: they spoke an alien language (Gaelic) which sounded violent, they lived in an environment which looked violent, they followed a tradition of militaristic clan behaviour which *was* violent; they made wild predations on their Lowland neighbours, they dressed in the outlandish plaid and they spent their time lolling about, obviously looking for mischief. What is more important, the Highlanders were mostly Catholic, and their loyalty was to the House of Stuart. There was only one cure for them, they had to be civilised: taught to speak English, taught Presbyterianism, taught the Calvinist value of hard work and taught to wear trousers. Barbarity, Jacobitism and Popery were to be replaced by 'religion and virtue'. The means to this end was the establishment of parish schools in the Highlands, paid for by voluntary subscriptions, and supported by the General Assembly.

In the 1720s these same civilised values still needed to be fought for. In both 1708 and 1715 there had been severe outbreaks of disaffection: the Jacobite rebellions. Whig power had remained intact, but the Scottish nation was clearly not yet united and at peace with constitutional monarchy. It was the successors of men like Carstares who now held office in Scotland – or such office as was left to hold there.[44] One of the most important of these was George Drummond, who held the post of Lord Provost of Edinburgh. He was Provost on six occasions, a total of some twelve years, and for the fifty years from 1715 to 1766 was never far from the centre of power in the capital, even when not in the chair. Drummond was the 'Godfather' of the town. And he was a committed Whig. In the university, still run by the Town Council (which had founded it) he continued remoulding the nature of the institution along the lines established by Carstares, such that it not

[43] On which see M. G. Jones, *The Charity-School Movement: A Study of Eighteenth Century Puritanism in Action* (London, 1964), chapter 6, 'Scotland: Charity and "Civilitie"', pp. 165–214.

[44] On how Scotland was run after the Union, see Alexander Murdoch, *The People Above: Politics and Administration in Mid-Eighteenth-Century Scotland* (Edinburgh, 1980); see also the essays in N. T. Phillipson and Rosalind Mitchison (eds.), *Scotland in the Age of Improvement* (Edinburgh, 1970).

only became by the late eighteenth century the most highly regarded university in the English-speaking world, but it could provide a congenial and secure home for the highly unorthodox speculations of the intellectuals of the 'Scottish Enlightenment'. Again, Drummond was the chief promoter of the scheme to build the New Town of Edinburgh. He was highly active, had a finger in every pie, and his name is associated with the promotion of the interests of both Edinburgh and Scotland. He was an improver. But he was also a Whig. He seems to have been present, in an active capacity, at every confrontation in his lifetime between Jacobites and the forces of law and order: Drummond was always with law and order, the established authority, the Whig values. For Drummond, as earlier for Carstares, the improvement of Edinburgh, and of the nation of which it was still the capital, was a political activity, and indeed a *party* political activity. The promotion of certain activities would reinforce the stability of Scotland, its unity under its rightful monarchs – those stemming from the 1689 Revolution – its peace, and its prosperity. The models to which Drummond looked, to promote change of a desirable kind, were not indigenous (unlike the Jacobites); he was prepared to look anywhere, most particularly to England, but also to the traditional home of the House of Orange, the United Provinces. All this is important here because Drummond was the person, on the Town Council side, who actively promoted the establishing of the Faculty of Medicine in the university in 1726, and his involvement in the project was wholehearted.

BOERHAAVE'S PEACE IN SCOTLAND

So much for the civilising of Scotland on foreign models for Whig ends. Let us turn to the medical dimension. Here Scotland was suffering from open warfare. It was a tale of shabby little squabbles and of fighting for influence and power amongst the Edinburgh medical men. Here too the adoption of Boerhaave-style medicine helped put to peaceful purposes the energies which were being dissipated in intra-professional warfare.

Sour relations between the medical men of Edinburgh went back to at least 1680, and by the early 1720s there had been little peace between them for over forty years.[45] The hostilities were between three groups:

[45] See Cunningham, 'Sydenham Versus Newton'; and my 'The Medical Professions and the Pattern of Medical Care: The Case of Edinburgh, *c.*1670–*c.*1700' in Wolfgang Eckart and Johanna Geyer-Kordesch, *Heilberufe und Kranke in 17. and 18. Jahrhundert: die Quellen- und Forschungssituation* (Münster, 1982), pp. 9–28.

there was the Incorporation of Surgeon-Apothecaries, the local guild, important in town affairs, who had ruled the roost until 1680; then there were the simple apothecaries, a loose grouping of druggists; finally, there were the physicians, who in 1681 had got themselves established as a Royal College, and who aimed to control medical practice in Edinburgh by the highest continental standards – in other words, they wanted medical practice to be controlled by themselves at the head of a three-tier hierarchy of practitioners. Battle was joined between the physicians and the Surgeon-Apothecaries, with the simple apothecaries siding with whichever party would serve their interests. In the course of this battle the physicians could usually call on support from the most powerful people in the land, such as the king and his ministers; while the Surgeon-Apothecaries had their main allies in Edinburgh, in the form of the Town Council. Hence we find that the physicians could get a royal charter for themselves, while the repeated attempts of the Surgeon-Apothecaries to get an equivalent one were defeated by the physicians. On the other hand, whatever the powers over the Surgeon-Apothecaries that the physicians acquired for themselves by the terms of their charter, the Surgeon-Apothecaries could carry on pretty much regardless, under the protection of their Town Council.

This squabbling over who should control whom, and over who was superior to whom in Edinburgh medical practice, had some quite extraordinary consequences. In protecting and advancing their respective interests and claims, the physicians in their Royal College and the Surgeon-Apothecaries in their Incorporation, made innovations which were to be longlived. Amongst these were the teaching of botany, of materia medica, of chemistry and of anatomy. Under various different titles and in various institutions, there were teachers – loosely called 'professors' – for each of these subjects in the town of Edinburgh by 1720. Every one of these teaching enterprises was the direct result of rivalry between the physicians and the Surgeon-Apothecaries. Indeed the existence of two groups teaching Boerhaave's doctrines in Edinburgh in the early 1720s was itself a continuation of the rivalry, for one group taught under the aegis of the Royal College of Physicians, while the other under that of the Surgeon-Apothecaries. The rivalry between the institutions was still as alive as ever.

There was a growing audience in Edinburgh for the medical teaching which was becoming incidentally available, some of it the captive audience supplied by the apprentices of the Incorporation of Surgeon-Apothecaries, some of it young Scots lads preparing themselves to go on to a period of medical study in London or at a continental university and then into the British navy or army. The most popular foreign university for Scots was Leyden. However, thanks to the work of Carstares it was by 1705 possible to graduate in medicine at the University of Edinburgh[46] – although it was not possible actually to study the subject there yet.

The medical person most instrumental in turning this rivalry to the seemingly peaceful purpose of creating a proper medical school was John Monro,[47] father of the first of the string of Alexander Monros. A surgeon-apothecary himself, he had acquired abroad – including at Leyden – an education which rivalled that of the best physicians. He rose to being head of his profession at Edinburgh: that is, Dean of the Incorporation. John Monro was also a Whig, having fought in William's army, amongst other things. Reputedly John Monro was a man of vision, who nurtured a long-term scheme to improve Edinburgh and Scottish standards of medical education to the continental levels he had experienced in his own youth. His Whig allegiance helps explain why John Monro would have held such ambitions to civilise Scotland. In his civilising mission, John used his son Alexander as the instrument. The model was explicitly the teaching of Boerhaave at Leyden, where Alexander was sent to pursue his own studies. It should be noted that there were no English models to follow, for medical teaching at Oxford and Cambridge was all but defunct, and while medical life in London was lively, there was no university there.

In a series of manoeuvres which need not detain us here,[48] John Monro (during the period 1719 to 1722) pushed his son to teach anatomy in Edinburgh; by a sleight-of-hand got the Town Council to recognise this position as that of a 'Professor'; through his friendship with George Drummond got the post recognised as a university one; and then, again with the assistance of Drummond, got four of the young Boerhaave students recognised as professors in the university as well.

> The old Gentleman [John Monro] seeing none undertaking to teach the other Branches of Medicine pushed his Son to teach the Theory and Practice of Medicine with Chemistry as well as Anatomy, and with a view to this made him in the Summer Time to comment on Boerhaave's *Institutions* and *Aphorisms* to his Prentices and some few other young Gentlemen . . . But when this Plan was near the Time of its Execution,

[46] Edinburgh University MS Da 1.31, f.60.

[47] The best source on John Monro is the autobiography of his son Alexander, printed as H. D. Erlam, 'Alexander Monro, Primus', *University of Edinburgh Journal* 18 (1954), pp. 77–105; see also R. E. Wright-St.Clair, *Doctors Monro* (London, 1964).

[48] For the details see Anderson and Simpson, *The Early Years.*

> others offered their service [1725], Dr George Martin undertook to teach the Theory and Dr William Graham the Practice of Medicine, and the same two Parts with the Chemistry were proposed to be taught by Drs Andrew Sinclair, John Rutherford, John Innes and Andrew Plummer... The Rivalship did not continue long, for the Patrons of the University appointed the last four named Gentlemen to be Professors there, and then the other two desisted from Teaching.[49]

Thus did the famous Edinburgh medical school get started in 1726.

The format in which the medical school was founded cut across the ancient rivalries between the Incorporation and the Royal College: it involved both surgeons (Alexander Monro) and physicians (the four other teachers), and it placed medical teaching in a neutral arena, the university. The teaching was available to students of both groups. And there was, and could be, no dispute about the content of teaching being offered, for it was exclusively that of Boerhaave – on which there was total agreement. Boerhaave continued to be taught for decades.[50] William Cullen, for instance, recalling his student days there in 1734–6, wrote 'I learned the system of Boerhaave; and except it may be the names of some ancient writers, of Sydenham, and a few other practical authors, I heard of no other names or writers on physic; and I was taught to think the system of Boerhaave to be very perfect, complete and sufficient.' When, as professor himself some twenty years later, Cullen began to differ from Boerhaave he was condemned as a whimsical innovator, and was warned by Provost Drummond that his behaviour was likely to hurt both himself and the university.[51] As in Leyden, so here in Edinburgh Boerhaave's doctrines brought in the students from everywhere, to the great profit of the town; and the students thus attracted – for Edinburgh had no religious tests – also found progressive teaching available there in other subjects too. If the Enlightenment means the promotion of free, open, rational modes of thought – the opposite of bigotry – then the foundation of the Edinburgh medical school is very properly to be seen as the start of the Enlightenment in Edinburgh. And the delightful irony about it is that the medicine taught there was the more tolerant and open, the more closely it was based on

49 Alexander Monro's account, printed in Erlam, 'Alexander Monro, Primus', p. 84. On Alexander Monro's teaching of anatomy see Christopher Lawrence, 'Alexander Monro *Primus* and the Edinburgh Manner of Anatomy', *Bulletin of the History of Medicine* 62 (1988), pp. 193–214. Graeme published *An Essay for Reforming the Modern Way of Practising Medicine in Edinburgh, Wherein it is Proved, That the Foreign Method of Paying Physicians with Small Fees at a Time, Would be of Great Benefit to the Nation, if it were Followed in Edinburgh, and in the Other Royal Burghs of Scotland, and do no Hurt to Physicians Themselves* (London, 1727); he then moved to London, where he published *An Essay on the Method of Acquiring Knowledge in Physick* (London, 1729).

50 A number of reprints of Boerhaave's works were issued in Edinburgh, such as the *Aphorismi* in 1744.

51 Thomson, *Life, Lectures and Writings of Cullen*, vol. 1, pp. 118–9.

the doctrines of just one man – as long as that man was Herman Boerhaave!

The typical product of this Boerhaavian teaching, and of the compromise that it made possible between the rival professions of physician and surgeon-apothecary in Edinburgh, was someone new: the 'general practitioner'. In his very person the general practitioner was a triumph of eirenicism with respect to the traditional division of labour and esteem amongst medical men: for he represented the best – the core of shared truths – of the roles, training and attitudes of the physician, surgeon and apothecary. These Edinburgh-trained men, these general practitioners, came to expect a new range of practice. The Union of England and Scotland of 1707 meant that England was open to them to practise in. But when they arrived there they found medical teaching, practice and professional organisation amongst the English chaotic, confrontational and discordant, for unfortunately that fierce race had remained relatively untouched by Boerhaave's soothing hand.

3

Georg Ernst Stahl's radical Pietist medicine and its influence on the German Enlightenment

JOHANNA GEYER-KORDESCH

German scholarship uses the term *Frühaufklärung* to designate a period roughly spanning the last decade of the seventeenth century until well into the reign of Frederick William I (1740+). These years are decisive in a number of ways: the 'new' philosophy begins to change the approach to nature, to scientific endeavour and to religion; knowledge as a fashionable pastime for an elite and knowledge as a tool for general improvement merge to create a new ideal, that of utilitarian knowledge, an important element of 'enlightened' thinking, common to both the goals of the new Prussian Royal Society (founded in 1700)[1] and to Pietist writings when they stress *Nützlichkeit*[2] (usefulness); the State consolidates itself as a regulatory agency in the lives of its subjects ('Absolutism');[3] and the initial potential of radical Protestantism for politico-social reform is subsumed after 1730 into a quiescent Pietism engaged in managing proper institutions for training good public servants.

My aim in this chapter will be to examine how the ideas on medicine of Georg Ernst Stahl (1659–1734) influenced early Enlightenment society. Stahl's active career began with his medical studies at the University of Jena (1679); his ideas increased in importance as he

[1] For the history of the Royal Society see: Adolf Harnak, *Geschichte der Königlich Preussischen Akademie der Wissenschaften zu Berlin*, vol. 1 'Von der Gründung bis zum Tode Friedrichs des Großen' (Berlin, 1900; Olms reprint, 1970). The intent to support practical projects determined the early history of the Society, pp. 105–75.

[2] As for example in the manuscript programmatic 'Fußstapfen' of A. H. Francke in which he sets out his reforms: 'Die Fußstapfen des noch lebenden und waltenden liebreichen und getreuen Gottes, zur Beschämung des Unglaubens und Stärking des Glaubens durch den ausführlichen Bericht vom Waysen-Hause, Armen-Schulen und übrigen Armen-Verpflegung zu Glaucha an Halle, wie selbige fortgesetzt bis Ostern 1701' (Halle, 1701).

[3] For which medical regulation is a good example, see J. Geyer-Kordesch, 'Court Physicians and State Regulation in Eighteenth-Century Prussia: The Emergence of Medical Science and the Demystification of the Body' in Vivian Nutton (ed.), *Medicine at the Royal Court 1500–1800* (in press).

became court physician to Johann Ernst von Sachsen-Weimar (1687–94), professor at the University of Halle (1694–1715) and first court physician to Frederick William I as well as *praeses* of the *collegium medicum* in Berlin (1715–34).

I will try to paint a less classical portrait of the period 1670 to 1730, using colours not often used, in the hope that the composition does not resemble that of a court-appointed artist. This means that I will stress the radical Protestant opposition to natural philosophy as it is expressed in Stahl's medical theory. It offered explanations on a medical basis for questions raised in psychology and theology in the aftermath of the 'scientific revolution'. Stahl maintained that sensory impressions, mental images and emotional perceptions were neither replications of objects nor sense-information which 'triggered' responses. The 'soul', in his work a term covering all perceptual processes, had the capacity to form images and incite emotion as well as to formulate an idea, and these combined processes effected physiological changes in the body. The unity of the body and soul, for which Stahl argues, directly challenged a somatically oriented medicine as well as post-Cartesian philosophy. To give an example: in his medical advice to General G. D. von Natzmer on how to overcome nausea and sleeplessness he disclaimed a somatic cause and recommended seeking psychological reasons in order to effect a cure.[4] In a case cited in the *Theoria Medica Vera* he describes symptoms of irritation and disturbed sleep for which there are no apparent conscious reasons, only stating that the patient had reacted subconsciously to textiles to which she was – in today's terminology – allergic.[5] The intention of Stahl's medical theory is to prove that subconscious perceptions affect the mind and the body as a unity. In this sense he expounds a holistic approach to cognition: 'intelligence' is for him the sum of sensory, imaginative, emotive and mental perception.[6] For Stahl there is no qualitative difference between conscious reasoning and unreasoned emotion. Both are agents which change the vital economy of the individual. Emotion is connected to reason as well as to the imagination: they are coordinated in the individual organism.

These ideas contrast sharply with mechanist and dualist assumptions. In his post-Cartesian Enlightenment philosophy, for example, Christian Wolff (1679–1754) divides the imagination into components

[4] Stahl's *consilium medicum* is reprinted in M. Stürzbecher, *Beiträge zur Berliner Medizingeschichte, Quellen und Studien zur Geschichte des Gesundheitswesens vom 17. bis zum 19. Jahrhundert* (Berlin, 1966), pp. 121–2.

[5] G. E. Stahl, *Theoria Medica Vera* (Halle, 1708), pp. 27ff.

[6] For Stahl's explanation of 'intellectus et voluntas' see *De Mechanismi et Organismi Vera Diversitate* in *Theoria Medica Vera*, pp. 1ff.

that are either subservient to reason (the ability to envision abstract concepts) or subservient to the passions (images that stir up feelings).[7] Stahl did not think that perception functioned in dichotomies.

When Stahl writes about the organism, he does *not* mean a body 'endowed with organs'. 'Organic' to him means a coordinated and integrated whole, the 'organism', adjusting to its environment both on a conscious and unconscious level (sensually, emotionally and mentally) with immediate physiological results. Thus Stahl's medical theory is essentially a theory of a holistic, self-determined 'organism'.[8] His understanding of the organism is not equivalent to nineteenth-century vitalism because he did not centre his theory on the function of specific organs in the body. His definition of the organism is encompassing, equating 'life' with the ability of the whole organism to organise change. The 'organ' of perception is not somatic at all: it is the sum of all perceptual processes, and he calls this the soul.

The decisive passages in Stahl's writings where he elucidates the meaning of his 'holistic organism' (my term) can be found in his main work, the *Theoria Medica Vera* (Halle, 1708). To quote Stahl:

> Everywhere one is conditioned to see only what the senses grasp, the material surface, the structural composition of bodies and their spatial relation to each other, but no one pauses for even a glance at the orderliness of motion, its energy, how it absolutely determines matter, its duration, its different composition, how it changes, and, above all, how motion culminates in purpose. Because of this no one seems even to have a notion of how everything is integrated (*Zusammenhang*), how all matter (*Körper*) is joined together in the world (*Weltganzes*) and no one realises, above all, how organic bodies are integrated in themselves, to serve special purposes. There is a great deal of truth in the proverb of the Greek physicians that the doctor must begin his work where the physicist leaves off.[9]

The organisation of 'life' (='*organischer Körper*') is based on holistic principles (integration) which refer to intelligent purpose. Stahl supports his view in his definition of motion:

> It is a false assumption to predicate that the character of motion is simply and immediately dependent on the composition of matter or on the material relation of various organs, and that motion operates on these terms, so that the correct 'state' (*Bestand*) of matter will maintain itself, that its decomposition will cause disorder of and by itself, and that an improvement of material conditions will restore the rules by which matter functions. These opinions are doomed to failure when confronted with (medical) experience, observations which can be made every day . . .[10]

7 Christian Wolff, *Vernünftige Gedancken von Gott, der Welt und der Seele des Menschen, auch aller Dinge überhaupt* . . ., revised and augmented third edition (Halle, 1725; 1720), pp. 467ff.

8 The introductory treatises to the *Theoria Medica Vera* explain the full import of this holistically conceived organism, especially *Disquisitio de Machinismi et Organismi Diversitate; De Vera Diversitate Corporis Mixti et Vivi.*

9 Stahl, *Theoria Medica Vera*, p. 31; see the German translation in Karl Wilhelm Ideler, *Georg Ernst Stahl's Theorie der Heilkunde* (Berlin, 1831). 10 *Ibid.*, p. 42

The ideas contained in these two statements, which are fundamental to Stahl's medical theory, fly in the face of Newtonian physics and Cartesian dualism. Stahl claims that medical experience justifies the view that living organisms (self-contained living beings) have recourse to an intelligent and will-ful organisation of physical processes (the soul). Contingent on these ideas is Stahl's view that illness is not primarily a product of chemical imbalance (*Iatrochemie*) or explained by humoural pathology.[11]

Stahl's penultimate statement on his idea of 'Organism' can be found in his treatise *De Vera Diversitate Corporis Mixti et Vivi . . . Demonstratio* (Halle, 1707) which was reprinted as a key introductory statement to the *Theoria Medica Vera:*

> Since every action that the soul carrries out through the body is 'organic' or, in other words, as the body with respect to the soul is nothing but a simple 'instrument'; it is unheard of – and there are no instances of – the 'action' of the superior cause *in an instrument* (or, as it is commonly called, the actuation of an instrument) ever being called by the name of LIFE by any school: it follows that no-one gets bogged down in confusion in saying 'organic body', when talking about 'Life'.
>
> For since in the strict sense this diversity of 'body' and 'organic' is very simple, anyone may understand without qualification and quite simply in that broad sense that there are two meanings of 'body' taken as a separate term: one insofar as it is *non organic*, that is, not organic *in its very act*; but another understanding should be given to '*Organic body*' when and whenever – indeed to express it more briefly and formally – INSOFAR AS it is organically *actuated* [i.e. body + soul].
>
> Hence this expression will never give occasion nor ground of error to anyone: 'the life of the organic body'. Provided that someone accepts the expression 'the life of the body, BECAUSE it is organic', 'the life of the body INSOFAR as it is organic' will be acceptable . . .[12]

[11] G. E. Stahl, *Dissertatio Epistolica de Motu Tonico Vitali Hinc Dependente Motu Sanguinis Particulari* (Jena, 1692); in German translation *Ausführliche Abhandlung von den Zufällen und Kranckheiten des Frauenzimmers, dem beigefüget . . . eine völlige Beschreibung des Motus tonici* (Leipzig, 1724), pp. 553ff.

[12] Cum autem omnis actio, quam anima *per* corpus exercet, sit *organica*, seu corpus in ordine ad animam sit simplex *instrumentum*; inauditum et sine omni exemplo sit, *actionem* causae superioris *in instrumentum*, sive *actuationem* vulgo dictam, *instrumenti*, ab ulla unquam schola VITAE nomine appellatam fuisse: nemo utique ita cespitabit in perplexa loquendi, *corpus organicum*, in sermone de *Vita*.

Cum enim *kurios* simplicissima sit diversitas haec, *corporis*, et *organici*; quilibet inde utique simplicissime etiam, quasi ipso crasso sensu comprehendit, quod diversa sit ratio *corporis* seorsim, quatenus *non organicum*, id est non *in ipso actu* organicum est: aliam autem considerationem deberi, *Organico*, quando, quamdiu, imo potius breviter et *formaliter*, QUATENUS organice *actuatur*.

Unde numquam homini errandi occasionem praebebit, nedum materiam, formula loquendi: *vita corporis organici*. Nisi enim accipiat, *vita corporis*, QUOD *est organicum*, accipiendum erit, *vita corporis* QUATENUS *est organicum* . . .' in Stahl, *Theoria Medica Vera*, pp. 113–14; see also the French translation of this passage in G. E. Stahl, *Oeuvres medico-philosophiques et practiques*, 5 vols., translated by T. Blondin (Paris, 1859), vol. 2, pp. 405–6.

In sum, Stahl wants it clearly understood that he differentiates between matter (or substances) and matter in its organic form. Matter is 'put into action' and this comprehensive teleological 'motion' – the body is constantly in motion, as Stahl says elsewhere[13] – is nothing less than life. 'Soul', 'life', 'nature' and 'organic motion' merge in their meaning to the extent that Stahl denies matter as the source of motion, or as a causal determinant of processes in the body. Because of his definition of the organic he has no trouble including emotion or mental images as active agents in changing the 'state' of the body. There can be little doubt that Stahl's definition '*vita corporis quod est organicum*' directly challenged mechanist and dualist philosophy. It was as upsetting to his contemporaries as it is difficult to understand after three hundred years of dualistic thinking about the mind and the body.

The point to remember is that an integrative view of the organism that intentionally seeks to avoid linear causal relationships will not harmonise with the attempt to define strict mechanical sequences as natural laws. Stahl was not interested in finding a specific irritability or sensibility of muscle reactions (as was Albrecht von Haller)[14] nor in designing a philosophically plausible construct which brought the soul and matter into existential harmony (like the Monads of Leibniz),[15] nor in a philosophical systematisation of terms and their definitions such as Christian Wolff's *psychologia empirica*.[16] He maintained, against the philosophical suppositions of his time, that the 'organic' was an adequate definition of living bodies as they assimilate sensory, emotional, imaginative and mental information.

It is of some consequence to eighteenth-century thought that Stahl's ideas were strongly opposed by the leading philosophers of his time, while also being essential to the interests of radical Protestantism. The latter found in his writings a defence of their own endeavours to maintain religious and political freedom. 'The spirit goeth where it

13 G. E. Stahl, *Negotium Otiosum, seu Sciamachia, Adversus Positiones Aliquas Fundamentales, Theoriae Verae Medicae a Viro Quodam Celeberrimo Intentata, sed Adversis Conversis Enervata* (Halle, 1720), as partially translated by L. J. Rather and I. B. Frerichs, 'The Leibniz–Stahl Controversy-II', *Clio Medica* 5 (1970), pp. 59–60.

14 Albrecht von Haller attacks Stahl's concept of 'soul' while not taking account of the problematic of the organism, on these grounds. See R. Toellner's explication of von Haller's views in 'Anima et Irritabilitas. Hallers Abwehr von Animismus und Materialismus', *Sudhoffs Archiv* 51 (1967), pp. 130–44.

15 For a brief overview and bibliography, see Jürgen Mittelstrass and Eric J. Aiton, 'Leibniz: Physics, Logic, Metaphysics' in *Dictionary of Scientific Biography* (New York), vol. 8, pp. 150–60.

16 The German vernacular version of Wolff's psychology in his *Vernünftige Gedancken von Gott, der Welt und der Seele des Menschen* (Leipzig, 1725).

will' was a fundamental precept of radical Protestantism.[17] If inspirational freedom has no place in nature, then it cannot create 'movement' in its own 'body'. The 'organic' life, the '*vita corporis quod est organicum*', has analogous meaning in radical religious movements dependent on inspirational guidance. Thus it is hardly surprising that Stahl's medical theory became a rallying-point for Pietism and that it was so strongly attacked by eighteenth-century medical men and philosophers.[18]

PIETISM AND THE ORGANIC UNITY OF BODY AND SOUL

My aim is to demonstrate how a medical *theory* was a substantial part of a socio-political movement. It is usual to show that medical contributions to social progress are to be found in health care issues, such as, for example, the founding and reform of institutions (such as hospitals), or in standards of professionalisation. But the practical reforms in medicine just mentioned came relatively late, in the latter half of the eighteenth century, and were an eclectic and pragmatic implementation of leading doctors' practical experience and knowledge.[19] When they were instituted they were a measure of the profession's importance for the State. Medical theory, however, drew on and influenced the structure of ideological processes.

In England after 1660 institutions such as the Royal Society were used to advantage in stabilising parliamentary monarchy. Utopian concepts, prophecies, eschatological expectations, the social visions of Ranters and Levellers, were curbed by an appeal to common sense, an intellectual preference for logic and proof, conveniently provided by the new elite of prominent natural philosophers.[20] Northern Germany in about 1670 was less 'advanced'. Not unified as a nation, and composed of sovereign territories with fairly fluid boundaries, these vied for talented professionals, enterprising inventors and alchemists, and they lured scions of aristocratic houses seeking their fortunes, and those Protestant exiles seeking a non-Jesuit education.

[17] Heinrich Bornkham, *Das Jahrhundert der Reformation* second edition (Göttingen, 1966).

[18] See my forthcoming book *Georg Ernst Stahl: Pietismus, Medizin und Aufklärung in Preußen im 18. Jahrhundert*, especially the chapter 'Zur Problematik der Rezeption Stahls: "homo acris et metaphysicus"'.

[19] Geyer-Kordesch, 'Court Physicians and State Regulation'.

[20] See the literature on the 'revolt against Enthusiasm': Georg Rosen, 'Enthusiasm "a dark lanthorn of the spirit"' *Bulletin of the History of Medicine* 42 (1968), pp. 393–421; John F. Sena, 'Melancholic Madness and the Puritans', *Harvard Theological Review* 66 (1973), pp. 293–309; George Williamson, 'The Restoration Revolt Against Enthusiasm', *Studies in Philology* 30 (1933), pp. 571–603; Truman Guy Steffan, 'The Social Argument against Enthusiasm', *Studies in English* 21 (1941), pp. 39–63.

This fairly mobile population made use of the needs of courts (to fill their administrative, medical and other posts) and educational institutions. Brandenburg-Prussia was underpopulated and welcomed the Huguenots after 1685 and the 'Salzburger Emigranten' after 1731. Migratory habits characterised the lives of prominent figures. It comes as no surprise, therefore, to find that there were supraterritorial concerns which shaped a pattern of visits, correspondence, and exchanges of information, irrespective of whose subject one really was. Pietism, a reform movement within German Lutheranism, began to assemble a clerical and lay following after 1670. German Pietism became an active force in Quedlinburg, at universities such as Erfurt and Leipzig (where considerable orthodox opposition forced confrontations), at the courts of Sachsen-Weimar and in Gotha-Eisenach, at Jena and in Halle and later in Berlin, including the Prussian Court.[21] The rise of early Pietism had a very different flavour to it than its later accomodation with the State. In the beginning it was of a piece with more radical Protestant movements whose representatives included the followers of Jane Leade, Jean de Labadie, Johann Wilhelm and Johanna Eleonora Peterson, Johann Georg Gichtel or Johann Conrad Dippel, Gottfried Arnold and other Separatists, and the Moravian exiles from Bohemia. As the Halle Pietists devoted themselves to educational works and supplied the infrastructure of the Prussian monarchy, they lost the loyalty of more radical men.[22] In contrast to the Halle Pietists the Moravians continued to harbour radicals in the sovereign territories of Nikolaus Ludwig Count Zinzendorff and the Counts Sayn-Wittgenstein.

Beliefs and ideas were at the core of Protestant radical endeavour which extended across all boundaries. Those dissatisfied with orthodox solutions believed that Reformation was a continuous task. The doctor and theologian Johann Conrad Dippel, never integrated into any group for long, was praised by radicals as greater than Luther himself because of his adamant criticism of the orthodox church.[23]

[21] The Pietist controversies regarding these places are variously described in Martin Schulz, 'Johann Heinrich Sprögel und die Pietistische Bewegung Quedlinburgs', theological dissertation (Halle, 1974); Gustav Kramer, *A. H. Francke, Ein Lebensbild* (Halle, 1880–2); Max Steinmetz, *Geschichte der Universität Jena 1548/58–1958*, 2 vols. (Jena, 1958–62; Johann Christoph von Dreyhaupt, *Ausführliche Beschreibung des Saal = Kreyses*, second part (Halle, 1750); Johann Just von Einem, *Das erbauliche Leben des christlichen Theologen Herr Caspar Johann Weidenheins* [Weydenhain] (Magdeburg, 1734).

[22] Gertrude Zaepernick, 'Johann Georg Gichtels und seiner Nachfolger. Briefwechsel mit den hallischen Pietisten, besonders mit A. H. Francke', in *Pietismus und Neuzeit* 8 (1982), pp. 74–118.

[23] Marint von Geismar (ed.), *Bibliothek der Deutschen Aufklärer des Achtzehnten Jahrhunderts*, vol. 2, 'Edelmann über Dippel' (Darmstadt, 1963), pp. 212ff., especially p. 217.

The climate of renewal was strong in Quedlinburg, in Jena, and at the Court of Johann Ernst von Sachsen-Weimar. Tensions arose between an orthodox clergy abetted by rulers interested in maintaining the usual – and useful – hierarchies, and radical Protestants instigating Bible discussion groups (*Konventikel*) in the face of clerical or aristocratic disapproval. Quedlinburg – a hot-bed of radical initiative – was relatively independent because it was ruled by an abbess.[24] In close proximity, Jena, Halle, Erfurt, Leipzig (all university towns with young theologians no longer primly and sedately orthodox) exploded into Enthusiasm. Gottfried Arnold, a leading radical, whose influential books advocated heretical and mystic traditions as the *true* Church, and who wrote much in the vein of Pietistic introspective literature, resided in Quedlinburg. He married the daughter of the Hofprediger Johann Heinrich Sprögel, himself caught up in a fairly vicious attempt by the orthodox to oust him for turning the flock into radical Enthusiasts. Sprögel and radical Pietists cared more for religion than for stability or the niceties of social snobbery. The underlying unease among those in power was electrified by the manifestations of radical Pietism: servant girls who prophesied, meetings where women, artisans, clergy and intellectuals mixed, preachers who took monarchs to task over their lifestyles, and a religious conscience which baulked at communion services with 'nominal' Christians. The Pietist preachers were notorious for not behaving as religious servants should: Philipp Jakob Spener had to leave the Dresden court for not condoning its immorality;[25] Sprögel was known to preach 'against high and low';[26] Johann Caspar Weydenhain, at the Pietist court of Johann Ernst von Sachsen-Weimar, described how he was worn out by fulfilling his mission to take everyone to task.[27] Heinrich Julius Elers, who ran the successful publishing house of the Pietists in Halle, spent a great deal of his time at the book fairs in Frankfurt-on-Main and Leipzig praying with all alike for the good of their souls at the back of his bookstall behind a screen.[28]

The obvious involvement of women in Pietist thinking and praying, in philanthropy and behind-the-scenes manoeuvring, is also an indication of how the authority derived from inner feelings broke the mould of the seen-but-not-heard housewife and mother. Female Pietists wrote books, were very stubborn on religious issues, defied

[24] Schulz, 'Johann Heinrich Sprögel'.

[25] On Spener, see Paul Grünberg *Philipp Jakob Spener*, 3 vols., (Göttingen, 1893–1906).

[26] Schulz, 'Johann Heinrich Sprögel', p. 37.

[27] Von Einem, *Das erbauliche Leben*, p. 14.

[28] Joachim Böhme, 'Heinrich Julius Elers, ein Freund und Mitarbeiter August Hermann Franckes', philosophy dissertation (Berlin, 1956), p. 104.

social conventions on marriage and organised religious communities. In the case of speaking-in-tongues of servant girls, the orthodox used these scandals to discredit inspirational behaviour.[29] Prophecies and visions favoured the revival spirit and not the orthodox.

Georg Ernst Stahl and Friedrich Hoffmann, next to Herman Boerhaave easily the two most important medical innovators on the continent, both studied in Jena while the events described above were holding Thuringia in thrall. Stahl, graduating in 1684, taught as *extraordinarius* in Jena and then became first Court physician to Johann Ernst von Sachsen-Weimar in 1687. While teaching in Jena and while at Court he practised among religious Enthusiasts. Both the Court at Weimar and the quasi-independent Quedlinburg (where he was consulted on medical matters) were reft with religious controversy.

The social milieu of Pietism, if not directly then certainly indirectly, helped create Stahl's willingness to jettison the mechanical and anatomical emphasis developed in medicine in the wake of the English Restoration and the ascendency of the medical teaching of the University of Leiden. In 1692 Stahl published a treatise which took him medically beyond the observations he had made on the nature of fevers.[30] Like Thomas Sydenham, Stahl thought fevers a part of nature's inherent capacity to heal. On this basis he rejected contemporary explanations for fever such as heat, friction or fermentation. Already he was aware of the importance of physiological 'motions' (dynamic changes in the body) for medical theory and therapeutics. In 1692 he went further: he challenged the mechanical concepts attached to the reception of William Harvey's circulation theory. In the 1692 treatise, *De Motu Tonico Vitali*, Stahl defends the assumption that the body must be 'intelligent' because the blood flow could be observed to 'move' to where it was physiologically needed.[31] In the event, this was the seminal insight that led to the *Theoria Medica Vera*, Stahl's full-blown exposition of physiology and pathology based on his concept of the 'organic body'.

In *De Motu Tonico Vitali* Stahl wishes to prove to his contemporaries that a vital movement within the fibres and the fluids of the body

[29] Schulz, 'Johann Heinrich Sprögel', pp. 96ff.

[30] Stahl, *Dissertatio Epistolica de Motu Tonico Vitali*; citations from the German translations of 1724 (note 11 above). On the fever theory see J. Geyer-Kordesch, 'Fevers and Other Fundamentals: Dutch and German Medical Explanations Circa 1680 to 1730' in W. F. Bynum and V. Nutton, *Theories of Fever from Antiquity to the Enlightenment* (London, 1981), pp. 99–120.

[31] Stahl, *De Motu Tonico Vitali* (German translation, note 11, above), pp. 589ff.

regulates the pulse and the distribution of the blood. He is here discounting any mechanical regularity in the circulatory activity of the 'pumping' heart.[32] He marshalls his proof by citing case-studies: these he gleaned, not surprisingly, from his treatment of emotional disturbance and the attendant 'breakdowns' of religious Enthusiasts who were his patients and, secondly, by the observation of irregularities in the menstrual flow of his women patients.[33] Added to these arguments from case-studies are Stahl's observations on the changes in the size of his own veins as they dilate or diminish according to emotional states.[34] In other words, Stahl's practical encounters with 'psychologically' alternating states (emotional irregularities which produce physiological effects) induced him to seek explanations outside mechanical principles. His close association with religious Enthusiasts forced the trained medical observer that he was – for Jena trained 'modern' doctors – to challenge iatrochemical and 'mechanist' explanations. Clearly, from the evidence of his cases, the body was following the soul. Stahl found that one could not deny this medically, and ideologically it was very appropriate: in effect Stahl had discovered a mode of argument on the basis of medical observation which could challenge materialist cause-and-effect explanations. Not only was the soul relevant, but it could be shown to organise matter. Emotions could not be discounted, and physiological change had to be seen as the product of perceptual, not mechanical, influences. Thus purely medical conclusions correlated with other truths: the mechanical philosophy which had heartened those wishing to rid philosophy of 'superstition' and which optimistically proposed different laws for 'mind' and body, was now challenged by a medical theory championing spontaneous self-organisation in the 'organism'.

Stahl had reintroduced the soul on modernistic terms. Following *De Motu Tonico Vitali* he wrote on medical subjects closely correlated to major debates on philosophical and religious themes. *De Passionibus Animae Corpus Humanum Varie Alterantibus* (1695) (on the passions of the mind variously affecting the human body) tried to establish a typology of physiological substructures and emotional types, an early try at psychological theory whose main intent was to establish the interaction between cognitive, emotional and physiological change. The explanatory base was one thoroughly opposed to mechanical thinking. In *De Vita* (Halle, 1701) and *De Differentia Rationis et Ratiocinationis* (Halle, 1701) he takes issue with dualistic notions of life, and with a form of rationality that equates reason with logic. For

[32] *Ibid.* [33] *Ibid.*, pp. 556ff., 586ff. and 608ff. [34] *Ibid.*, pp. 599–601.

Stahl *intellectus* is *not* the same as the ability to transform the 'objects of intelligence' into abstract ideas. As he writes in *De Mechanismi et Organismi Vera Diversitate* (Halle, 1707), the agents of the soul at work in the instrument of the body are *intellectus et voluntas*, the former capable of perception ('intelligence' in its broadest sense), the latter giving the 'organic' process its meaningful direction. Knowledge and purpose are thus the primary forces at work in the body.[35]

Stahl states that structures and composition (for example, the chemical substances in the body) do not sufficiently explain the ordered and purpose-directed interplay of process (=life) in living beings.[36] Himself no mean advocate of logical thinking, he states that processes and their interaction must presuppose the organisation of the whole. The organism is composed of processes using matter and these processes are *a priori* dependent on intelligence.[37] In *De Differentia Rationis et Ratiocinationis* he clearly states that intelligence cannot be philosophically reduced to conscious reasoning.[38] Hence it is admissible and even necessary, as Stahl's medical experience showed, that the 'material' of the body thinks: sensual information translates into reactions *and* into the active creation of feelings, apprehensions, intuition, knowledge and thought. A continuity of sensation, emotion and knowledge, as validated by experience, cannot be philosophically partitioned into separate concepts; 'reason' cannot be opposed to 'corporeal phantasy', 'ideas' opposed to 'sensation' and 'passion', the one invalidating the other because the 'mind' is superior to the 'body'. The attack on dualism and on material cause-and-effect explanations is Stahl's unifying theme from *De Motu Tonico Vitalis* (1692) to the summary treatment of his ideas in the *Theoria Medica Vera* (Halle, 1708).

'The life of the body which is organic' expresses what Stahl was trying to achieve: it is nothing less than a substantiated theory (based on case observations and medical logic) that the soul and the body are a unity. Life is organic and life is the active soul working within the structures and substances of the body. Its limit, but not its essence, is the body.

This mode of thinking was greatly irritating to proponents of the 'new' philosophy of Descartes and of Newtonian physics, who were

[35] See Stahl, *Theoria Medica Vera*, pp. 1–5. [36] *Ibid.*, pp. 66ff.

[37] Stahl, *Negotium Otiosum*, in the translation of Rather and Frerichs, 'The Leibniz–Stahl Controversy-II', p. 59.

[38] G. E. Stahl, *Propempticon Inauguralis de Differentia Rationis et Ratiocinationis, et Actionum, quae per et Secundum Utrumque Horum Actuum Fiunt in Negocio Vitali et Animali* (Halle, 1701; second edition 1710; third 1712).

determined to discover 'laws' and to pronounce both man and the universe predictable. The tremendous normative power of such abstractions as the idea of the 'reasonable' and of 'laws of nature' were the product of dualistic thinking and the mechanical cause-and-effect philosophy. That these assumptions came to be seen as synonymous with reality is the achievement of the secular philosophy of the Enlightenment.

No one was more sensitive to the coming ice age of reason than radical Enthusiast Protestants. It is impossible to retrace the *exact* links between Stahl's dedication to 'organic' explanations, and early radical Pietism. But the essential congruence of Stahl's medical theory with the religious views, aims and thinking of Pietists is plain to see. They also provided practical support. In 1694 Stahl's teaching and the content of his treatises were rapidly integrated with the nascent Pietist movement in Halle.[39]

THE VISION OF GOD AND NATURE

The integral connection of Stahl's ideas on medicine with the reform movement of Pietists in Halle, allows one to see the development of Stahl's theory from 1692 to 1708 as part of a larger ideological constellation. As a reform movement Pietism was interested in securing freedom from orthodox religious domination. Enthusiasts were critical of enforced dogma and church authority. For them 'piety' meant that an inner conversion, an emotionally tangible 'idea' of God, individualistic as it may be, was more important than the articles of faith. Religion had 'to touch the heart' as Christian Albrecht Richter expressed it.[40] Similar to Stahl's idea that matter was 'moved' and organized by the soul, Pietists thought that the natural could be changed by spiritual rebirth. Philipp Jakob Spener distinguishes the natural from nature that is reborn.[41] Even history was subject to divine intervention. 'Nature' like 'matter' was an 'outward' manifestation, an 'instrument' only, open to surprising variations. Pietist thinking went in the direction of the Lutheran definition: God is the unmoved Mover of all creatures.[42] This expresses the essential tension of all mystically

[39] See J. Geyer-Kordesch, 'Georg Ernst Stahl: Pietismus, Medizin und Aufklärung in Preußen im 18. Jahrhundert', Manuscript of Habilitationsschrift (Münster, 1988), pp. 150ff.

[40] Christian Albrecht Richter, *Trauer- und Trost-Reden* (Halle, 1723), which reprints the relevant letter to 'Jungfer Rosciin und deren Schwester'.

[41] See the very interesting treatise on nature and grace, which Spener claimed was the result of discussions in the Pietist Bible-reading circles (*collegia pietatis*): Philipp Jakob Spener, *Natur und Gnade, Oder der Unterschied der Wercke so aus natürlichen Kräften und aus den Gnädenswürckungen des h. Geistes herkommen ...* (Frankfurt am Main, 1687).

[42] Cited from Bornkamm, *Das Jahrhundert der Reformation*, p. 334.

oriented forms of religion: a striving for God within the forms of the naturally tangible. Enthusiast religion could not forfeit the tension between the spiritual and the natural, otherwise – along with other religions – it would not fulfil its redemptive mission. Pietism did not share the contemplative goal of some monastic orders – its political impact was far too worldly.[43]

The ideological environment of early radical Pietism was cosmosophic, theosophic and *naturmystisch*: they believed that knowledge of nature pointed to knowledge of God. August Hermann Francke, for example, intended to popularise the writings of the mystic tradition, including works which the Catholic church devoutly wished to remain in oblivion.[44] Meditation to the point of ecstasy was not unknown among the Moravians, a particular group of whom valued the cult of the wound – the wound from which flowed the blood of Christ as he was pierced on the cross.[45] The writings of Jacob Böhme were of particular interest to radical Pietists and were reissued through the efforts of Johann Georg Gichtel and had a strong influence on Gottfried Arnold.[46] The metaphorical structure of Enthusiast religious writing depended upon the identification of the natural with the spiritual, as, for example, hunger and erotic love as descriptions of spiritual states.[47] As literary historians have remarked, the use of erotic metaphors in some Pietist hymns would bring more than a blush to the cheek. The expression of Enthusiastic religious feeling was in bodily, sensual terms. Love of God was to be 'tasted' and 'felt'.[48] The same unity applied to the apprehension of nature: the sensual knowledge of the world was a direct insight into the transcendental. The embodiment or incorporation of the spiritual essence in nature was such a key assumption of radical Protestants that much of the polemic they vented against mechanism attacks its reductionist principles.[49] Mechanists and atomists are chided for the 'imbecile' belief that a

[43] Carl Hinrichs, *Preußentum und Pietismus, Der Pietismus in Brandenburg-Preußen als religiös-soziale Reformbewegung* (Göttingen, 1971).

[44] Böhme, 'Heinrich Julius Elers', pp. 160ff.

[45] This veneration of the 'wound' was especially associated with Nikolaus Ludwig Count Zinzendorf's son, Christian Renatus.

[46] Eberhard Pältz, 'Jacob-Böhme', *Theologische Realenzyklopädie* 6 (Berlin, 1980), p. 752; Martin Schmidt, 'Gottfried Arnold', *Theologische Realenzyklopädie* 4 (1979), pp. 136–40.

[47] This is especially true of the hymns. Christian Friedrich Richter wrote a number of important Pietist hymns. See also August Langen, *Der Wortschatz des deutschen Pietismus* (Tübingen, 1954; second edition 1968).

[48] Johann Samuel Carl uses exactly these words, *Zeugnisse von Medicina Morali*... (Büdingen, 1726): 'de paedagogia cordis', p. 19.

[49] Johann Conrad Dippel, *Weg-Weiser zum Liecht und Recht*... (no place given, 1704), pp. 29ff.; *Die Krankheit und Arzney des thierisch-sinnlichen Leibes* (Frankfurt, 1713), pp. 8ff.

materialist analysis would yield an answer about how nature or the body functions.[50] The educational reforms pleaded for by the radical Protestant and Stahlian, Johann Samuel Carl, not only argued in favour of dropping the elite Latin language, but also advocated that while learning the 'alphabet' of nature (i.e., its 'outward' manifestation) the *sense* of the language, its spiritual meaning, should be taught.[51] In a time when Pietists were receptive not only to the mystical tradition, but were also familiar with Judaic teaching on the hidden meaning of letters and numbers,[52] it seems very logical that they would not accept the ideology of mechanism and dualism.

In the context of this ideological interpretation of nature, the focus of medical arguments was not solely on health or social hygiene. Nor were radical Protestants keen on castigating the flesh in the sense of medieval self-flagellation. 'Flesh' is a singularly materialistic term, derived from Greek dualistic thinking, but having no conceptual equivalent in a set of ideas that views the body and soul as one. Good health was regard highly among Pietists and it was argued for, but with respect to psychosomatic health as the determinant of spiritual growth.[53] After all, radical Protestantism took the position that the body as well as the soul would be resurrected at the Last Judgement. In this life the body was the instrument of the soul and was absolutely necessary for all good works as well as being the essential 'vessel' of thought and feeling. The point is that thought and feeling – in which spiritual growth develops – are psychosomatic in origin: the idea of the unity of body and soul as Stahl explained it in his theory.

Christian Friedrich Richter, the populariser of Stahl's *Theoria Medica Vera*, wrote one of the most widely disseminated books of the early Enlightenment, his *Höchst-Nöthige Erkenntniß des Menschen* (The Most-necessary Knowledge about Mankind) (Leipzig, 1709).[54] It

[50] Dippel, *Die Krankheit und Arzney*, pp. 89ff.

[51] Johann Samuel Carl, *Vorstellungen von Dreyfacher Einleitung in die Medicin, Dem Decoro Medici zugegeben* (Büdingen, 1723): 'Erste Vorstellung Encyclopaediae medicae Hodegus et Methodus Synthetica de Paedagogis cordis', pp. 7–28 (despite the title, a German-language treatise!).

[52] Knowledge of Jewish religious teaching and, of course, of the Hebrew language were characteristic of Halle Pietism. Many radical Pietists were familiar with the Caballa. For example, Dippel, *Die Krankheit und Arzney*, pp. 10ff.; pp. 54ff. See also E. Benz, *Die christliche Kabbala* (Zürich, 1958).

[53] Christian Friedrich Richter, *Die Höchst-Nöthige Erkenntniß des Menschen sonderlich nach dem Leibe und natürlichem Leben, oder ein deutlicher Unterricht* . . . (Leipzig, 1709; citations from the 6th edition, 1719): 'Vorrede vom rechten Gebrauch des Leibes und der Kräffte des natürlichen Lebens'.

[54] *Ibid.* On the many editions of the *Höchst-Nöthige Erkenntniß*, see Eckard Altmann, *Christian Friedrich Richter (1676–1711), Arzt, Apotheker und Liederdichter des Halleschen Pietismus* (Witten, 1972).

should be seen together with the *Theoria* as a statement of radical Protestant thought, comprising on the one hand an attempt to reform and advance knowledge (the *Theoria*), and on the other a popular *breviary* of bodily and sensory management. In seeing these books as a unity the ideological intention becomes apparent. Stahl initiates a medical theory which stresses individuation: the individual soul, for good or evil, active with the body. Richter applies this non-mechanist formula to Pietist *Seelenführung* (management of the soul). The introduction states that the images formed in the soul in life are the images which will constitute that person for eternity. The images formed in the soul are thus the spiritual vision of the individual and constitute his or her religious achievement.[55] If the inner vision, as Richter argues, is directed toward the attractions of life (lust, love, riches, power, etc.), then the vision of 'God' in the soul is lost.[56] For Richter (and by implication, for radical Enthusiasts and Pietists) spiritual growth is not possible without mental images. Richter departs from his use of the German vernacular at this point in his introduction, and used the word *Idea*.[57] Richter was theologically, philologically and medically educated and he used this word advisedly. *Idea* is a transliteration of the Greek 'to see' and stresses the visual aspects of thinking. *Idea* here does not mean 'abstract universal concepts' nor is it synonymous with 'the object of conceptual thought'. *Idea* was not yet divested of its sensual imagery. This is quite important because then *Idea* has the emotional power of poetry: it 'moves' persons in a sensually tangible form. The image, as a sensory composite the product of the imagination, is inseparably linked with the emotions in the *Seelenlehre* (psychology) of Pietism. While Cartesian philosophy was intent on separating the 'passions' from 'pure' thought (a singularly static representation), Stahlian medical theory and Pietist *Seelenführung* were busily entwining the two as psychologically active agents. It seemed to the Pietists a fact of fundamental importance that for good or ill what happens in the mind happens in the psychosomatic transactions of the senses, the imagination, and the emotions (which generally can be called 'feelings', as in the German, non-translatable term, *Gemüthsbewegung*).

Spiritual growth, in the view of Pietism and the traditions which fed it, is inexorably linked to imagination and emotion. When Stahl chides the followers of Cartesian dualism for their attempts to create an inviolate island of reason, he mentions the mental 'attractions' which pitch men into despondency, over-optimism, melancholy, fear, timid-

[55] Richter, *Höchst-Nöthige Erkenntniß*, pp. 18–22. [56] *Ibid.*, pp. 22–3. [57] *Ibid.*, p. 18

ity etc.[58] His ideological adversaries on the other hand were trying to convince men that reason, defined as the ability to abstract and deal with ideas logically, would vanquish the dangers of unruly subjectivity. Christian Wolff described man as either 'free', when in use of his reason, or a 'slave', when subject to his passions.[59] Richter, as a convinced Pietist, was concerned to popularise Stahl precisely because Stahlian medical theory shows how the body and the soul 'move' together, thereby giving substantial support to the idea that emotion and mind are to be seen holistically. Religious radicals were very shy of the notion that 'pure' reason could lead to spiritual growth.

For radical Protestantism in Germany, Stahl's holistic medical theory was essential. Otherwise the basis for its message of an inspired, naturally tangible vision of God and nature (i.e. via the body as the instrument of the soul) could not be legitimated. To the extent that mechanism and dualistic approaches to the body mind problem were not able to cope with the psychology of images and the emotions, Stahlian medical theory remained influential. This is in evidence throughout the eighteenth and nineteenth centuries. The world view of radical Enthusiasm ran counter to the enlightened ideology lauding man's autonomy through reason, because a holistic psychology seemed to them a more truthful explanation of man's (and woman's) nature.

One must not fall prey to 'enlightened' viewpoints and think that radical Protestants were being less 'free' in rejecting reason as the sole arbiter of what counted as freedom. They wished to be 'free' on other terms, namely in the pursuit of a spirituality based on the activities of the soul: perception, feeling, imagery. In the years which saw the publication of the *Theoria Medica Vera* and the *Höchst-Nöthige Erkenntniß*, it was not the Enlightened who were being sent to prison, but radical Protestants such as Johann Conrad Dippel and Stahl's student, Johann Samuel Carl.[60]

ANTIMECHANISM AND THE ENLIGHTENMENT

Stahl's medical theory gained ground between 1694 and 1715, the years of his tenure as professor at the University of Halle. His ideas spread

[58] G. E. Stahl, *De Scriptis Suis ad hunc Diem Schediasmatibus, Vindiciae Quaedam, et Indicia* (Halle, 1707); translated into German: Ideler, *Georg Ernst Stahls Theorie der Heilkunde*, p. 1.

[59] Wolff, *Vernünftige Gedanken von Gott*, pp. 298–9.

[60] In 1706 a new attack on Pietism is launched, Dippel defends radical claims in polemical form and is sent to prison. He escapes to Holland. At the same time Carl is forced to live covertly because he is under ecclesiastical persecution for 'heterodox religious views'.

rapidly, although a flavour of unorthodoxy quite naturally attached to them. As indicated above, his medical theory, where it defended anti-mechanist and anti-dualist positions, bolstered and enlarged the ideological position of radical Protestantism. But Stahl's sphere of influence was larger than radical or Enthusiast circles. Luminaries of the early Enlightenment were carefully keeping informed of what he wrote. Leibniz's interest can be traced to before 1700, and later culminated in a published exchange with Stahl on questions of the relation of the soul to the body, the *Negotium Otiosum* (written 1712–15, published in 1720). Christian Thomasius, Professor of Jurisprudence in Halle and a figurehead of opposition to traditionalist views, used Stahlian ideas in his reassessment of Cartesianism.[61] Thomasius also engaged two doctoral candidates of Stahl, Johann Jacob Reich and Christian Weissbach, in his battle against the persecution of witches. Johann Franz Buddeus (Budde) Professor of Moral Philosophy in Halle, one of the most learned and historically underrated mediators between moderate and radical Protestants, was keen on Stahlian ideas.[62]

Christian Wolff could hardly overlook Stahl, a faculty colleague and later a member of the commission which recommended the termination of Wolff's teaching at Halle. Hardly any of the medical mandarins of the early Enlightenment could ignore Stahlian theory or therapeutics, although they could, as in the case of Herman Boerhaave, somewhat disingeneously proclaim they did not know what he meant. In Berlin, always sensitive to the intellectual climate in Halle, Stahl was well known. Influential members of the court were patients of Stahl, including the highly regarded General G. D. von Natzmer. After 1715 Stahl was installed as first physician to the King and president of the *collegium medicum*, the administrative body in control of medical practitioners in Brandenburg-Prussia.

Stahl's influence in Germany was both ideological and practical. The alliance with the ideological goals of radical Protestantism, as expressed in his medical theory, countered a rationalist philosophy and prepared the ground for Vitalism and Romanticism. The late-eighteenth-century discussions of nature in the writings of Albrecht von Haller, Herder and Kant refer back to questions of teleology and

[61] Thomasius, Johann Franz Buddeus and Stahl edited and wrote the highly controversial periodical *Observationes Selectae ad Rem Litterariam Spectantes* (Halle, 1700–5); A reassessment of Cartesian dualist philosophy was given in C. Thomasius, *Einleitung zur Sittenlehre . . .* (Halle, 1692; seventh edition, 1726).

[62] Buddeus was involved in the Pietist rejection of Wolff's philosophy and worked with Stahl on the *Observationes Selectae*.

the problem of essences and appearances in nature as they were formulated and discussed at the beginning of the century between Leibniz and Stahl and in the vitalist–mechanist debate between Pietists and the secularised philosophy propagated by Christian Wolff. The political and judicial advances of the Enlightenment in Brandenburg-Prussia in respect to 'natural law' were probably influenced by Stahl's criticism of Aristotelian concepts of nature and his views of psychology. Christian Thomasius's familiarity with Stahl and his ideas in Halle indicate that medical and judicial reform were linked on a theoretical and practical level. Unfortunately these are questions which have not received proper scholarly attention.

Stahl's medical theory can be seen as a major reference point for the ideological development of the early Enlightenment. Mechanist and dualist philosophy defined its terms against this background, and those opposed to Rationalism discovered *psychological* arguments more to their taste in the wake of Stahl's medical theory. The Stahlian school of physicians (among them Johann Daniel Gohl, Michael Alberti, Ernst Anton Nicolai, Johann Gottlieb Krüger, Johann August Unzer) advanced medical claims that turned the later Enlightenment toward Sensibility (as in Jane Austen's opposition between 'Sense' and 'Sensibility').

In a poem congratulating one of Stahl's medical students on the completion of his doctorate, the following lines were used to explain the ideological value attached to Stahl's theories of medicine by his contemporaries:

> Wohl dem: der bey dem Schwarm der Blinden solchen findt,
> Der helle sehen kan, und uns zurechte weiset!
> Wohl dem! der auf der See mit dem Compasse reiset!
> Und der den Faden hat im falschen Labyrinth.
> Wohl dem! der einen Grund von festem Stahle leget,
> Auf dem der Bau gesetzt, den nicht der Sturm beweget.[63]

(How fortunate, he who finds among the multitude of the blind the man who can see clearly and who can warn us. How fortunate the man who travels across the seas equipped with a compass and who has found the thread to guide him through a false labyrinth. How fortunate the man who lays a firm foundation of steel (Stahl) on which to build the house that no storm will move.)

This laudatory characterisation of Stahl in the published *Carmina* in honour of the doctorate of Georg Sigmund Liebezeit, published in 1713, is slightly unusual, although typical for the time in the choice of metaphor. Laudatory remarks on a medical teacher do not always

[63] Georg Heinrich Ayn, *Der Dreyfache Grund zur Gelehrsamkeit . . . als . . . Georg Sigmund Liebezeit . . . sich den wohlverdienten Doctor=Hut . . . auffsetzen ließ* (Halle, 1713).

name him as clairvoyant ('*helle sehen*') in regard to a multitude seen as blind. Stahl's theory is called a compass by which to cross oceans and as the thread to follow when escaping from the 'false labyrinth'. His house is not one to be torn asunder by storms: it possesses a foundation of 'solid steel' ('*festem Stahl*'). Such praise points to his being judged in a different light than the normal praise for the competent teaching of a medical canon. The poem highlights Stahl's role in the defence of something new and essential. It lends credence to the claim of his having found answers to troubling questions.

THE INFLUENCE OF STAHL

There is much historical truth in this contemporary 'occasional' poetry whose images record nothing more than what Stahl was known for among his contemporaries. From Stahl's own writings it is clear that he attempted a reform of medicine on the basis of a new theoretical framework, constructed also to influence practical therapeutics, and that he was forced to defend his theory from the beginning.[64]

In view of bibliographical research, it is impossible to maintain the idea either that Stahl's influence was minor or that it receded with the advance of the century. The annotated Latin bibliography of Stahl's publications by Johann Christoph Goetz, printed in a second edition in Nürnberg in 1729, lists some 700 items, dividing into 284 writings by Stahl and 420 *ad mentem Stahlii*.[65] A compilation of medical publications either reissuing, translating (into German), or compiling Stahlian principles and therapeutics after 1729 shows no significant decline in interest by mid-century. After 1750 the debate on Stahlian theories continues to be relevant for the medical books written by a third generation, the central questions posed by Stahl being discussed on only slightly shifted philosophical ground.

Beyond the intellectual debates of the late seventeenth and the eighteenth century, which are fundamental to any understanding of modern scientific development, Stahl's writings also became part of the concern for popular instruction. Outside the medical faculties of the universities, which were small and which trained relatively few

[64] G. E. Stahl, *Programma quo Vindicias Theoriae Verae Medicae a Superfluis, Alienis, Falsis Opinionibus et Suppositionibus ex Incongrua Anatomiae, Chymiae, & Physicae, Tractatione & Applicatione Prognatis, ut Physiologia Positiva Demonstrativa Asseratur & Stabiliatur, Publicis Ordinariis Lectionibus & Privatis Petentium Exercitationibus Anatomicis Chymicisque Prosequi Indicat* (Halle, 1694).

[65] Johann Christoph Goetz (Goetzius), *Scripta D. Georg. Ern. Stahlii, aliorumque ad ejus mentem disserentium* (Nürnberg, 1729).

doctors, competence in medicine seemed to depend heavily on reading books. The compilations of medical knowledge, the description of remedies, indeed the setting out of pattern of symptoms, were intrinsically linked to knowledge gained from books. Even though direct practical experience in medicine was not lacking, contrary to what is often disparagingly maintained about the 'theoretical teaching' of medicine at the universities, medical transactions were based on description, on oral communication (even via a third person), or they assumed written form (the *consilia medica*). Reference points for medical expertise were the medical textbooks and medical compilations, especially the *observationes clinicae*, these being integral to medical discourse and to medical learning. To undervalue the influence of publications in the eighteenth century is to misunderstand practical didactics as well as its meaning for the transfer of knowledge. Because of the importance of medical literature as the basis for the exchange of knowledge and as an influence on the practice of medicine in the eighteenth century, it is important to record the translation of major medical works.

The publication of the *Theoria Medica Vera* in 1708 led to an immediate 'translation' into the vernacular German by the Pietist physician Christian Friedrich Richter. In 1709 the *Höchst-Nöthige Erkenntniß des Menschen* went into print in Leipzig. The German translations and books loosely using Stahl's theory and cases were popular enough to all reach several editions. To trace these editions shows how Stahl's medical theory and therapeutics permeated eighteenth-century thought. The Pietist medical books,[66] the first genre to popularise Stahl in German, all reached many editions: Richter's *Höchst-Nöthige Erkentiß* going into a nineteenth edition in 1791; Weissbach's *Wahrhaffte Und gründliche Cur* into its ninth edition in 1764; Kundmann's *Abhandlung vom Verstande des Menschen* a second edition in 1720; Forbinger's *Der vernünfftige Medicus* a third edition in 1735; Reich's *Anweisung zur Gesundheit* a third edition in 1738. Almost all of the Eyssel translations of Stahl's treatises went into third and fourth editions, marking an interest in Stahl that extended well into the 1740s.

At the beginning of the nineteenth century two translations into

[66] Christian Weißbach, *Wahrhaffte und Gründliche Cur, aller dem menschlichen Leib zustossenden Kranckheiten . . .* (Straßburg, 1725); Johann Christian Kundmann, *Kurtze Abhandlung vom Verstande des Menschen vor und nach dem Falle* (Budissin, 1716); Samuel Forbinger, *Der vernünfftige Medicus, in der Physiologie, Pathologie und Praxi . . . nach der berühmten Herrn D. Stahls Methode* (Leipzig, 1717); Johann Jacob Reich, *Anweisung . . . zur Gesundheit*, second edition (Büdingen, 1738).

German of the *Theoria Medica Vera* (whose second Latin edition appeared in 1737/8) were published: Wendelin Ruf's *Theorie der Heilkunde*, with a preface by Kurt Sprengel, was printed in Halle in 1802 and Karl Wilhelm Ideler's *Theorie der Heilkunde*, published in Berlin, appeared in 1831. Both contain the important theoretical treatises and the physiology and pathology, but neither mark the passages they did not translate, and hence are not reliable as faithful renderings of Stahl. Ludwig Choulant republished the entire *Theoria Medica Vera* in Latin in Leipzig in 1831–3.

My work in tracing the prevalence of Stahlian ideas in the eighteenth century shows to what extent his medical theory was discussed and how widespread was his influence.[67] Stahl uses medical evidence to challenge some of the fundamental concepts of the new philosophy and Newtonian physics: the definition of motion, the qualitative difference between mind and matter, the emphasis on reason to the detriment of sentiments and the passions. His championing of the imagination as a creative element in the psyche's holistic construction of perception is most certainly important for Romanticism. In sum, Stahl's medical theory presented the case for a very different view of the unity of body and soul (his theory of the organism) which was alien to ideas of mechanical cause-and-effect relationships based on matter acting on matter or the hierarchical view that reason alone was man's ultimate recourse for justifying his actions. The idea of the 'organic body' appealed to radicals who had to withstand the authority of the State and established church hierarchies. It correlated with their need to legitimise the inspirational freedom of the spirit. As the political terrain of Absolutism shifted and radical Protestantism adopted quietistic methods or as religious radicals emigrated to the New World, the socio-political influence of the medical theory was lost. In the medical sphere, however, it retained its impact as medicine took up questions of vitalism, of the role of the nervous system or of the imbalance of the mind (psychiatry).

[67] See my forthcoming book (note 18 above).

4

Sickness and the soul: Stahl, Hoffmann and Sauvages on pathology

ROGER FRENCH

If a single word had to be chosen to characterise the intellectual history of the eighteenth century, it would be 'enlightenment'. The aim of this book is to look at medicine in the period. What then, was 'enlightenment' medicine? What place can such a business as medicine have in the broad sweep and the detail of the historian's picture of the century? 'Enlightenment' for the eighteenth century surely meant a new confidence in Reason. As the seventeenth century grew more distant so its different passionate perceptions of God were replaced by a reasoned natural theology or deism. Man's revealed duty became a rational Natural Law. When science replaced natural philosophy at the end of the century there was no necessary place left for God in the scheme of natural things.[1]

Medicine could not remain unaltered by these changes. Indeed, it was shaped – as it always had been – by the natural philosophy that underlay it. And it was only by the beginning of the eighteenth century that the home of natural philosophy, the university arts course, had ceased to depend on late commentaries on Aristotle. In their place – and this is arguably the most radical change since the very introduction of Aristotle into the *studia* some 500 years earlier – came various embodiments of the doctrines of Natural Law and the physical principles of Descartes and Newton. This chapter examines some changes in medicine that occurred in consonance with these dominant and determinant changes. But rather than examining the 'Newtonising' of medicine or education, we shall follow the changes that followed the – after all more important – changes in religious commitment. It was

[1] See the argument by Andrew Cunningham that science – and scientific medicine – is not older than the nineteenth century and involved the disappearance of God from natural philosophy: Andrew Cunningham, 'Getting the Game Right: Some Plain Words on the Identity and Invention of Science', *Studies in History and Philosophy of Science* 19 (1988), pp. 365–89.

their perception of soul that linked these two fields of men's thought – religion and medicine.

PIETISM AND PATHOLOGY

There was a German saying of the eighteenth century: 'Whoever goes to Halle comes back either a Pietist or an atheist.' This aphorism can serve both to introduce this chapter and to conclude it, for we shall begin with the passions of the Pietists and end with the disappearance of God from medical thinking.

The University of Halle was founded at the end of the seventeenth century by Frederick III of Brandenburg-Prussia. It was a Pietist foundation. Uniquely in Europe the Halle Pietists found they were supported and protected by the State.[2] The State in turn found that the educational and commercial activities of the Pietists had beneficial effects that could be used in the development of an absolutism of rule that led to the military State of Frederick William, and after 1740 of Frederick the Great.[3]

The Pietists Philipp Jakob Spener and Augustus Hermann Francke were involved in the setting up of the 'Frederican' university. The theology teachers, among them J. Breithaupt, were chosen from those who shared Spener's views. But no great uniformity of belief was stamped on the young university. As important in its founding as Francke was the great liberal jurist Christian Thomasius. The medical teacher was Frederick Hoffmann, who, although undoubtedly a Pietist, disliked religious Enthusiasm and gave his religion a markedly rational and natural character. The arrival of Christian Wolff in 1706 greatly strengthened these enlightenment strands in the education available at Halle, and these are undoubtedly the 'atheism' of the saying quoted above. Wolff's natural theology aroused the opposition of the Pietists in 1721 but was welcomed by Hoffman.

To see how Pietism relates to pathology, we must look at its nature a little more closely. Its roots are normally traced to the mystical and passionate religious writings of Böhme and Arndt. For many it remained a religion of emotion rather than reason, centred on direct experience of God, which reason could never attain. This 'Enthusiasm' made advances where the orthodox Lutheran church was seen as over-

[2] For a stimulating account of this relationship, see Mary Fulbrook, *Piety and Politics. Religion and the Rise of Absolutism in England, Württemberg and Prussia* (Cambridge, 1983).

[3] K. S. Pinson, *Pietism as a Factor in the Rise of German Nationalism* (New York, 1934); Fulbrook, *Piety and Politics.*

concerned with refining the doctrines of the Reformation and correspondingly over-logical, disputational and scholastic. It was a call for a new reform and was based on a personal 'rebirth', a moment of spiritual conversion. Nowhere was this call more effective than in Halle, where the destructive effect of war and pestilence had rendered the population, at least in the eyes of Francke, demoralised, inebriated and immoral. Pietists believed in practical Christianity, and Francke began by excluding from communion those of his flock who refused to be 'born again'. He continued with attacks on orthodox pastors and ultimately set up a variety of schools for the improvement of the population, that is, for the spread of Pietism.

In intervening to settle the social disturbances caused by such actions, Frederick as Elector and then king, found that there were a number of advantages in supporting the Pietists. A Pious and practical born-again population, and more to the point, army, was more obedient; the commercial activities of the Pietists in publishing and chemical preparation of medicines brought money into the State; the powers of the guilds and of the local Estates were clipped: in making Pietism the new orthodoxy with himself at the head, the ruler of Prussia secured for himself, as Francke shrewdly pointed out, a nation of honest and faithful servants, and thus a rule that tended ever more to absolutism.

It increasingly came to be the case in Prussia that a profession of Pietism was a necessary qualification for employment by the State. This was particularly so in Halle, where Francke's schools and the university were the chief instruments of propagating Pietism. (By 1717 universal school education was imposed in Prussia, and by 1727 all training theologians had to spend at least a year in Halle.) So when Hoffmann, the medical teacher at Halle, began to look for a colleague to share the teaching, it is likely that he looked for a Pietist. The new teacher was Georg Ernst Stahl. He had written to Hoffman, recalling their past friendship in Jena and expressing an interest in the new university.[4] Indeed, there seemed a considerable parallel between the two: born in the same year, they had been at school together, were both medical men with a strong interest in chemistry, were both Pietists and had been selected by the same university to teach the same subject. Yet Stahl's system of medicine was so fundamentally different to Hoffman's that their opposition was the archetype of the disputes between the 'animists' and 'mechanists' that recurred through most of the century.

[4] This account is taken from the biography of Hoffmann at the beginning of the first volume of the collected works. See note 11 below.

This difference seems to have arisen ultimately from the nature of Stahl's Pietism, less 'enlightened' and more Enthusiastic than Hoffmann's.[5] In Enthusiastic Pietism, the moment of rebirth, conversion and the subsequent spirituality, were essentially individual experiences variously described as direct experience of God or as having Christ (or Arndt's 'temple of God') within one. The soul or spirit was essential in such communication that linked God to the physical body of man. It was in this communication that real, spiritual life existed. Even the 'enlightened' Pietist Hoffmann declared that the 'born again' Christian (*homo regenitus*) had two lives, spiritual (in communication with God)[6] and physical. As a self-proclaimed 'mechanist' he held that physical life was simply the regular appearance of the motions that derived from the motion of the heart, and that this was precisely paralleled by the moral actions arising from the heart of the spiritual life, the soul. And, he says, it is in the soul that we may see 'vestigia' of the image of God.[7] Stahl, in contrast, whose medical beliefs were based on *organismus* rather than *mechanismus*, and whose Pietism may have been more inclined to radicalism and Enthusiasm, conflated the spiritual and physical lives and derived all motions from the heart of the spiritual life, the soul.

The point Hoffmann makes in comparing his own beliefs with those of Stahl (as its title announces)[8], is that what Hoffmann perceived as Stahl's mistakes at the level of fundamental theory result in bad practice of medicine, that is, in bad pathology and therapeutics. So what was a Pietist pathology? And how did Hoffman's differ from Stahl's?

The difference between the two was simple and fundamental. For Stahl the soul was dominant. It had cognisance of all the motions of the body by *intellectus* and gave them direction by *voluntas*. Body and soul were thus indivisible, a unity. In illness the cognisant functions of the soul could become so misdirected that the disease took on a lethal

[5] On Stahl see J. Geyer-Kordesch, 'Georg Ernst Stahl: Pietismus, Medizin und Aufklärung in Preußen im 18 Jahrhundert,' Manuscript of Habilitationsschrift (Münster, 1988).

[6] F. Hoffmann, *Opera Omnia Physico-Medica*, 6 vols. (Geneva, 1749–53): for the *homo regenitus* see his *Meditationes Theologicae, Quibus Summa Religionis Christianae Brevite et Perspicue Traditur* (1737) in the *Supplementum* to the *Opera Omnia* (1749), part 1, first pagination, p. 62. The spiritual life in which one is joined to God is discussed in his *Dissertatio Theologico-Medica de Officio Boni Theologi ex Idea Boni Medici*, in *Supplementum*, vol. 3, p. 57

[7] Hoffmann's *Exercitatio de Optima Philosophandi Ratione* is to be found in the *Supplementum*, part 1, p. 3.

[8] *De Differentia Doctrinae Stahlianae a Nostra in Pathologicis et Therapeuticis*, in *Supplementum*, part 2, p. 9. This was not published in Hoffmann's lifetime, no doubt, as its editor observes, to avoid open controversy with Stahl in Halle.

course. For Stahl the primary and irreducibly vital action of the soul in the body was the generation of blood. Blood and the other material components of the body were, above all, highly putrescible, and the outstanding paradox of physiology was how the soul preserved them from decay during the lifetime of the individual. No mere mechanism could do this, but only imposed and salutary motion from an incorporeal source and with beneficial purposes. Stahl's pathology centres on the tendency of blood to become denatured in the body.[9]

But Hoffman could not interpret Stahl's doctrine in this way, as a modern historian might.[10] Instead he saw his opponent through the eyes of a mechanist, selecting and distorting points of Stahl's teaching that seemed significant to, and objectionable to, his own doctrine. Thus to Hoffmann, the soul in Stahl's doctrines moved the inert matter of the body, and did so not by union but by imposition. In illness, said Hoffmann, the Stahlian soul perceived the noxious agent or cause, and generated bodily motions to evacuate it. It followed (in Hoffmann's interpretation) that the effect of poisons on the body was not chemical or in any way corporeal, but was the anxious recognition by the soul of the danger, and its subsequent efforts to remove it. If the danger should be too great, continues Hoffmann, the Stahlian soul gives up the effort and the body dies. Stahl further maintained (concluded Hoffmann) that while the soul's intention was always good, yet in putting it into practice the soul sometimes makes mistakes, perhaps selecting an inappropriate time or place for evacuation. It was then the duty of the Stahlian physician to understand and help to achieve the soul's intention. All these points then, as we shall see below, were selected for refutation by Hoffmann as being significantly opposed to mechanism; but by the same token Hoffmann can see them only in mechanist terms.

Hoffmann's objection to Stahl's pathology at the level of practical medicine is that it makes nonsense of one of the doctor's principal weapons, his management of the non-naturals. Diet, exercise, regimen, the effects of airs, waters and places could have no effect on the body if the soul chose to ignore them. The very effects of medicines themselves were called into question on the Stahlian assumption that,

[9] Stahl's doctrine of sanguification can be seen in his early thesis, *Dissertatio Physiologico-Medica de Sanguificatione in Corpore Semel Formato* (Halle, 1704). While at Halle he published (1706) *Disquisitio de Mechanismi et Organismi Diversitate*, also published in Choulant's edn of the *Theoria Medica Vera*, which contains his pathological doctrines and a convenient 'Brief Repetition of Physiology': L. Choulant, *Georg Er. Stahl Theoria Medica Vera* (Leipzig, 1831–3).

[10] I am indebted to Dr Geyer-Kordesch (personal communication) for this authoritative summary of Stahl's doctrine. I am also grateful to her for many useful suggestions, many of which I have used in this chapter.

as composed of matter and thus passive, they had no innate powers. But to justify his own pathology and therapeutics Hoffmann had to go back to the foundations of his beliefs.

HOFFMANN THE ENLIGHTENED PIETIST

There is no doubt of Hoffmann's Pietism. His pupil and biographer makes much of the *pietas* of his early education, of that of his parents and that of his wife.[11] He was a friend of Spener, and joined with Breithaupt in setting up a school for youths. After his wife died and he was himself approaching eighty he wrote a summary of his Christian beliefs, a tract on 'physico-theology' and a comparison between the roles of physician and theologian. We have already met his *homo regenitus*, the true Pietist, and we can see more Pietism in his *Medicus Politicus*,[12] a series of rules that begins '*Medicus sit Christianus*': the doctor should be a Christian. But a Christian is not merely one who understands Christianity, but one who (like the Pietists) practises it. Besides, in matters of (Pietist) religion, understanding – reason – can have but limited powers, like an eye without a telescope.[13] Correspondingly, the doctor must not be an atheist. Hoffmann has in mind (in his own terms) the 'practical' atheist, who knows there is a God, but who does not live in accordance with his precepts. (It is only 'theoretical' atheists who deny the existence of God.) We can guess that Hoffmann's view of practical atheists was a Pietist view partly of the orthodox Lutherans and partly of any other group that did not practice the Pietist form of Christianity. His sadness at the abuse of private confession[14] is surely that of a Pietist, akin to the desperation at empty and formal Lutheran confession that drove Schade to a nervous breakdown.[15]

But although a Pietist, Hoffmann was antagonistic to the radical, Enthusiastic side of Pietism. Rule 4 of his *Medicus Politicus* is 'The doctor is not superstitious', where 'crass superstitions' are listed as *Enthusiasmus*, *Fanaticismus* and *Quakerianismus*. (Perhaps these are the 'inspirational and insane' theologies that he elsewhere[16] attributes to disease of the brain.) All these, says Hoffmann, involve the belief

[11] Hoffmann, *Opera Omnia Physico-Medica*, vol. 1. The text is prefaced by a short biography by J. H. Schulze.

[12] The *Medicus Politicus* begins a new pagination p. 240 of the *Supplementum*, part 1.

[13] Hoffmann, *Meditationes Theologicae*, p. 63.

[14] Hoffmann, *Dissertatio Theologico-Medica*, p. 58.

[15] Fulbrook, *Piety and Politics*, p. 161.

[16] Hoffmann, *De Optima Philosophandi Ratione*, p. 4.

that the spirit is part of God, and so such superstitious people believe that God lives within them and vouchsafes revelation directly to them. Hoffmann lays the blame for this belief on Platonism (as the Pietist Spener had done) but it is perhaps the Hermeticism of the Florentine Platonists that Hoffmann has in mind rather than classical Plato.[17] No, declares Hoffmann against the idea of personal revelation, our theologians more correctly identify revelation as double, the light of nature and the light of grace. The latter is found in the sacred word of the Scriptures and the sacraments; and the former is found in nature.

It is his searching for this 'light of nature' that makes Hoffmann an enlightened Pietist. He was appointed in Halle to a chair that was not simply medicine, but also of natural philosophy. His inaugural oration upon taking up his duties was 'On Defeating Atheism by Reference to the Skilful Structure of the Body'.[18] This set the note for the rest of his long life, in which natural philosophy had the purpose – by exposing the relationship between Creator and His skilful Creation – of bringing man to respect and fear God.[19] Hoffmann felt this to be a Pietist tradition, for he tells the reader[20] that Spener himself had expressed to him the divine nature of natural philosophy and regretted that he had no longer the opportunity to pursue it. But (Hoffman continues) Spener had clearly impressed it upon his sons, one of whom became the first professor of experimental physics and mathematics at Halle. In old age Hoffmann argued that natural philosophy was the best way to promote piety and he recalled from his youth not only the great advances made in astronomy, anatomy, chemistry and 'physico-mechanics' but also, in particular, English natural theological writings: Derham, Stillingfleet, Ray, Boyle.[21] From within what amounts to a Pietist version of a tradition of natural theology Hoffmann grasped eagerly the 'natural law' of Wolff after the latter's arrival in Halle, as an example of the 'laws of nature' by which God governed the universe. Wolff became a close friend.

Natural philosophy was fundamental also to Hoffmann's medicine: it was natural philosophy which underpinned the theory of medicine; and the practice of medicine was part of his Pietist following of God's precepts. Indeed, Hoffmann was conscious of a great parallel between

[17] See Spener's *On Hindrances to Theological Studies* in P. C. Erb (ed.), *Pietists. Selected Writings*, The Classics of Western Spirituality Series (New York, 1983), p. 68.

[18] Schulze's biography in Preface to Hoffmann, *Opera Omnia*, p. vii.

[19] Rule 5 of the *Medicus Politicus*. [20] Hoffmann, *De Optima Philosophandi Ratione*, p. 5.

[21] The English, he noted were generally disposed to be silent on their philosophical activities and novelties until one had broken down their conversational reserve with an account of one's own. See the preface to the *De Optima Philosophandi Ratione*.

the good physician and the good theologian. The cure of the body and the 'cure of souls' are the same kind of activity (*salus* is equally 'health' and 'salvation').[22] Both medicine and theology are theoretical and practical; the theologian's theory is the revealed word and that of the physician is the laws of nature, or in Hoffman's terms, mechanism.

ACTIVE MATTER

We are now in a position to follow Hoffmann's critique of Stahl. The first and most fundamental difficulty he found was that Stahl appeared to him to insist that matter was inert (and motion quite separate from matter). As we saw above, this was not the case. Hoffmann saw, in what he thought was Stahl's view, the great danger of atheism: if matter is purely passive, then all motion must come directly from God. But to say that *corporeal* motion comes from God is to fail to distinguish the Creator from the Created and so to slide towards the atheism (said Hoffmann) of Descartes and Spinoza. A Cartesian–Spinozan natural philosophy, he continued, also denies the possibility of spiritual action in corporeal bodies, a topic of great importance for the Pietist. In place of this Hoffmann insisted that God[23] in making the world had created corporeal bodies external to Himself, together with motion, which was neither material nor immaterial, but simply the operations of things. God gave to all matter a power of motion or resistance whereby all bodies interact, move and produce all the qualitative aspects of existence and life itself. All action is by contact and the ways that bodies interact are simply God's natural laws, the Will of the Creator remaining in things since the Creation. These laws have been in operation since Creation, asserts Hoffmann, which means that God is not continuously generating motion for the world. It would not be pious, said Hoffmann, for every motion in the world, such as a dog biting a man, to be ascribed to the direct action of God.

Hoffman had worked out this fundamental position before the end of the seventeenth century, after the dispute between Leibniz and Sturm on the passivity of matter. In an exchange of letters with Hoffmann[24] Leibniz agreed with Hoffmann's assertion that anything purely passive could not even receive the power to move, and so could not exist (since everything is mobile). A recipient and retentive force is necessary in any body for it to move. All these actions, God's laws,

[22] Hoffmann, *Dissertatio Theologico-Medica*, p. 57.
[23] The 39th *Differentia* between his doctrines and those of Stahl.
[24] The Leibniz correspondence is printed at p. 49 of the *Supplementum*, part 1, first pagination.

were for Hoffmann (in 1699) mechanical. (He may have been prompted to think of these by Boyle, whose use of the term he mentions, perhaps in a personal conversation.)[25] By *mechanismus* Hoffmann meant at its simplest natural necessity: when fire is applied to wood, the wood necessarily burns. When a complex of such causes produces effects that are purposeful, this for Hoffmann is also mechanism, but more perfect. At this stage of his life, *organismus* was no more than other people's term for such mechanism within organic bodies. The true opposite of *mechanismus* for Hoffmann was *moralismus*, actions proceeding from the will. Indeed, it is often a mistake to translate *mechanismus*, as used by Hoffmann and his contemporaries, as 'mechanism', and a worse mistake to infer in the absence of the term that they meant 'machine-like'. 'Natural necessity' would be a better translation, and one that could be used equally of the exponents of Natural Law, who shared a terminology about natural necessity and related matters with the medical men.[26] It is said that Wolff's enemies in Halle argued before Frederick William that Wolff's doctrine of natural necessity meant that no deserting soldier could be punished if he had acted involuntarily. (One can see why the king preferred to be advised by Pietists.)

MECHANISM, STRUCTURE AND MOTION

So Hoffmann's position was that matter was innately mobile. Chemical actions, the intestine motion of water in dissolving solids, elasticity, momentum, resistance, equilibrium, reflection: all were God's laws or secondary causes and all were expressed in the wide range of topics available to Hoffmann in early-eighteenth-century natural philosophy: statics, hydraulics, hydrostatics, mechanics, optics. The interaction of fluids and solids in the body in accordance with these laws made structure very important for the physician who wished to understand the actions of the body. While structure and function had always had in

[25] See also Schulze's biography in Preface to Hoffmann, *Opera Omnia*.

[26] What was taught at Halle may be conveniently found in M. H. Otto, *Elementa Iuris Naturae et Gentium una cum Delineatione Iuris Positivi Universalis* (Halle, 1738). This is the second part of a treatise on divine law, and was designed for the young, no doubt in the university or one of Francke's schools. Drawing on Grotius, Pufendorf and Wolff, it shows how a 'natural' consideration of God lay behind the law of nature and nations as much as it did behind medicine. Like Hoffmann's 'best means of philosophising' its goal is human happiness by means of understanding. Its moral precepts are those recognised by the medical man as consequences of the rational soul's awareness of its Creator. 'Natural' actions in man are those that occur *mechanically* by virtue of structure and of a force created by God and implanted in matter.

Galenic medicine and Aristotelian natural philosophy a close and elaborate relationship, yet at the level of, for example, the similar parts there was no indication in structure (they were homogeneous) of the action (it was qualitative) they possessed. For the mechanist, on the other hand, every action and every use depended on the *shape and size* of parts – particles of moving fluids or combined particles of the containing solids. It was for this reason that Hoffmann recalled the great advances made in anatomy, and it was for the same reason that his own teaching at Halle was characterised by his biographer and pupil as based on anatomy that was to be learned by personal inspection. Indeed, Schulze, the pupil, sums up Hoffmann's medicine in a way that cannot be improved on for our purposes: the anatomical structure 'works' by God's eternal laws, and airs, waters, places and medicines necessarily act on the body by the natural laws that govern the innate activity of their matter. It was thus, says Schulze (in his biographical note), that Hoffmann's medicine stood in opposition to Stahl's doctrine of a freely acting, intelligent and mobile soul, for like others[27] what Schulze saw in Stahl's doctrine of unity of body and soul was primarily the autonomy of soul.

Stahl's soul was 'mobile' in the sense of generating the motion of the animated body. Faced with this, Hoffmann seems to have felt the need to demonstrate the source of motion as located in a *mechanical* body. Developing the argument of this inaugural oration (that the mechanical structure of the body was a proof of the existence of God) he produced a dissertation in 1731 to demonstrate that the body was a machine that exhibited perpetual motion.[28] No man-made machine, said Hoffmann (despite an active investigation among his contemporaries), has true perpetual motion, that is, continues to move and will re-start if stopped, without any external aid, until its parts decay. (His objection to Stahl's doctrine was that the soul was an 'external' source of motion, an unneeded metaphysical intrusion.) Hoffmann's argument is that the human body demonstrates perpetual motion in that the effect of a moving cause becomes in turn a cause with a subsequent effect. The cycle starts in the heart and motion is transferred successively to the fluid contents of the arteries, the brain, the nerves and back to the heart, the effect becoming the cause. Although his explanation involves a respired and active material ether, the essential means

[27] For example, Robert Whytt (classified to his indignation by Haller as a Stahlian). See R. K. French, *Robert Whytt, the Soul and Medicine* (London, 1969).

[28] *Dissertatio Medica de vera Perpetui Mobilis in Homine vivi Idea* (1731): *Supplementum*, part 1, second pagination, p. 195.

whereby the motion lost by friction of the circulating fluids is replaced is the skilful structure God has given the muscles: it is here that the increased resistance of the smaller vessels to the circulating fluids results in a very great motion of the muscle. The importance of anatomy emerges here too: Hoffmann congratulates himself on living in an age when improvements in anatomy make it possible for him to refute what he (elsewhere) sees as the retrogressive and Aristotelian animism of Stahl. In particular the anatomy of fine structure shows that the body is a machine, with its columns, levers, springs, wedges, pulleys, bellows, sieves and presses. The doctor who recognises these and knows the laws of motion, concludes Hoffmann, will also recognise how the machine can break down, and so knows the essence of pathology.

PATHOLOGY AND STRUCTURE

Galen had said that disease was disordered function. The notion translated readily into mechanistic terms because function could be understood as the consequence of the natural laws of motion. It was the motion of clearly perceptible and intelligible parts, that is to say, structure: a mechanistic pathology related disease closely to structure. For the purposes of discussing the eighteenth century, I want to call this the Boerhaavian model, as set out in his *Institutiones*.[29] Diseases are classified as the parts of the body are classified. There are diseases of the solid simple parts, of the organs, of the humours and of 'systems' of solids and humours. Boerhaave's classification was followed by, for example, Jerome Gaub and Robert Whytt.

But despite the wide use of Boerhaave's texts in the earlier eighteenth century, not everyone adopted the mechanical-structural-functional view of disease. Stahl's view that 'disease' was an attempt by the soul to throw off a noxious cause found a parallel in many writers. The Hippocratic 'healing power of Nature' could be used instead of 'soul' with the same effect. And this effect was to loosen the ties between disease and structure. The efforts of the soul or nature need not be localised, and, if localised, might not be predictable. If the soul acted directly upon the body, there would be no perceptible, intelligible chain of (mechanical) events located in structure. The soul did not need the five simple machines of early-eighteenth-century mechanics, or any combination of them, to achieve its effects. Indeed, the very question of

[29] H. Boerhaave, *Institutiones Medicae in Usus Annuae Exercitationis Domesticos* (Leyden, 1727), pp. 342ff.

the locatability of a spiritual and immaterial entity was disputable, and disputed. The result was that while the 'mechanist' had a ready-made 'map' of the body in which to locate his knowledge of diseases, the 'animist' had none. He had to classify his diseases in a different way. It is suggested below that this helps to explain why one of the best known animists of the eighteenth century was also the first great nosologist.

DE GORTER AND THE CLASSIFICATION OF DISEASE

First I want to look at a figure who is less well known and who also came to construct a kind of nosology. This is Johannes de Gorter, the ordinary professor of medicine at Harderwijk.[30] His inaugural oration, given in June 1726, is an attempt to overcome what he sees as the neglect of medical practice. Disappointed that the theoretical medicine of the schools, so subject to hypothesis and novelty, had not properly prepared him for practice, he here advocates a better system, based on arranging and indexing medical aphorisms for ready use in practice. De Gorter compares the state of practical medicine as a discipline unfavourably with that of botany, and proceeds to improve the former by means of the latter; that is, he adopts an ideal of botanical classification in arranging his aphorisms. Aphorisms, terse and irrefutable, will make the practice of medicine, he says, certain and stable, just as the characteristics of plants have been used in botany. Classification by genera, classes and species allows the botanist to identify plants quickly by their taxonomic characteristics, and to fit newly discovered species into the framework: so should the physician readily be able to recognise the disease from the features of the aphorism, and to fit new aphorisms, derived from experience, into their proper place, that is, where they are related to their neighbours in the classification.

The first step in the proposed system was to be to write down all aphorisms that dealt with cause, effects, symptoms, predictions or method of cure. This would compose a 'nursery' or *sylva* (the model is no doubt Bacon's) in which each 'plant' is set down with no preconceived hypothesis, but as observed. Each of them is then numbered for easy reference. Then by means of an index, related aphorisms could be grouped into genera. Finally tables were to be constructed listing the classes and species within the genera. The purpose was to construct a

[30] J. de Gorter, *Medicinae Compendium, in usum Exercitationis Domesticae . . ., Pars Prima* (Frankfurt and Leipzig, 1749). The *Pars Secunda* is in the same volume, at the end of which is the *Oratio Medica Inauguralis de Dirigendo Studio in Medicinae Praxis sive de Tabulis pro Disciplina Medica Concinnandis.*

cumulative body of information: the operator of the system was advised to underline in each observation, or aphorism, all important words, which were to go into the index. This was so arranged that additions could be made in alphabetical order. As the system grew so the coverage became more comprehensive: a genus (in the first table) might be for example 'pain', which was to have six classes – location, type, causes, symptoms, methods of cure and change. Class one might be 'chest', which then in table two breaks down into species, like rib-pain or clavicle-pain.

We can learn a little more from de Gorter about eighteenth-century attempts to classify disease. As we see in Martin's chapter on Sauvages in this volume, some inspiration for the attempts came from Bacon, and more from the botanists. Five years or so before Sauvages was classifying diseases on the model of the botanist Tournefort, de Gorter was using a botanical method that brought him into contact with Linnaeus, at whose graduation (in 1735) in Harderwijk de Gorter acted as sponsor; at that time de Gorter's son David joined Linnaeus on botanising expeditions.

Twenty-four years after his inaugural dissertation de Gorter was ready to put his observations and reading to the test of his system. But it had changed in the interval. It was no longer a classification of aphorisms. Perhaps they have served their purpose and have turned this *System of Medical Practice* into a kind of nosology of disease.[31] Half of it is concerned with general diseases after the Boerhaavian model (see above) and the other half is particular diseases, where the numbered paragraphs approximate to species of disease and seem to be derived from the original numbered aphorisms. The basis of classification is function or location; groups of diseases are 'titles', not classes. His modest hope is 'to open a little window to the true names of diseases', and the cross-referencing by which this is achieved also enables the reader to discover from the listed symptoms and locations a suitable remedy, even if he does not know the name of the disease.

In short de Gorter has used a botanical technique not so much to classify disease entities in the way that Sauvages was to do, but to refine and make more practical the picture of disease as disordered function. There is one particular in which, during the course of his life, he departed from the strict Boerhaavian model, as others also did. In 1730, four years after his inaugural oration he gave another, on the soul in

[31] J. de Gorter, *Praxis Medicae Systema* (Frankfurt and Leipzig, 1755). The earlier botanical ideal had largely been lost from this work. There is no evidence that de Gorter allowed Linnaeus's work to influence him.

medicine.[32] Unlike Boerhaave and Hoffmann, de Gorter said that the soul has 'automatic or vital' motions in the body, such as that of the heart and intestines; or it can at least affect such motions. His devotion to medical practice, the subject of most of his writing, later convinced him that there were hidden things in the body that could not be explained on the basis of chemistry, mechanics or hydraulics, but which come from 'distinct laws of life'. He first formulated what he called General Laws and had his son David defend them in a thesis in 1732, and later discovered Special Laws. By reason of these he was obliged to withdraw from the usual mechanical explanation, *qua recedo a consueta explicatione Mechanica.*[33] The critical case was secretion, where the particles and pores of the mechanists had replaced the old faculties. But to de Gorter secretion was essentially a *vital* motion, following laws that were not found in non-living systems. There had to be, he concluded, an active principle in the body. Certainly, he said, such things had not been admitted in discussion until now, but this was because the chemists and physicists had succeeded in closing the door and holding up the progress of knowledge.

This was a personal conversion for de Gorter, a reaction against the campaign for mechanism typified if not started by Boerhaave's oration on the topic. Similar reactions were recorded by Whytt in Edinburgh, Sauvages in Montpellier and Rosetti in Padua, in the 1730s and 1740s. Rosetti indeed presents himself as part of a campaign to reintroduce the Hippocratic principle of movement, the *enormon.* This term was also used by Gaub, whose system of animistic pathology was partly adopted by Whytt in lecturing on pathology in Edinburgh in the 1760s. The choice of the term seems a deliberate one by animists in their campaign against mechanism.[34] What was common to the animist alternative was that the lower soul(s) of seventeenth-century doctrines was abandoned. Where the passivity of the animal machine made an energetic soul a necessary part of theory, to identify that soul (as the animists did) with the immortal soul of Christian doctrine drew

[32] J. De Gorter, *Oratio de Animi et Corporis Consensione Mirabili tam in Secunda Quam Adversa Valetudine* (1730) bound and probably published again with his *Oratio de Praxis Medicae Repurgatae Certitudine*, 1729 (Frankfurt and Leipzig, 1749).

[33] J. De Gorter, *Opuscula Varia Medico-Theoretica* (Padua, 1751): the fifth of the *Exercitationes Medicae Quinque* in this collection seems to date from the 1730s and is entitled *De Actione Viventium Particulari*, p. 130.

[34] J. S. Rosetti, *Systema Novum Mechanico Hippocraticum de Morbis Fluidorum, et Solidorum, ac de Singulis Ipsorum Curationibus. Opus Theorico-Practicum* (Venice, 1734). For Boerhaave's orations, see E. Kegel-Brinkgreve and A. M. Luyendijk-Elshout (translators and eds.) *Boerhaave's Orations* (Leiden, 1983).

medicine and religion together in a satisfactory way. Rosetti identified the Hippocratic *enormon* or *impetum faciens* with the divine breath breathed into the body of man. It was for religious rather than physiological reasons that the soul was held to be perfect: it is not damaged by disease, said de Gorter, and any apparent vices – the subject matter of pathology – came from the body.[35] Gaub and Whytt both claimed that even in cases of drunkenness it is the body that is affected, not the soul.[36] Likewise in therapeutics, medicines act on the body, not on the soul. Where practice renders complex motions habitual and almost unconscious, it is the body, said de Gorter, not the soul, that becomes used to the actions. In all this the way in which the body and soul interact remains unknown, and is attributed directly to God.[37]

A characteristic of eighteenth-century animism in the period after Stahl was that the soul was generally thought to be super-added to a mechanical body. It was a rigorous use of mathematics to prove that the machine of the body could not produce its own motion that convinced Sauvages and Whytt that there must be an additional, non-material source of movement. In contrast the mechanists' arguments were generally qualitative, not mathematical. They were statements of faith in a principle, a faith that de Gorter questioned. A large proportion of such arguments was concerned with circulation and the hydraulics of the various fluids and vessels. Guerrini has pointed out the importance of secretion for Cheyne,[38] and we can recall the experiments of Stephen Hales and the equally well-known calculations of the force of the heart by Borelli, Keill and Bernouilli, together with the hydraulicism of Pitcairne and the Newtonians, to locate de Gorter's experiments. He did not deny the laws of mechanics and hydraulics, but insisted that vital motions rose above them. The proof was experimental: attach the cut (upper) end of the carotid artery of a living dog to a tube of warm water raised to the height to which the heart would send the blood, and the water, de Gorter found, comes down the tube and passes through the brain. But with a dead dog, not twice the height forces water through the brain. Nor in the dead animal can water be compelled to pass through the kidneys, the liver or the pancreas: secretion is a *vital* process.[39]

[35] De Gorter, *Oratio de Animi*, p. 32 and *Praxis Medicae Systema*, p. 28.

[36] Whytt's unpublished notes for lectures on pathology, Edinburgh University MS Gen. 745D.

[37] De Gorter *Opuscula Varia Medico-Theoretica* (of which that on secretion appears to date from 1727), p. 148 and *Oratio de Animi*, p. 32.

[38] See A. Guerrini's chapter on Cheyne in R. K. French and A. Wear, *The Medical Revolution of the Seventeenth Century* (Cambridge, 1989).

[39] *De Actione Viventium Particulari*, p. 132.

ANIMISM AND NOSOLOGY

There is a good case against ismism – the excessive use of -isms in historical discussion – and it is something of an -ism paradox that the eighteenth-century 'mechanists' generally described the body in non-quantitative terms whereas the 'animists' used mathematics to demonstrate the need of a soul to power the machine of the body. The paradox is that Sauvages's concept of the body as a machine was so firm that, by analogy with all machines known to him, the body needed an 'external', non-mechanical, source of motion. We can if we wish call him a mechanist because he thought the body was a machine, but in his own eyes it was the soul that moved the machine that was more important. He called himself and his kind *animistes* or, where they were concerned with the Hippocratic healing power of nature (or *enormon*), *naturistes*.[40] I adopt this terminology in this chapter. Sauvages's use of the terms indeed seems to belong to the language of propaganda, a language he shared with, and used to support, those who agreed with him, and which he used against those he thought to be in error. His letter to Whytt shows that he carried on this battle until at least two years before he died. We can, without historical distortion, describe a battle between mechanists (*machinistes*, *méchaniciens*, said Sauvages) and animists from approximately the 1730s to the 1760s.

I want to conclude this chapter with a rather more speculative connection between animism and nosology in the case of Sauvages. This suggestion is that, believing that the action of the soul was an important part of explanations about how the body worked, Sauvages could not accept the largely mechanical account of disease which located disease tightly to a structure-function 'map' of the body. He had to seek other ways of relating diseases together.

Sauvages's reaction against mechanism occurred at some point before he began teaching an animistic physiology in the 1730s.[41] His medical education had been at Montpellier, from 1722, where Astruc, Chirac, Deidier and Chicoyneau were Regius Professors of Medicine. It was in this form of mechanism that Sauvages began to find the need for a non-mechanical source of motion, and we can gain some notion of this mechanism by looking at texts and particularly theses produced at this time.

[40] S. Hales, *Haemastatique, ou la statique des animaux*, translated by Sauvages (Geneva, 1744). The translation is heavily annotated; these terms appear for example in the final footnote.

[41] R. K. French, 'Sauvages, Whytt and the Motion of the Heart. Aspects of Eighteenth-Century Animism', *Clio Medica* 7 (1972), pp. 35–54.

In such theses Astruc was concerned with the cerebral location of the senses and intellectual operations, with the glands, fibres and pores of the brain and their motions. While it is the soul that perceives and reasons, yet the quality of its perceptions and judgements is determined by reflections, tensions, elasticity, consonance and tone – God-given – within the tissues of the brain: in a word its *dispositiones*, which can be represented diagrammatically.[42] Likewise sensation is effected by the transfer of motion from the perceived object to the spirits and fibres of the brain. Again the mechanism of the action is represented geometrically.[43] Astruc's 'mechanical brain' resembles that of Thomas Willis, or more precisely, that of his source, Willis's Montpellian counterpart, Raymond Vieussens. Astruc's colleague Deidier had adopted a Willisian-chemical explanation of muscle action, and retained a liking for chemical explanations in the age of Newtonian mechanism.[44] Astruc was equally mechanical in his dissertation of 1736 in which he claimed that the sympathy of the parts of the body was owing to connections between nerves in the material *sensorium* of the brain.

The disputes about sympathy are not unimportant for our story. It was obvious that the parts of the body cooperated for the good of the whole, and mechanist and animist alike could quote Hippocrates on the unity of the living body: *confluxionem unam, conspirationem unam, consentientia omnia esse*.[45] The mechanists, like Astruc and Hoffmann, claimed that the source of such collaboration lay in the structure of the body, so wisely and skilfully put together by God. But to others it seemed that mutual cooperation in the working of the body and mutual suffering in disease (the origin of the doctrine is in Galenic pathology) implied some level of mutual sensitivity of the parts, some feeling that a machine would not have.

When Sauvages began to teach at Montpellier he too was among the disputants of theses on mechanism,[46] along with the Chicoyneaus, father and son. The body is a hydraulic machine: Galenists, chemists and Paracelsians are all in error. Life consists in the continuation of circulation, which sets in motion a libration – a dynamic equilibrium –

[42] J. Astruc (*proponens*), *Quaestio Medica de Naturali et Praeternaturali Judicii Exercitatione* (Montpellier, 1718). (Chicoyneau and Deidier among the disputants.)

[43] J. Astruc (*praeses*), *Dissertatio Medica de Sensatione* (Montpellier, 1720). (With Chicoyneau and Deidier.)

[44] A. Deidier, *Quaestio Medica de Motu Musculari* (Montpellier 1699). See also his *Institutiones* as note 51.

[45] J. Astruc, *An Sympathia Partium a Certa Nervorum Positura in Interno Sensorio* (Montpellier, 1736).

[46] J. Bajollet (*proponens*), *Vitae ac Mortis Animalium Conspectus Medico-Mechanicus* (Montpellier, 1735).

between the fluids and solids of the body. 'Function' is simply 'motion of the organic parts' and relates to 'faculty' just as 'actual force' (mass in motion) relates to 'virtual force' (mass at rest). The language is that of the mechanism which (because no machine can move itself) proved to Sauvages that there was a super-added, energetic soul.[47] In a hydraulic machine all depends on the pump, and Bajollet, the student speaking for Sauvages, presents the calculations of Borelli and Keill on the force of the heart and sets up the problem of finding the force of blood in the aorta (where *vis* is mass multiplied by speed). This is almost certainly Sauvages speaking through his student, but there is yet no place given to the soul.[48] To judge by dissertations of his students, Sauvages's conversion to animism seems to have happened in the following year (1736).[49]

But Sauvages had hit on the idea of classifying diseases like plants during his stay in Paris in 1730 and 1731, before becoming an animist. He communicated the notion to Boerhaave, who (not surprisingly, if my claim about the structure-function 'map' is right) thought that it would be very difficult to put into practice.[50] But Sauvages was not deterred and the result of his efforts helped to secure him the chair in Montpellier.

What Sauvages had done at this early stage and even before he became an animist, I believe, was to separate disease from pathology. That is to say, pathology was a major item in early-eighteenth-century divisions of medicine, alongside physiology and semiotics as theoretical, and hygiene and therapeutics as practical. Some such division was general, the theoretical subjects at least usually being treated in eighteenth-century style as the Institutes of Medicine. Pathology normally[51] treated causes, disease and symptoms as an assemblage 'against nature' and damaging to function. To classify diseases in the botanical manner, that is, from their appearances alone, was to take them out of their causal relationship ('predisposing' and 'proximate' were the simplest of a number of causes) and away from the structure-function 'map'. It seems likely that this is what Sauvages was doing in the 1730s; and when he became an animist, to see disease as an attempt of the soul to throw off the offending cause, was another reason to delocate

[47] R. K. French, 'Ether and Physiology' in G. N. Cantor and M. J. S. Hodge (eds.), *Conceptions of Ether: Studies in the History of Ether Theories*, (Cambridge, 1981), pp. 111–34.

[48] N. Cambray, *Dissertatio de Vita Humani* (Montpellier, 1738).

[49] Sauvages sent some of these theses to Whytt in seeking his support. See note 41 above.

[50] For biographical details see L. Delarbre, *Etude sur Sauvages, ses oeuvres et sa doctrine* (Montpellier, 1880).

[51] See for example A. Deidier, *Institutiones Medicinae Theoricae, Phisiologiam et Pathologiam Complectens* (Paris, 1731).

disease (see below). In some ways Sauvages's early attempt at classifying diseases was paralleled by what De Gorter had done two or three years before, that is, to take diseases out of their theoretical context and seek a relationship between them as entities. De Gorter's modest claim to be helping in the nomenclature of diseases is central: one of the botanists' purposes was to agree upon names. Moreover all medical men were aware that the literature from the Greeks onward contained disease entities; asthma, pleurisy, angina and so on. These often appeared in the literature without immediate references to a (generally Galenic) causal system, which would otherwise have supplied a rational and morphological 'map' to provide their mutual relationships.

SAUVAGES THE ANIMIST

For Sauvages the animist the soul was primarily the non-material source of motion for the body machine. This doctrine appears most formally in his *Elementa Physiologiae*,[52] of which the opening postulate is the scholastic dictum that man consists of body and soul united. Life is presence of soul (not continued circulation); the active powers of the soul are the will, voluntary motion, habitual (unconscious) motion: at least in the edition of 1755 Sauvages uses the terms *enormon* and *impetum faciens*, which look like part of a new campaign on the part of the animists to identify the soul with the Hippocratic healing power of nature (they were used too by Rossetti, Gaub and Whytt). It is precisely because the body is a true hydraulic machine that it needs such an immaterial supply of motion to replace that which is lost through friction, inertia and attraction. The 'useful effect' of any hydraulic machine, concludes Sauvages, can never be more than one seventh of the force put into it by its moving power.

So for Sauvages the soul is not only that by which we live, the immortal principle of the Scriptures and the church fathers, but it is also the motor of the body and, moreover, the 'nature' of Hippocrates. He expresses this identification first in the aggressively titled dissertation defended by Labroquère in 1740: *Medical Dissertation on the Cause of Vital Motions, Where is Justly Restored to Nature, or the Soul, what Ill-Conceived Mechanism has Usurped.*[53] The soul is the

[52] F. Boissier de Sauvages, *Elementa Physiologiae.* I have used the edn of Amsterdam, 1755 and have been unable to verify that it is similar to the Toulouse edn of 1742.

[53] F. Labroquère (*defendens*), *Dissertatio Medica de Motuum Vitalium Causa. Ubi, quae Pravus Mechanismus Usurpaverat Natura seu Animae iure Restituuntur* (Montpellier, 1740). Republished by A. von Haller in *Disputationes Anatomicae* (Göttingen, 1746–51), vol. 4, p. 483.

spiraculum vitae breathed by God into Adam (as set out in Genesis and discussed by Augustine and Aquinas); it is the principle of understanding and motion (Aristotle) and the defender of the body (Hippocrates); quoting Cheyne, mechanism is 'mere jargon and ignorance'. Much up-to-date reading has gone into this dissertation (a surprising number of English authors are represented). Its text is headed *Natura Rediviva*, the proclamation on which his animist campaign was founded, a campaign he continued for nearly thirty years. The reason that he found Stephen Hales's *Haemastaticks* so interesting that he had to translate it into French, was because it was direct experimental evidence that he could use in arguing that the hydraulic, Newtonian machine of the body could not work without *La nature, ou cette puissance mouvante qui anime nos corps.*

NOSOLOGY

For Sauvages disease was partly the way in which the soul elected to heal or rid the body of a noxious agent. I suggest that a nosology became possible, if not necessary, when disease was no longer regarded as disordered function and so was no longer 'mapped' on the structure-function perception of the body. But for Sauvages the body was very much a machine, and one that could be so successfully investigated by mathematics that its structure-functions could be shown to demand a soul as a source of motion. So how was his concept of disease freed from this so as to make a nosology possible?

The answer may be that he *redefined* 'pathology' to correspond to his animist physiology. Sauvages's pathology was divided into aetiology and nosology, and into the first of these he put what had made up Boerhaavian pathology – the 'vices' of the simple and complex solid and fluid parts. But these are *not* now disease entities, for it is Sauvages's nosology that lists these and their symptoms. Sauvages has abandoned the Galenic notion that disease is disordered function, and his *Pathologica Methodica*[54] is based, he claims, on the ancient sect of Methodists, whom Galen had attacked. Sauvages opens his proem by denying the Galenic view that pathology deals with the contranaturals: cause, disease and symptom (in which disease is disordered function). What can such a term as 'contranatural' mean? demands Sauvages. Indeed, what is 'nature' in this context? Sauvages of course fancied he had a more properly Hippocratic notion of what nature was, and

[54] F. Boissier de Sauvages, *Pathologia Methodica seu de Cognoscendis Morbis* (Amsterdam, 1752).

disliked the Galenic view. And if we agree with the *vulgares Pathologi* (says Sauvages) who use 'contranatural', that 'nature' is the interrelated system of the world as created by God, then even the worst diseases are natural in following the laws of nature (and the will of God). No, concludes Sauvages, distinctions between naturals, non-, contra- and preternaturals are figments of dialecticians. The vomiting that follows excessive drinking is in accordance with nature in ridding the body of the noxious cause; it is neither contranatural nor preternatural; instead, it is an action of the soul, for which support could be found among the animists and elsewhere. Categories like contranatural and preternatural are best forgotten, concludes Sauvages, and it is best simply to treat that of 'nature'.

So for Sauvages, pathology is not a study of the contranaturals. Nor is disease a disordered function: an analysis of disordered function normally proceeded from cause to disease to symptom, a chain that varied with the medical system of the proponent. Sauvages gives examples of how a Galenist, a Boerhaavian and a Stahlian would define 'pleurisy', and argues that all such explanations are little more use than explaining to a peasant what a magnet was by talking about helical pores. The peasant, like a medical student, would grasp the essence by a demonstration of the appearances: the magnet attracts iron, pleuritic patients are acutely feverish, suffer pains in the side, cough, and breathe with difficulty. No causality is involved, no systems are required for explanation and little morphology is needed on which to map a disordered function. It is here that Sauvages claims to be following the ancient Methodists, in recognising a series, *congeries*, of symptoms that constitute the disease. The disease is indeed recognised by its symptoms; and since symptoms were the end, and in a sense accidental, result of a chain of events, then their anatomical location (particularly when the *congeries* was large) was less important than in the disordered function of the Boerhaavian model.

ANIMISM AND NATURAL LAW

For the animists it was the soul that moved the machine of the body and so it was the soul that determined what motions were employed in ridding the body of noxious agents, thus producing the appearances of disease. Sauvages's reading included not only Stahl and two authors, Nenter and Juncker, recognised as having adopted Stahl's doctrine, but now also Christian Wolff of Halle. This mid-century discussion of pathology, the *Pathologia Methodica* is informed by Natural Law and

Natural Religion: the perfection of man is the concord of all his actions, moral and natural, in health and agreement with God's will; in the wonderful *machina* of the body, created by God, nothing can be changed without damaging that perfection; God has accordingly made an active, intelligent, sentient principle, devoted to the care and preservation of the body, the soul. In this 'school pneumatology'[55] the soul is said by Sauvages to have three faculties, cognition, appetite and motion. These operate on the moral and rational level as well as on the sensitive or natural. In both cases Good is perceived and pursued and Evil is avoided: moral Good is rational, it awakens the rational appetite and so leads to appropriate actions; on the natural level things necessary for the body's preservation are pursued, and things threatening it are avoided or rejected. The mind is not conscious of the soul's activity at the natural level – '*non appercipimus*, to use the words of Wolff' says Sauvages.[56] And it is the action of the soul at this level which is responsible for all the basic physiological activities, from swallowing to the beating of the heart, as well as for the pathological motion by which noxious causes are eliminated from the body.

In this way Sauvages, the animist and nosologist, has bound together into a satisfactory whole an enlightened Natural Religion, Natural Law, an apparently hypothesis-free Methodism and his earlier rejection of mechanism. But more: the soul acting in this way in the body is what Galen meant by 'nature' as the mover of the body, and what Hippocrates meant by 'the healing power'.[57] It is, too, the soul of church doctrine. The soul's intentions are always good, but (as Stahl said) sometimes its material instruments are imperfect. The physician's duty is to know the soul (nature) and to help, for example (says Sauvages) by encouraging evacuation of the noxious agent through the proper places. The physician must also be on hand (he adds) on the occasions when these natural actions result in harm, just as a man who is fighting for his liberty or life cannot expect to escape damage.

SUMMARY AND CONCLUSION

This chapter argues that the particular political circumstances of Halle encouraged a particular form of reformed religion. This Pietism in turn played a large part in determining who was chosen to teach medicine at the new university. But for all their similarities the two medical

[55] An example of school pneumatology is F. Hutcheson, *Synopsis Metaphysicae, Ontologiam et Pneumatologiam Complectens*, fourth edition, (Glasgow, 1756).

[56] Sauvages, *Pathologia Methodica*, p. 17. [57] Sauvages, *Pathologia Methodica*, p. 33.

teachers there developed systems that could scarcely have been more opposed. Their differences seem to have arisen because their individual preferences within their shared religion were at opposite ends of a spectrum that ran from explicit 'Enthusiasm' that was claimed to surpass reason, to an 'enlightened' Pietism that depended on reason. Enlightenment as a characteristic of the eighteenth century is here contrasted to a passion in religion that rose late in the previous century. The differences are reflected perhaps most intensely in the question of the soul, which was many things: the Enthusiastic Pietist's communication with God, the Rational Principle of the enlightened rationalist, the principle of life for the physician. The differences between Hoffmann and Stahl are characteristically those of the mechanists and animists who campaigned against each other in different European locations: at Halle they centred on pathology. Pathology was morbid physiology (and not yet morbid anatomy) and therefore it was located in a network of theory, largely about causes. This chapter discusses some reasons – some little known, others speculative – why diseases should have become divorced from a tight adherence to a structure-function causality and treated as entities that could have, or needed, other and perhaps classificatory relationships with each other. Both de Gorter and a little later Sauvages adopted a botanical technique for classifying disease, and both rejected the mechanistic physiology of the earlier part of the century. It is tentatively suggested that these two actions are related, the connection being the animism discussed earlier in the chapter.

Finally, some attempt must be made to fulfil the promise made at the beginning of the chapter that it would end with the disappearance of God from medicine. We have seen how the passionate, personal experience of God of the practitioners of Enthusiastic religion contrasted strongly with (and ultimately vanished before) the reasoned and moderate beliefs of the enlightened. Natural Law, Natural Religion, Natural Theology, the true heirs of the position held in education by Aristotle, all in their different ways restricted the ways in which God was seen to act in eighteenth-century man's perception of the natural world. By the end of the century the process in some circles – scientific circles – was complete, and an increasingly de-christianised Natural Philosophy had become a godless science.

5

Sauvages's nosology medical englightenment in Montpellier

JULIAN MARTIN

INTRODUCTION

François Boissier de Sauvages (1706–67), the celebrated Montpellier medical professor, is commonly remembered by historians of medicine for his attempts to classify diseases ('nosology') and for espousing a 'vitalist' approach to the understanding of the human body. He is remembered both as a principal medical exponent of Linnaean enthusiasms for classificatory schemes and as part of a continental tradition of medical philosophy which rejected strictly mechanical explanations of the animal oeconomy.[1] I wish to suggest that this characterisation is an unsatisfactory one: Boissier de Sauvages was not the man the historiography of medical ideas has led us to expect. Sauvages's 'nosology' did not stem from Linnaeus and he is not well described as a 'vitalist'. On the contrary, Sauvages's medical researches display his idiosyncratic amalgam of Baconian reform, botanical method and Newtonian 'mathematical physick'. Moreover, when Sauvages used the term 'nosology', he was describing not simply his classification of diseases but the entirety of his medical reform programme. I propose, therefore, first to discuss the local origin of this unlooked-for mixture of philosophical allegiances, and then to describe Sauvages's programme for the classification of diseases and his devotion to Newtonian natural philosophy.

Acknowledgement: I wish to express my thanks to Andrew Cunningham: his advice and attentions have proved invaluable.

[1] See, for example, Lester S. King, *The Medical World of the Eighteenth Century* (Huntington, 1958) and 'Boissier de Sauvages and Eighteenth-Century Nosology', *Bulletin of the History of Medicine* 40 (1966), pp. 43–51; E. Haigh, 'The Roots of the Vitalism of Xavier Bichat', *Bulletin of the History of Medicine* 49 (1975), pp. 72–86.

A MEDICAL STUDENT AT MONTPELLIER

François Boissier de Sauvages was the sixth son of a Languedoc seigneur of small means but ancient lineage. His father, a Captain of the Regiment of Flanders, was determined that François would pursue a profession and he pushed his son to excel in his studies at the local school in Alès. In 1722, at the age of sixteen, François matriculated in the University of Medicine of Montpellier. Why Sauvages père (or fils) decided upon medicine in particular we do not know, yet, given their reduced circumstances, a career in medicine was a reasonable choice.[2]

Montpellier was famed as a great medical school from the later middle ages onwards, and a complex medical community existed in and around the city and the university. Next to the royal administration of Languedoc, medicine was the principal service industry in Montpellier: professors, private physicians, surgeons, apothecaries, apprentices, university students, hospitals and the sick had been a constant feature in the city for centuries. When Sauvages arrived in 1722, the university could boast an impressive panoply of physician-professors, large medical libraries and a dozen senior medical teaching posts. The medical school had wealth, fine buildings, international prestige and a long tradition of royal favour and patronage.[3]

During the early eighteenth century, there was no unanimity of medical opinion or philosophy in Montpellier's medical faculty. In addition to those who accepted the usual *practice* of medicine, that is to say, the traditional 'Galenic' medicine taught in early modern universities, Montpellier also had men keen to espouse more recent medical doctrines. The sweeping reformation of the science of medicine proposed initially by Francis Bacon and then (in differing ways) by Thomas Sydenham and Giorgio Baglivi had advocates at Montpellier. So too did Cartesian mechanical medicine and even the latest vogue – the 'mathematical physick' of Archibald Pitcairne, James Keill and the

[2] See 'Sauvages', *Biographie Universelle (Michaud) ancienne et moderne*, vol. 38 (Paris, 1865); E-H. de Ratte, *Eloge de M. De Sauvages* (Montpellier, 1770); and L. W. B. Brockliss, *French Higher Education in the Seventeenth and Eighteenth Centuries: A Cultural History* (Oxford, 1987), especially chapter 8.

[3] See Louis Dulieu, 'Mouvement scientifique Montepellierain du XVIIIè siecle', *Revue d'Histoire des Sciences* 11 (1958), pp. 230–49, *La Chirurgie à Montpellier de ses origines au début du XIX siècle* (Avignon, 1975), *La Médecine à Montpellier: La Renaissance* (Avignon, 1979) and *La Médecine à Montpellier: L'époque classique. Première partie* (Avignon, 1983); and Colin Jones, 'Montpellier Medical Students and the Medicalisation of Eighteenth-Century France' in R. Porter and A. Wear (eds.), *Problems and Methods in the History of Medicine* (London, 1987), pp. 57–80.

London Royal College of Physicians.[4] Sauvages gravitated toward the most famous and well-established professors at Montpellier, Antoine Deidier, François Chicoyneau and Pierre Chirac, and during the four years he spent under their tutelage, he assimilated much of their individual passions and interests into his own outlook and expectations.

Sauvages found great encouragement for his youthful love of mathematics from Deidier, the Professor of Chemistry, an early French follower of Isaac Newton's natural philosophy. Deidier (d. 1746) had been elected a Fellow of the Royal Society of London in 1722, and he believed that Newton had shown that the Creator had made the world in number, weight and measure and that mathematics was the language of Nature. Archibald Pitcairne had carried Newton's reasoning into medicine, successfully showing physicians that the human body contained an intricate series of fluids and conduits that could be understood by application of Newton's hydraulics. Deidier impressed the truth of this upon his pupils by means of repeated demonstration in his experiments upon animals. Through the study of the mathematical principles of mechanical action (especially the hydraulics of Newton's *Principia Mathematica*), Deidier believed that the physician, like the astronomer, could come to know the truth of the nature of things. The 'ingenious' physical speculations and 'hypotheses' of the Cartesians, the chemical philosophies of the German physicians and the *humours* of traditionalist physicians were, for Deidier, crude and futile attempts to explain the causes of the animal oeconomy, which now were truly revealed by what the English called 'mathematical physick'.[5]

François Chicoyneau (1672–1752), the hereditary Chancellor of the University and the Professor of Anatomy and Botany, was fascinated by the study of botany and materia medica.[6] His special joy was the Royal Gardens at Montpellier, which had been reorganised when Chicoyneau was young by the great Montpellier botanists, Pierre Magnol (1638–1715) and his pupil Joseph Tournefort (1656–1708). Chicoyneau's enthusiasm for botany and his conviction of its impor-

[4] See T. M. Brown, *The Mechanical Philosophy and the Animal Oeconomy* (New York, 1981); Andrew Cunningham, 'Sydenham Versus Newton: The Edinburgh Fever Dispute of the 1690s Between Andrew Brown and Archibald Pitcairne', *Medical History*, Supplement no. 1 (1981), pp. 71–98; and R. J. J. Martin, 'Explaining John Freind's *History of Physick*', *Studies in History and Philosophy of Science* 19 (1988), pp. 399–418.

[5] See 'Deidier', *Biographie Universelle*, vol. 10 (1852); R. Williamson, 'The Plague of Marseilles and the Experiments of Professor Anton Deidier', *Medical History* 2 (1958), pp. 237–59.

[6] See Dulieu, 'Mouvement scientifique Montepellierain', and *La Chirurgie à Montpellier*.

tance for physicians rubbed off on young Sauvages. As a young doctor, he would need to learn a great deal about the identification of plants, and about their medicinal parts, properties, limitations and preparation. Yet the Montpellier Royal Gardens offered more than a collection of the plants a physician would need to recognise: the very arrangement established there was designed to mirror that in the natural world. Chicoyneau believed that the naming of the plants and their arrangement in the garden displayed the order, structure and relation which God had created in the plants.

The third Montpellier physician who deeply impressed young Sauvages was Pierre Chirac (1650–1732), who felt he had a mission to reform the art of medicine and had a method for doing so.[7] Chirac wished to make medicine the equal of other disciplines of natural philosophy which he believed had undergone great advancement in recent decades. Compared with mathematics, chemistry, astronomy and physics, Chirac believed medicine lacked solid philosophical foundations. He despaired of doctors' wranglings over theories and of the inconsistencies of their attempts to heal the sick. Chirac demanded that doctors emulate the wisdom of Hippocrates (i.e. the Hippocrates of *Epidemics*, and *Airs*, *Waters*, *and Places*) and *observe* the sick. He wanted patient, cautious and meticulous observations rather than a rush to dogmatic positions about *causes* after minimum reflection upon particulars (as he considered the Cartesians and the German chemical physicians to do). If medicine was to be reformed and advanced, then physicians must return to the ways of the ancient Hippocratic 'school' and eschew the idle speculations of partially informed hypothesisers. Chirac was engaged in an ancient argument here, but he also sought to follow the advice of Francis Bacon, which (as we shall see) had been repeated more recently by Giorgio Baglivi (1668–1707), and to establish a grand information-gathering network among physicians, who would pool their observations of the sick and the therapies they employed in order that a body of tried and true remedies could be established.

There is no reason to think that Sauvages would have had any difficulty in accepting the teachings of these three professors simultaneously. Botany and mathematics were searches for order, structure, classification and regularities, and similarly, the Newtonian medicine and chemistry of Pitcairne, Keill and John Freind was directed toward revealing the laws and order of the natural world. If the world was

[7] See 'Chirac', *Biographie Universelle*, vol. 8 (1844).

created by God in number, weight and measure, it was also built in order, structure and relation. Chirac's Baconian demand for reform of the art of medicine was capable of being construed as a comparable plan for order, measured precision and immutable laws to replace ingenious personal speculations about medical practice and 'the animal oeconomy'.

BAGLIVI'S DE PRAXI MEDICA

While a student, Sauvages read Giorgio Baglivi's *De Praxi Medica* (1696). Whether it was Deidier, Chicoyneau or Chirac who introduced him to the book, we do not know, but it was a revelation for young Sauvages. Baglivi's call for a sweeping medical reform galvanised Sauvages into action. Yet Sauvages could not have been so deeply moved by Baglivi's text if he had not recognised so much of himself in it. Sauvages was being trained in Montpellier in such a way that Baglivi seemed to have been articulating his own beliefs; without being 'primed', it is unlikely that Sauvages would have been fired by Baglivi's words.

In *De Praxi Medica*, having bewailed the present state of medical theory and knowledge, and having dismissed the hypothesising of the Galenists, the chemists and the Cartesian mechanists, Baglivi declared that the truths about the natural world were to be uncovered through mathematics, and by mathematical inquiries we would come to know the workings of the body

> since the human body in its structure, and equally in the effects depending on this structure, operates by number, weight and measure; it operates thus by the wish of God, the highest Creator of all things, who, so that the framework of the human body should be accommodated more suitably to the capacity of the mind, seems to have sketched the most ordered series of proportions and motions in the human body by the pen of Mathematics alone.[8]

Yet Baglivi had not written his book merely to state his allegiance to mathematical natural philosophy and to condemn the present state of the art. He was convinced that he had a positive contribution to offer toward the advancement of medicine, not in its theoretical sphere (Newton and Pitcairne, he declared, were showing physicians how to proceed here) but in its practical application, that is, in the advance-

[8] *De Praxi Medica ad Priscam Observandi Rationem Revocanda* (Lyon, 1699 edn), I, vi, 2, p. 29. Baglivi, a pupil and assistant of Malpighi, was Professor of Anatomy at Rome from 1696 and a Fellow of the Royal Society of London from 1697. A very free anonymous translation of *De Praxi Medica* appeared as *The Practice of Physick* (London, 1704). Translations from Latin in this chapter are mine.

ment of knowledge about the actual practice of curing the sick. For Baglivi such a reformation would take place in two stages: the first, which he called *medicina prima*, involved the creation of 'Histories of Diseases', and the second stage, the *medicina secunda*, was actual 'Methods of Cure' of particular diseases. Most of *De Praxi Medica* was devoted to a discussion of *medicina prima*, which Baglivi considered to be the necessary foundation of a reform of 'Methods of Cure':

The history of diseases is a science *sui generis*, nor does it derive its principles and its augmentation from anywhere else but from the most wholesome and purest fountains of nature alone ... Or, to speak more plainly, the entire history of diseases depends on a diligent and patient description of those things which the learned Observer has recorded concerning the invasion, progress and exit of diseases; and that which he has observed, he will set forth plainly in his pages, adding nothing from his own opinions, nothing from the precepts of books or of other sciences.[9]

The grand plan for constructing 'Histories of Diseases' was something which Baglivi had found in the works of Francis Bacon. Bacon had claimed that the creation of 'Histories' was the essential and fundamental stage in the advancement of any science.[10] By the term 'Histories', Bacon was referring to the collection of a mass of careful observations of things, both as they are, and through active experimentation upon them. This data would then be collated with comparable information from other investigators and scrutinised until a body of particular 'instances' free of falsities and dubiousness was ready for a process Bacon called *Induction*, which would produce insightful knowledge about the principles of Nature. In *De Praxi Medica*, Baglivi offered explicit directions for the development of a History of Diseases which were faithful in most respects to the methodological demands of Bacon's *Novum Organum* (1620) and *De Augmentis Scientiarum* (1623):

In making a history of any disease, four things are most especially necessary: firstly, the infinite acquisition of particular observations. Secondly, an arrangement of them. Thirdly, their maturation and consideration. Fourthly, at last, the extraction from them of precepts and general axioms.[11]

In the first place, if one was to acquire 'particular observations', one could not turn to books for them; it required personal active inquiry:

[9] *De Praxi Medica*, I, v, 4, p. 22.

[10] See *Instauratio Magna* (London, 1620), especially *Parasceve ad Historiam Naturalam et Experimentalem*, in R. L. Ellis, J. Spedding and D. D. Heath (eds.), *The Works of Francis Bacon* (London, 1858), vol. 1, pp. 393–411; and my '"Knowledge is Power": Francis Bacon, the State and the Reform of Natural Philosophy', unpublished Ph.D. thesis (Cambridge, 1988), chapter 5.

[11] *De Praxi Medica*, II, iii, 2, p. 174.

> Therefore, since the assistance of books contributes little to the perfect and stable history of diseases which is to be worked out in medicine, it is necessary to pass to those things which inhere more closely to nature, viz., experiments, observations, dissections of dead bodies, gardens of simples, chemical furnaces, whatever things by variously observing, by separating and torturing nature, open up for us true notions of nature.[12]

Record every observation made, instructed Baglivi (echoing Bacon), and act like a magistrate: make judgements upon the information extracted from the 'witnesses' rather than be swayed by fine theories and pleadings. Although the study of particulars is 'perplexed by fallacious similitude of things and signs, entanglements of causes and an ambiguity of ways', the careful historian of diseases could rest assured that all the particulars he compiled were either 'antecedents, concomitants or consequents of the disease'.[13]

Baglivi proposed that the particulars be arranged under headings that were at once formal and traditional: diagnostics, prognostics, various sorts of causes (but not Aristotle's formal, material or final causes), the non-naturals (diet, exercise, air, sleeping and watching, repletion and inanition, the passions of the mind), the seasons of the year, the symptoms (constant and inconstant), the remedies used (successful or not) and the outcomes (happy or fatal). Within these categories, which he called 'Articles of Inquisition', Baglivi expected to locate all the 'antecedents, concomitants and consequents of the disease'.

The third stage of the construction of a History was one of 'mature digestions', making 'an orderly and digested body of those particulars which formerly lay straggling and unparcelled', culling out falsehoods and making qualifications. This work prepared all the materials of observation for the final stage: the arrival at 'general precepts', or 'Aphorisms'. 'Aphorisms', said Baglivi, 'are like indicators of a royal road . . . [they are] secure and stable in overcoming difficult cures of diseases.'[14]

Up to this point, Baglivi was faithfully following Francis Bacon but now, in the details of proceeding to 'general precepts', he differed significantly. Speaking for his 'Interpreter of Nature', Bacon had stressed

> then, and only then, may we hope well of the sciences, when in a just scale of ascent, and by successive steps not interrupted or broken, we rise from particulars to lesser axioms, and then to middle axioms, one above the other; and last of all to the most general.[15]

[12] *De Praxi Medica*, I, vi, 9, p. 42. [13] *Ibid.*, II, iii, 5, p. 180. [14] *Ibid.*, II, iii, 6, p. 180.
[15] *Novum Organum*, I, Aphorism 104: in *Works*, vol. I, p. 205.

Baglivi, however, argued

After the Observer has exercised himself sufficiently (and more) in the abounding forest of observations, and has truly learnt the Alphabet of the nature of diseases, he ought not to fly to the most general things in a compendious and precipitate way (impassable to nature and liable to disputes), but he ought to reach them gradually and in succession, by ascending and descending, by penetrating sufficiently into the mass of particulars, and afterwards *deduce* from them middling propositions and axioms.[16]

In other words, Baglivi was proposing a not wholly Baconian method for the final construction of a History.

Sauvages was unaware of, or untroubled by, Baglivi's signal deviation from Bacon over 'induction', and he pounced upon other remarks Baglivi made about the method for classifying and for the construction of 'middling terms'; in particular this passage:

Certainly we justifiably place this among the great *desiderata* of our Art: that every individual disease should be subdivided into as many species as there are primary diseases by which they are fostered or violent and constant causes by which they are produced; and that the characteristic signs of each species should be set forth with the primary history of each species, and a suitable and stable method of cure for each, for this reason especially, that we see this done by the botanists, who under the general name of any plant, for instance, the Thistle, comprehend many species of thistles; and are so sedulous in describing the magnitude, figure, colour, taste, and other accidents of the plant, by which they may distinguish one species of thistle from another.[17]

This passage is from Baglivi's chapter entitled 'Preliminaries Calculated for the History and Division of Causes of Diseases', and *Causes*, Baglivi had declared, were one of the 'Articles of Inquisition', i.e., a category of consideration during the second stage of the construction of a History. Yet Sauvages immediately took Baglivi's remarks here to be applicable to the method of arranging a History of Diseases as a whole. And why not? What Baglivi had said seemed to fit admirably with the method of the botanists, as Sauvages understood it.

THE BOTANISTS' METHOD: TOURNEFORT

When Sauvages was a student at Montpellier, the study of botany was dominated by the work and principles of the university's great botanist, Joseph Tournefort (1658–1708). Stung by criticism from the English botanist, John Ray, Tournefort had written several defences of the validity and pre-eminence of his method of classifying plants. His method was the most sensible one, he declared; that is to say, it was the

[16] *De Praxi Medica*, II, iii, 6, pp. 180–1. My emphasis.
[17] *De Praxi Medica*, II, ix, 3, pp. 223–4.

one accepted by the best botanists of recent centuries.[18] In his *Elémens de Botanique, ou méthode pour connoître les plantes* (Paris, 1694), Tournefort proclaimed:

It is absolutely necessary, in this science, to gather into groups those plants which resemble one another, and to separate them from those which they do not resemble. This likeness ought to be drawn solely from their immediate signs of relationship, that is to say, from the structure of some one of their parts, and one ought not to pay attention to remote relationships that can be found between certain plants, such as the similarities of [medicinal] virtues which they have, or the places where they grow.[19]

This classifying, or gathering of resemblances, was not only a true and natural classing of living things, but it verged on a religious duty for the conscientious natural philosopher:

The Author of Nature, who has allowed us the liberty of giving the names we please to the genera of plants, has impressed a common character on each of their species, which must serve to guide us in ranging them in their natural places.[20]

Each species of plant, then, has invariable signs by which we are to recognise it for what it is, and (just as Adam did) we can thereby distinguish and name the species. Such distinctions lie not in our imaginations but are truly in the species themselves. For Tournefort (echoing Aristotle and Theophrastus), the invariable characteristic, the 'essential character', was the fruit and flowers of the plant. Because the final cause or purpose of the plant is to reproduce itself, its essential nature is best evidenced in its reproductive parts. Other considerations are not to be ignored, yet they can never supplant the essential sign in making classifications. Under the weight of the attacks of John Ray, who (with his friend John Locke) rejected the use of a principal sign on the grounds that any such key was unknowable by men, Tournefort agreed that

when the flower and fruit are not sufficient for the correct distinguishing of genera, then not only should all the other parts of the plants be called upon for aid, but also their abnormalities (*affectiones*), mode of growing, physical character and external appearance.[21]

This is a far cry from conceding epistemological ground to Ray, but Tournefort agreed that if the preferred indicator was deemed insuffi-

[18] See P. R. Sloan, 'John Locke, John Ray, and the Problem of the Natural System', *Journal of the History of Biology* 5 (1972), pp. 1–53.

[19] J. Tournefort, *Elémens* (Lyon, 1797 edn), vol. 1, p. 60; my translation. [20] *Ibid.*, p. 70.

[21] Tournefort, *Institutiones Rei Herbariae. Editio Altera* (Paris, 1700), vol. 1, p. 61. And see his *De Optima Methodo Instituenda in Re Herbaria . . . Epistola. In qua Respondatur Dissertationi D. Raii de Variis Plantarum Methodis* (Paris, 1697).

cient in itself, then a consideration of *everything* else could substitute for the key indication.

Not only was Tournefort engaged in the work of distinguishing species from species, but he was also making more complex classifications. In classical logic, it was a commonplace to group species further into genera and then into higher, more inclusive genera. Although faithful to this procedure, Tournefort was the first botanist to name these higher groupings not *genera* but *sectiones* and *classes*. Eventually, he distributed 10,146 *species* of plants into 698 *genera*, these into 107 *sectiones* and these into 22 *classes*. So, 'naming' the plants required not only the ability to see the characteristic sign of a species which God had put in the plants, but also a careful attention to the rules of logic. To arrange the species of plants into genera and then into higher categories did *not* involve a speculative arrangement of the true and natural groupings (the species). Because they were based squarely upon God's given indicator, the fruits and flowers, the botanist's labours would produce nothing artificial; the result would be a revelation of the structure, order and relation hidden within the world of the plants.

'NOUVELLES CLASSES DES MALADIES'

Boissier de Sauvages published his first book at the age of twenty-four. It was the first fruit of his decision to follow Baglivi (and Chirac and Chicoyneau) towards a reformation of medicine. *Nouvelles Classes des des Maladies dans un Ordre à celui des Botanistes, comprenant les Genres et les Espèces de toutes les Maladies, avec leurs signes & leurs indications* (Avignon, 1731) was 450 pages in small type, representing several years of hard work dedicated to creating a History of Diseases and furthering a reformation of the art of medicine:

> si l'on a jamais eu besoin d'étudier l'Histoire des Maladies, c'est aujourd'hui que cette étude est devenue necessaire; la fureur des systemes qui flâtent tant l'imagination, ayant fait presque oublier l'étude de la nature & negliger la connoissance des Maladies.[22]

Sauvages was aware that his book represented a new departure for medicine. Not only was he actually preparing a History of Diseases, as Baglivi had called for, but he was the first physician to adapt the botanists' classification scheme to a programme for creating such a History.

Nouvelles Classes has a formal structure that belies the passion with

[22] *Nouvelles Classes*, p. 3; I quote accents and spelling throughout as in the original.

which it was written. It opened conventionally enough with a dedication, an introductory essay of some twenty pages, a table displaying the *Classes of Diseases*, a reproduced letter to Herman Boerhaave (the celebrated Leyden Professor of Medicine) with Boerhaave's brief reply to Sauvages, wishing him good fortune. The 400-odd pages which follow describe some 2,400 *Species* of diseases, in rigid accord with the classificatory structure (*Classes*, *Sectiones*, *Genera* and *Species*) which Sauvages had adopted from Tournefort.

Each *Class* of diseases was introduced with a short general description of the Class itself – the constant visible symptoms shared by the *Species* of diseases found here, and their shared key characteristics – and in some of these Class headnotes Sauvages offered a description of the causes of these species of diseases, again in broad terms. A heading *Sectio 1* then followed, and after a general description of the species of diseases grouped here and their key characteristic, came a discussion of each *Genus* of diseases which were gathered under this *Sectio*, in much the same format, one after another. With each *Genus* of disease he listed, Sauvages gave a summary of its constant visible symptoms, sometimes gave cautions against confusing it with another, seemingly similar, *Genus*, and occasionally provided a recommendation about treatment. Below this statement were listed all the species of disease he knew about and deemed appropriate to group here. After this followed *Sectio 2* with the same format and so on throughout the book; we can illustrate this with a chart.

Class I Morbes Febriles
(general discussion pp. 33–44)
Sectio I Febres Intermittentes
(general discussion pp. 34–6)
Genus 1 'Quotidiana'
(general discussion pp. 36–7)
Species pp. 37–9
– Q. Regularis simplex. Sydenham
– Q. subintrans. Gabelkofer
– Q. duplex. Sennert.
– Q. triplex. Primirosii
– etc.
Genus 2 'Tertiana'
(general discussion pp. 39–40)
Species pp. 40–44
Etc.

Within this structure Sauvages distributed all 2,400 species of diseases, provided 'slots' thereby for the placement of any he would find later, and made claims about the relationships (or lack of them) that existed between species of diseases. Sauvages's book is a 'work in progress', a 'snap-shot' of his research to date, and he made the provisional status of the scheme perfectly clear in his introductory essay. Yet however provisional *Nouvelles Classes* was in its structure and fine details, Sauvages had set out for himself a huge research programme, with its own internal logic, methods and problems to be solved. By unravelling some of the discrepancies that exist in the text as printed in 1731, we can see how Sauvages had chosen to work on his research project and see as well how his classificatory plans had continued to change.

Sauvages took it for granted that Tournefort's principles of classifying were the ones to employ in the construction of the Histories of Diseases Baglivi had called for in *De Praxi Medica*. Sauvages knew he would need a characteristic sign of the species of diseases in order to follow the botanical method and here Baglivi provided the clue.

'For every disease there is not a fictitious, but a certain and peculiar nature', wrote Baglivi, and it has 'constant natural qualities [*passiones*], as the characteristic signs of diseases may be called'. These 'constant natural qualities' were 'sometimes manifest and obvious to our senses, and sometimes obscure', and thus Baglivi was all the more insistent upon the collection of every particular observation.[23] Sauvages, however, concluded that the visible signs of diseases were sufficient to allow him to begin classifying as the great botanists did. In other words, he regarded the visible signs (or 'visible symptoms') of a disease to be, for taxonomic purposes, equivalent to the (obviously visible) 'fruit and flowers' used by the botanists.

Baglivi had spoken repeatedly of *species* of diseases, and regarded them as the fundamental unit the historian would work with. In using this terminology, Baglivi was accepting, or so he thought, the opinion of Thomas Sydenham, 'the embellisher and ornament of our profession', that such entities as *species* of diseases actually existed. Sydenham (1624–89) had been making the point that diseases were indeed entities in their own right – 'specific entities' – and had argued against the opinion prevalent among his own contemporaries that each disease was a condition individual to each patient and therefore requiring an individualised treatment.[24] But because Sydenham and Baglivi spoke of *species* of diseases and praised at the same time the botanists' method of classifying, Sauvages concluded that there were

[23] *De Praxi Medica*, I, ii, 3, p. 7 and I, ii, 9, p. 10.

[24] See Andrew Cunningham, 'Thomas Sydenham: Epidemics, Experiment, and the "Good Old Cause"' in Roger French and Andrew Wear (eds.), *The Medical Revolution of the Seventeenth Century* (Cambridge, 1989), pp. 164–90.

species of diseases like species of plants and that he should inquire about them and classify them as the botanists did.

Thus any patient whom Sauvages observed would provide him with a series of constant symptoms, and by gathering these he could provide himself with a check-list of the characteristic signs of a species of disease. For example, Sauvages described the constant symptoms of the species he entitled *Cynanche vera simplex antiquarum Bonet* to be: a swelling of the tonsils, a pain in the throat, a chill followed by heating, a desire to vomit and a 'continual fever' for as much as one or two weeks. Yet, as his name for this species suggests, Sauvages did more: he also consulted medical books and extracted symptoms from the case-histories they contained. Baglivi had expressly forbidden this approach, and had called for years of careful observation of patients. Young Sauvages saw no reason to wait so long.

Sauvages spent the 1720s labouring to coordinate suites of constant symptoms into species of diseases, using both his own observations and those in medical books. Yet it would not have taken him long before he was confronted with another problem: how was he to organise the species he was gradually uncovering among all the symptoms of diseases? Clearly, according to Baglivi's prescriptions for making a History, he had to begin making 'general axioms' and 'middle propositions', that is, to begin making higher categories upon the mass of information he was collecting. And, as Tournefort had done in botany (but no physician had yet contemplated doing), Sauvages decided to build his 'middling propositions' and 'general axioms' in the form of *Classes*, *Sectiones* and *Genera* raised upon his *species* of diseases. The result was that Sauvages's History of Diseases was both a compilation (following Baglivi's plan) and a classification based on the *essences* of diseases (following Tournefort's method).

Sauvages accepted Baglivi's advice 'to keep the ancient division into Acute and Chronical': here was the principle upon which he made his first division of the species of diseases. He took Acute, conventionally enough, to refer to diseases which were likely to be very dangerous and perhaps fatal, and he took Chronical to encompass all those which appeared to be a constant but not fatal condition. Examining his two very large groups of species of diseases, Sauvages believed that he could see differences among the species in the group 'Acute' and differences among those in the group 'Chronical'. He decided the group Acute fell into four different sorts of species of diseases, and a similar number could be found in the group Chronical. This division involved judgements about key differences between species of diseases: which symptom from among the suite of constant symptoms that constituted a species was to become the telling indicator when comparisons between species were made?

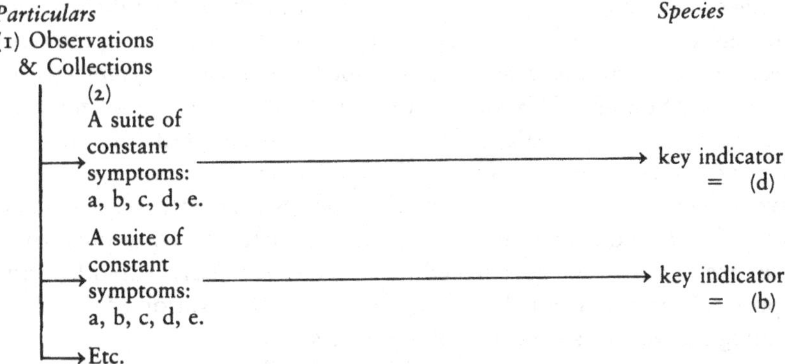

For example, Sauvages decided that Acute diseases comprised four groups he called 'Fevers', 'Inflammations', 'Evacuations' and 'Paralyses'. 'Inflammations' all had a fever associated with them but Sauvages justified their distinction from 'Fevers' on the ground that the fever here was less 'essential', less 'primitive', than the inflammation itself. This presupposes that Sauvages had apportioned priority to a certain one of the constant signs; he then was able, in Baglivi's terminology, to rise to 'general axioms'. This helps explain why Sauvages entitled his book not 'Nouvelles Espèces' but 'Nouvelles *Classes*'.

After finding eight Classes of diseases in this manner, Sauvages began to look at the species of diseases *within* a particular Class: what was there about these species that could distinguish them into smaller groupings? When Sauvages had uncovered an answer to this question, he could separate the species into *Sectiones*. He then repeated the procedure with each smaller grouping of species, the *Sectio*: what was there here that could distinguish them into smaller groups? The answer would provide the criterion by which *Genera* were discovered among the species of a *Sectio*.

The final, formal arrangement of this long process of sifting and checking, of induction then deduction, on to a continuous series of printed pages foists an illusion upon the reader of *Nouvelles Classes*. The illusion is that Sauvages proceeded from constant symptoms to Species and then to *Genera*, to *Sectiones*, and finally to *Classes*: that is, in a continuing series, as Francis Bacon had demanded a History be devised. But Sauvages actually worked from constant symptoms to

Species, and then to *Classes*, and from these to *Sectiones* and finally to *Genera*: that is, as Baglivi had suggested a History should be devised. Subsequent to the real work, Sauvages had arranged his results in a logical subordination for his presentation of them. The differing methods can be illustrated in a chart:

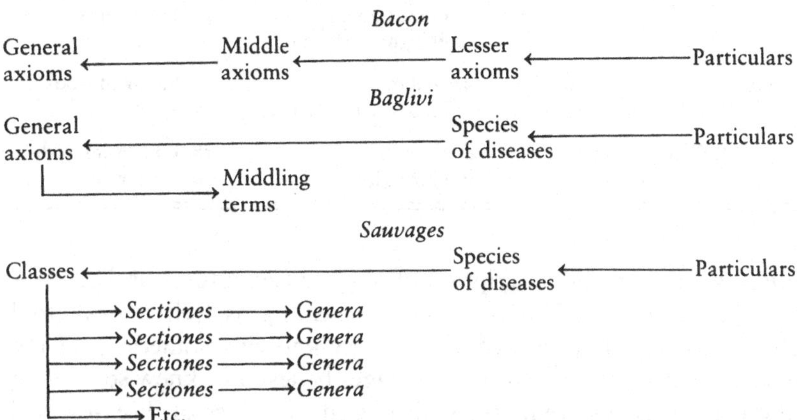

After constructing his classification, Sauvages began a process of critical re-examination of his History. Some *Sectiones* contained far too many species (and therefore too many *Genera*); some *Genera* were in *Classes* where they seemed upon reflection to be problematical. He reviewed the criteria he had employed for various divisions of species in the hopes that certain anomalies could be resolved in this manner. His efforts at this stage are illustrated by the tentative intrusions he introduced into the second *Sectio* of the Class 'Evacuations' (see table 5).

These three new divisions, which were not part of the formal *Classes–Sectiones–Genera–Species* arrangement, were late interpolations into the introductory tables of *Nouvelles Classes*: they are not reflected in the text itself. We find in this, and in other such discrepancies, confirmation for Sauvages's claims about the unfinished state of his researches. Nonetheless, *Nouvelles Classes des Maladies* illustrated not only the current state of Sauvages's inquiries but the principles and methods with which he was operating.

Sauvages did not mind presenting an unfinished work; he believed he already had made a large step toward fulfilling the hopes of Baglivi and Chirac for a refounding of knowledge of diseases upon a sure base of 'Histories of Diseases'. Yet Sauvages was not only presenting a

Table 5. *Morbi evacuatoria*

Sectio 2: Evacuatoria albi vel limpidi

Genus:		
1. Cathorhosi	8. Epiphora 9. Fluxus-aurius 10. Phlegmatorhagia	11. Coryza 12. Ptyalismus
2. Serosi	13. Diabetes 14. Incontinentia urinae	15. Sudor-morbosos
3. Lactei, Chilosi, Purulentia	16. Vomica 17. Fluor-albus	18. Lochia-immodica 19. Gonorhaea

History – the careful description of observed symptoms of diseases – but, following Tournefort, he was presenting as well the essential characteristics of species of diseases. By knowing something of the essence of a species of disease, Sauvages believed he knew something about its *cause* as well, and with regard to causes of diseases, had embarked upon his researches already full of Newtonian presuppositions about the working of the body.

In the headnotes to each of the Classes of diseases, Sauvages listed not only the essential common symptoms of all the species in this particular Class, but their (hydraulic) common cause. Common to them all, then, was a certain form of curing. For example, in all the species grouped under Inflammations, there was a vast local increase in the amount of blood; they all shared at least one common line of cure: a bleeding. So, Sauvages was able to see himself as engaged not only in fulfilling Baglivi's call for a *medicina prima* (Histories of Diseases) but also in promoting a *medicina secunda* (Methods of Cure).

Nouvelles Classes des Maladies greatly pleased Sauvages's former teachers at Montpellier. In the autumn of 1731, he was elected into the Société Royale des Sciences de Montpellier and in 1734, he was appointed Professor of Medicine at the University. Judging from the stream of treatises and essays which he wrote after being given his chair, Sauvages was an energetic scholar with a wide range of research interests, but he continued to work steadily on his first research project.[25] In 1739, 1752, 1759 and 1763, he published the results of his

[25] A listing of his works can be found in L. Dulieu, 'François Boissier de Sauvages', *Revue d'Histoire des Sciences* 22 (1969), pp. 303–22.

re-examinations of the classificatory scheme employed in *Nouvelles Classes*. He regarded the project as a cumulative programme: each version which he published represented some alterations on the one it superseded. Every version of his classificatory scheme represented for him an increment in the advancement of the art of medicine. *Nouvelles Classes*, nevertheless, was arguably Sauvages's most impressive achievement: his arrangements of diseases were, after all, '*nouvelles* classes'. No one before him had classified diseases in this manner and here he had devised all the classifications which he employed in later research. His subsequent works on the Histories of Diseases were logical extensions of his initial labours. In them, he expanded the number of species of diseases, refined his descriptions of earlier ones, and puzzled over the criteria for division and distribution he had used in *Nouvelles Classes des Maladies*.

Sauvages's most celebrated work was the five-volume *Nosologia Methodica* of 1763. Since 1731, when Sauvages had written *Nouvelles Classes* in unpolished Languedoc French, European natural philosophers had been taken as by storm by the classificatory enthusiasms of Carl Linnaeus. Investigation has shown the debt Linnaeus owed to Sauvages's *Nouvelles Classes*,[26] but contemporary readers had eyes only for Linnaeus's *Genera Morborum* (1735) and his later works. When Sauvages published *Nosologia Methodica*, classification had become all the rage and his book benefited from it, going through many editions and vernacular translations before the end of the century, yet the enterprise of classifying diseases (among so many other things) was by this time associated indelibly with Linnaeus. Not surprisingly, Sauvages's youthful book was largely forgotten, but his *Nosologia Methodica* displayed little alteration from the conclusions he had arrived upon in 1731. This can be illustrated most conveniently in a table (see table 6).

The most important change in the organisation of the Classes of diseases since 1731 had occurred in 1763 in the Class 'Paralytiques'. Here Sauvages adopted new criteria for the division of the species of diseases within this Class. In 1731, Sauvages had declared 'la paralisie est un privation [*sic*] du sentiment & du mouvement ou de l'un des deux', and accordingly he distributed the species into three *Sectiones*: 'Universelles, ou soporeuses'; 'particuliares organes du mouvement'; and 'particuliares organes de sens de nature'. In 1763, he employed five

[26] F. Berg, 'Linné et Sauvages: Les rapports entre leurs systèmes nosologiques', *Lychnos* 16 (1956), pp. 31–54.

Table 6. *Classificatory changes within a class of diseases*

1731(1)	1731(2)	1739	1752	1759	1763
Fievres	—	—	—	—	—
Inflammations	—	—	—	—	—
Evacuations	—	—	d	—	—
Paralytiques	—	—	b	—	h
Douloureuses	—	f	—	—	—
Spirituelles	b	—	a	—	b
Cachetiques	b	—	a	c	—
Convulsives	c	e & g	—	c & f	—

1731 (1) = the actual text of *Nouvelles Classes* (1731)
1731 (2) = the chart prefaced to the text
1739 = *Pathologia Methodica* (Montpellier, 1739)
1752 = *Pathologia Methodica* (Amsterdam, 1752)
1759 = *Pathologia Methodica* (Amsterdam & Lyon, 1759)
1763 = *Nosologia Methodica* (Amsterdam, 1763)
(—) = no alteration on previous text
(a) = a return to 1731 (1)
(b) = a *Sectio* split into 2 *Sectiones*
(c) = 2 *Sectiones* split into 4
(d) = 2 *Sectiones* combined into 1
(e) = 5 *Sectiones* combined into 2
(f) = an existing *Sectio* dropped
(g) = a new *Sectio* added
(h) = a major rearrangement involving new criteria for division of a Class.

Sectiones, and the criteria of division were more complex. Sauvages chose to distinguish the species of diseases in this Class in accordance with his beliefs about 'forces', 'facultés', 'mouvements libres & des mouvements vitaux'; that is, in accord with his beliefs about the nature of the human body in general and not solely on the basis of visible characteristics of diseases. This might be taken as indicating Sauvages's 'vitalism', yet there is another explanation: Newtonian natural philosophy.

NEWTONIAN NATURAL PHILOSOPHY

It is true that, like those eighteenth-century physicians described as 'vitalists', Sauvages had always been resolutely opposed to Cartesian physicians. The opening sentence of *Nouvelles Classes* was a direct attack upon them and their 'fictions, systemes, hypotheses, des idees chimeriques & des jargons inconnus'. Thirty years later, Sauvages continued to attack the 'Mechanical Sect':

> The principles established by the mechanists are so far removed from the true principles of mechanics, they are so erroneous, that none of them seems fit to be preferred to the principles of the ancient Galenists . . .[27]

But while a severe critic of Cartesian mechanists, Sauvages was a firm believer in *Newtonian* natural philosophy, mechanics and medicine. In *Nouvelles Classes*, he declared

> Je conviens que les belles découvertes qu'ont fait Baglivi, Bellini, Pitcairn, Keill, Newton, Boerhaave, Michelotti, Bernoulli, par l'application des Mathématiques à la Physique & celles des Anatomistes, ont developés bien des secrets de la nature.[28]

In the 1760s, Sauvages's admiration for a Newtonian medicine was as strong as it had been in his youth; mathematical physics was necessary for a 'sure theory of the human machine':

> the truest theory of all is produced from Anatomy, experimental Physics, and the store of mathematical Philosophy together.[29]

From Sauvages's remarks we can draw the conclusion that if an eighteenth-century physician accepted that arguments from mechanics belonged in sound medical philosophy, it did not mean that he was an admirer of Descartes and his followers:

> recent Moderns proclaim before everyone . . . that they want the animal oeconomy to be ruled or, what is the same thing, governed by blind fate, and this charming theory, they decorate with the name 'mechanics', even though utterly contrary to the mechanics approved in the Academies of Sciences.[30]

Sauvages was asserting that all the ideas 'received in the Academies' were *Newtonian* ones, and that mechanics was only part of natural philosophy, not everything, as it seemed to be with Cartesians.

Cartesian philosophers, who tried to find a physical, material explanation for all natural phenomena, were commonly perceived as skirting dangerously close to disbelief in God; dedicated Newtonians were quick to accuse them of pride, impiety, and even atheism. Newtonian natural philosophy, however, was expressly a 'God-centred' enterprise. Newtonians claimed that through the application of mathematics to the study of natural phenomena one could discover God's Laws

[27] *Nosologia Methodica Sistens Morborum Classes Genera et Species Juxta Sydenhami mentem et Botanicorum Ordinem* (Venice, 1773 edn), vol. 1, p. 2.

[28] *Nouvelles Classes*, p. 2. [29] *Nosologia Methodica*, p. 4. [30] *Ibid.*, p. 2.

of Nature because He had created the world in number, weight and measure, and therefore their natural philosophy was honourable and dedicated to a pious end. Indeed, Newton's 'Forces', especially 'Attraction' (or 'Gravity') were repeatedly attacked by continental mechanists, most notably by Leibniz, as the intrusion of undemonstrated 'occult' forces or causes into natural philosophy. Newton's champions responded by arguing that on grounds both of logic and of piety there must always be undemonstrated 'simple causes' in natural philosophy. Similarly, in Newtonian medical philosophy there was room for (indeed a need for) unanalysable, undemonstrable 'forces' or causes of diseases.[31]

James Keill, for example, had written his *Account of Animal Secretion* (1708) in the hope of demonstrating the harmony between the workings of the animal oeconomy and the principles of Newtonian natural philosophy. He relied heavily upon Newton's 'Attraction' and, by positing 'attractive forces between the constituent particles of the secreted fluids . . . [Keill] used these forces to circumvent certain theoretical difficulties'.[32] In 1724, the young Newtonian physician Henry Pemberton had declared that God had established

> such Principles of Action, as might most compendiously produce the infinite number of Operations in Nature, though by what means any of these Effects can most easily be brought about consistent with the rest, we can in no wise pretend to be proper judges.[33]

Several years later, Pemberton wrote

> It was no trifling discovery, that the contraction of the muscles of animals puts their limbs in motion, though the original cause of that contraction remains a secret, and perhaps may always do so.[34]

Sauvages's beliefs about 'des mouvemens vitaux' and about the soul itself, in support of which he wrote several physiological treatises attacking Cartesians, were in complete accord with the general principles of Newtonian medical theory. He was convinced that the human body was composed of the soul and the 'machine of the body' together:

[31] See John Freind, *Praelectiones Chymicae* (Amsterdam, 1709), and 'Praelectionum Chymicarum Vindiciae . . .', *Philosophical Transactions* 27 (1710–12), pp. 330–42; and Roger Cotes's famous preface to the second edition of *Principia Mathematica* (1713). For a general discussion of what was deemed to be at stake here, see Simon Schaffer, 'Godly Men and Mechanical Philosophers: Souls and Spirits in Restoration Natural Philosophy', *Science in Context* 1 (1987), pp. 55–85.

[32] T. M. Brown, 'From Mechanism to Vitalism in Eighteenth-Century English Physiology', *Journal of the History of Biology* 7 (1974), pp. 179–216, at pp. 187–8.

[33] Pemberton, 'Introduction Concerning Muscular Motion' in J. Jurin's and R. Mead's edition of William Cowper's *Myotomia Reformata, or an Anatomical Treatise on the Muscles of the Human Body* (London, 1724), p. lxviii.

[34] *A View of Sir Isaac Newton's Philosophy* (London, 1728), p. 16.

'Man is composed of a living and motile soul, and a hydraulic machine, united together.'[35] While the soul controlled the body, it did so not in any mystical or supernatural way, but in accordance with knowable laws of nature. In Sauvages's opinion, a knowledge of mechanics certainly was important if a physician was to understand the animal oeconomy, and yet, even if mechanics could explain the observed workings (i.e. the phenomena) of the body, it could *not* explain the *causes* of the phenomena. The principles that mechanics necessarily took as given were the 'forces', or 'causes': these could only be explained by God.

'ON THE CAUSE OF VITAL MOTIONS'

In 1740, Sauvages published a treatise in which he argued for the importance of the role of the soul in the workings of the human body. Not only did Sauvages repeatedly attack Cartesian mechanist physicians, but *On the Cause of Vital Motions* was a self-consciously Newtonian enterprise: its formal structure and its very terms of argument derived directly from Newton's *Principia Mathematica*. In the course of his argument, Sauvages appealed to 'Newtonian principles', referring repeatedly to the British Newtonian physicians Pitcairne, Cheyne, Keill, Arbuthnot, Hales, Jurin and Wainewright. Moreover, this treatise was organised like Newton's *Principia*, with the argument laid out in the form of 'Axioms', 'Corollaries', 'Lemmas', 'Propositions' and 'Scholia'. The key terms Sauvages employed were 'Bodies', 'Effects', 'Phenomena', 'Velocity', 'Power', 'Forces' and 'Potency' – all of which echo the *Principia Mathematica*. Sauvages explained 'Effects' and 'Motion' in strict accordance with Newton's three 'Axioms of Motion':

> Effects are proportional to their causes, and the quantities of the motions correspond proportionally with their moving causes. An effect or Phenomenon is a change in the position or motion of the Body or the Soul, for as long as it is produced.[36]

Sauvages had begun to build his general theory about the workings of the human body around Newtonian laws of motion. We obtain philosophical knowledge of the true motions of bodies, wrote Newton, from the mathematical analysis of the apparent properties and effects on and in bodies; 'Forces' explain for us these true motions. A 'force',

[35] *Nosologia Methodica*, p. 20.

[36] *Dissertatio Medica de Motuum Vitalium Causa* (Montpellier, 1740), paragraphs 1 and 2: reprinted in A. von Haller (ed.), *Disputationum Anatomicarum Selectarum Volumen* (Göttingen, 1749), vol. 4, p. 487. Cf. *Principia Mathematica*, ed. and trans. F. Cajori (Berkeley, 1934), p. 13.

or 'potency', wrote Sauvages, was the power to exercise motions, either the motions of bodies or 'the motions of cognition'. Similarly, and regarding the soul, Sauvages believed that the 'principal attributes' of the soul were 'motive potencies' (or 'principles of motion') and that these produced all the phenomena of motion in humans.

The detailed argument of the treatise began with the mathematics and hydraulics of the 'forces' and velocities of the blood circulating in the body and of the pumping action of the heart. The editor of Newton's *Principia* had declared that 'no mechanical account ... of the most simple cause is to be expected' and had then asserted 'certainly there *are* primary properties of bodies; and these, because they are primary, have no dependence on the others'.[37] Similarly, in *On the Cause of Vital Motions*, Sauvages wished to prove not only 'that the vital motions are not automatic' (i.e. mechanical), but that 'the Primary Origin of Motion is from a Hypermechanical cause'. Sauvages argued

since the velocity sufficient for a fluid contracting the heart cannot be given to it by our machine, though wonderfully made ... [and] as no fluid in the body is circulated more quickly than the blood itself in the aorta, and since the soul gives the necessary velocity to the fluid contracting other muscles, then it seems very probable that the soul can in fact give to the nervous fluid contracting the heart that velocity that it actually has; since there is no other cause of motion in man than the machine and the soul, nor is any effect produced without an equal motive potency.[38]

Having proposed that 'the motion of the heart is maintained by a motive potency, not an automatic force', Sauvages explained an 'Automatic force' to be

that which continues the motion of the body or a machine when once a motion has been impressed upon it, without any new application of the motive potency. Thus, a football, once struck, continues its motion for some time.[39]

Sauvages was continuing to follow the *Principia* very closely indeed: his 'automatic force' was Newton's 'Impressed Force'.[40] The 'motive potencies', therefore, played a role in Sauvages's explanations of the animal oeconomy which was perfectly analogous to the role played by the 'Vis insita', or 'Innate Force of Matter', in Newton's explanations of the natural world as a whole.[41]

Sauvages described the soul and its faculty 'Nature' not only in the language of the *Principia* but in its central concepts. The thought that 'Nature' was the defender of health was an ancient one but Sauvages

[37] R. Cotes, 'Preface', *Principia Mathematica* (ed. Cajori), p. xxvii.

[38] *De Motuum Vitalium Causa*, paragraph 55; in Haller, *Disputationum Anatomicarum Selectarum Volumen*, pp. 498–9. [39] *Ibid.*, paragraph 56, p. 499.

[40] See *Principia Mathematica*, 'Definition IV', p. 2. [41] See *Ibid.*, 'Definition III', p. 2.

was employing the concept in terms of Newton's 'Innate', or 'Inertial Force':

As the Soul more ardently covets life or health, so it protects its body and the proximate and remote causes of its health more earnestly and with greater care and anxiety, and *with efforts proportional* to the degree of danger.[42]

Sauvages had published *On the Cause of Vital Motions* as part of his assault upon those physicians – the 'Cartesians', as he called them – whom he regarded as deviants from the pious tradition of natural philosophy in which he saw himself. It would appear from the available evidence that Sauvages was faced with strong opposition at Montpellier from such men.[43] This helps explain the belligerence of his repeated criticisms of Descartes and his impatience with Leibniz as well. Leibniz had been a persistent critic of Newton himself and he was deemed by Sauvages to be just as suspect of error as Descartes:

Those who are pledged to the Illustrious Descartes seem to concede nothing to the liberty of man, but continually introduce the omnipotent God for the pursuit of all ideas and motions. I do not intend to open verbose disputes but they should be careful . . . they do not cast Man and themselves into passive machines. Those who pursue the pre-established Harmony of the celebrated Leibniz seem to attribute everything to fate, which is ridiculous.[44]

No historian, to my knowledge, has characterised Newton, or Pitcairne, as a 'vitalist'; why then Sauvages, a devout follower?

In the first section of *Pathologia Methodica* (1759), Sauvages discussed the Faculties of the Soul, the 'philosophical nature' of the parts of the body, and defined both 'Health' and 'Diseases'. The Faculties 'discover everything which is appropriate for the welfare of the machine of the body, and what is harmful to it'. There were six Faculties of three different sorts:

Knowledge = (1) *Instinct* (or 'Sentiment'): produces 'indistinct' ideas via the sense organs.
(2) *Judgement*: produces 'distinct' ideas (Man only).

Desire = (3) *Sensitive Appetite* ('Cupidity'): relies on the Senses.
(4) *Rational Appetite* ('Will'): relies on the Judgement.

[42] *De Motuum Vitalium Causa*, paragraph 84; in Haller, *Disputationum Anatomicarum Selectarum Volumen*, p. 509. My emphasis.

[43] Dulieu, 'Mouvement scientifique Montpellierain', and Jones, 'Montpellier Medical Students', in Porter and Wear (eds.), *Problems and Methods*.

[44] *De Motuum Vitalium Causa*, paragraph 75; in Haller, *Disputationum Anatomicarum Selectarum Volumen*, p. 506. *De Motuum Vitalium Causa* is not an isolated example; for instance, in *De Animae Imperio in Cor* (1760), Sauvages employed similar Newtonian arguments and attacked the same, 'Mechanist', enemies.

Movement = (5) *Nature*: to carry out motions ordered by (1) or (3).
(6) *Liberty to choose*: to carry out motions ordered by (2) or (4).

Like this framework for understanding the causes of human actions, Sauvages's definition of the 'parts' of the body was peculiar to himself. And although some of the terms he employed, such as 'Crasis' and 'Similar Part', were used by the Ancients, Sauvages's use of them owed little to Hippocrates or Galen and much more to his Newtonian convictions.

The 'parts' of the body were either 'solid' or 'fluid' and in each category were 'imperceptible' parts and 'perceptible' parts. The 'perceptible' parts were composed from the 'imperceptible' ones (which he alternatively called 'elementary' or 'similar'). These 'imperceptible' parts were joined in a particular 'crasis' (or 'constitution') by means of physical causes, for example, by 'Gravity', 'Adhesion', 'Elasticity' and 'Putrefaction'. We understand the 'structure' of the 'perceptible' parts by asking about 'mechanical' causes such as 'Magnitude', 'Figure', 'Number', 'Form' and 'Situation'.

Sauvages then declared that 'Health' was 'the mutual accord of all the actions, above all, the natural actions, the functions, excretions and the mechanical and physical qualities'. A 'Disease' was 'a battle of Nature with morbific matter', and was the 'effect' produced by two opposed causes: the morbific matter itself and the 'vital forces' (which we can conceive as the action of 'Instinct', the 'Sensitive Appetite' and 'Nature'). Thus the 'Crisis' or 'judgement' of the disease was the last great effort of Nature to overcome the morbific matter.

Sauvages wrote a great deal more about the animal oeconomy, yet, even with this brief survey, we can see that he was determined to combine Newtonian convictions about natural philosophy with an understanding of the nature and functioning of the soul, which he construed in the language and terms of Newton's *Principia*. Sauvages was no more a 'vitalist' than any early-eighteenth-century Newtonian. Newtonians, no less than putative 'vitalists', were perfectly ready to employ 'undemonstrated simple causes' and to attack strict mechanists as impious and simplistic.

'NOSOLOGY'

In the later eighteenth century, several physicians produced books which they entitled or referred to as 'Nosologies'. Sauvages has been regarded as the principal inspiration of this 'tradition' because of his *Nosologia Methodica* (1763). Nosology is generally understood in the historiography of medicine in a modern medical fashion, as a synonym for the 'taxonomy' or 'nomenclature' of diseases. It has been remarked that:

Nosology means the classification of disease, something we now take so much for granted that we do not even think about its origin.[45]

Sauvages's *Nosologia*, moreover, has been dismissed as 'a rather pathetic tissue of inconsistencies and inadequacies, failing in all its intended goals',[46] and therefore 'when we read Sauvages, we feel that a brilliant mind has gone astray'.[47] But if it is true that Sauvages's was 'a brilliant mind', can it also be true that he was so stupid as to produce a 'pathetic tissue of inconsistencies'? We shall find ourselves less puzzled if we ask whether modern definitions of 'nosology' describe what *nosologia* meant to Sauvages. The answer, simply put, is that they do not.

Nosologia for Sauvages meant simply 'knowledge of diseases', exactly what its two Greek roots suggested. In the *Prolegomenes* to *Nosologia Methodica*, Sauvages wrote that his 'nosology' was of two sorts: 'Historical' and 'Philosophical'. The final purpose of both was the same – to make diseases known to us by our *combination* of proper Histories of Diseases and a truly 'philosophical knowledge' about the nature of the human body and diseases. 'Historical knowledge' relied upon what Sauvages repeatedly called his 'symptomatic method': the *historia* of constant symptoms of a disease joined with a careful (and botanical) classification of these constant symptoms. 'Philosophical knowledge', however,

does not stop, as does the Historical, in a simple knowledge of the fact, but, in going further, it makes known the reasons for the fact . . . Philosophical nosology, therefore, is the skill (*habitus*) of demonstrating what is asserted about the principles, causes and relations of diseases; the Greeks call it etiology.[48]

The *scientia* of natural philosophy was the knowledge of the nature and causes of things. *Nosology*, declared Sauvages, was the 'science of diseases', and by 'science', he assured his readers, he meant a rigorous 'manner of demonstrating what we assert about diseases'. And

for demonstration there needs to be set up a reasoning process built on indubitable experiences or historical 'facts', definitions, axioms and propositions demonstrated from elsewhere; therefore, for Nosology are necessary: definitions of diseases, their

[45] King, *Medical World*, p. 193.
[46] King, 'Boissier de Sauvages', p. 47.
[47] King, *Medical World*, p. 214.
[48] *Nosologia Methodica*, p. 19.

historical descriptions, and sure principles drawn from the anatomists, chemists, hydraulicists and mechanists.[49]

Nosology, then, was simply the sort of inquiry that Sauvages had spent his life engaged upon, and the central features of which we have outlined above.

CONCLUSION

Just as it is for scholars in our own day, Sauvages's education was crucial in forming his convictions. By looking at Chicoyneau, Deidier and Chirac – and botany, Newtonian philosophy, Baconian reform and Baglivi – we can uncover a great deal about Sauvages's concerns and the nature of his work. Sauvages was no more *bound* by his education than we are; certainly, what he *did* was due to his native intelligence, his energy and his circumstances, but it is equally certain that his education while a young man provided him with beliefs, methods of inquiry and intellectual authorities which he never abandoned.

Although he was a very early adherent to Newtonian natural philosophy in France, and battled for it against critics within his own university, Sauvages never saw himself or his medical convictions as avant-garde in any way. Newtonian natural philosophy was for him an uncovering of truths about God's natural world and Sauvages believed it to be in full accord with the wisdom of all the best physicians. He was convinced that his battle for a major role for the soul in the working of the human body was an act of conservation of true natural philosophy rather than any sort of innovation. In Sauvages's eyes, the opponents of Newton and Pitcairne were not simply criticising a rival contemporary hypothesis (as such critics often portrayed it). They were, he said, 'freethinkers', 'Moderns', who were attacking responsible natural philosophy. During his lifetime and in the generation after his death, Sauvages was a celebrated physician. Why this was so cannot be pursued here, beyond suggesting that it may have been the mid-eighteenth-century French enthusiasm – the 'Enlightenment' enthusiasm, if you will – for Newtonian natural philosophy, Baconian natural histories and Linnaean classifying that made Sauvages and his research programme seem perfectly 'up-to-the-minute'.

Insofar as the French Enlightenment can be characterised by a desire for 'improvement', by the reform of the sciences, and by a fascination

[49] *Ibid.*, p. 7.

with English philosophy, then Sauvages indeed was an Enlightenment figure. Yet this study of a provincial (rather than Parisian) scholar and of how he happily combined Bacon and Newton with his other local concerns may serve as a salutary illustration of the complexities which face the historian of the sciences when examining eighteenth-century French natural philosophers and medical men.

6

Honour and property the structure of professional disputes in eighteenth-century English medicine

DAVID HARLEY

The Reputation and Character, which every Honest Man wishes to maintain in the World, is so dear and tender in his own Eye, and of such Consequence to his Family and Friends, that when we find ourselves openly attack'd in our good Name, or privately vilified by Slander, or evil Reports, and oblique Insinuations, we cannot too publickly, or too firmly repel the Injury

Archibald Cleland[1]

From Galenic phlebotomy to modern obstetrics, medicine has always been prone to disputes, which have often helped to define a new theoretical posture or a new form of practice. Albergati, in his famous treatise on the resolution of private hostilities, called on his readers to imitate physicians but it was certainly not their ability to handle disputes amicably that he had in mind. Most published disputes were dressed in public-spiritedness and intellectual justifications, yet the personal battles that lay behind them could be extremely vitriolic. English medicine after the Restoration saw a wide variety of long-running disagreements, often centring on the College of Physicians, which was repeatedly attacked by chemists, apothecaries and physicians with degrees from universities other than Oxford and Cambridge.[2]

Although the medical practitioners of eighteenth-century England are only beginning to be the subject of detailed research, it has long

[1] A. Cleland, *An Appeal to the Publick* (London, 1743), sig. A2r.

[2] Fabio Albergati, *Trattato . . . del Modo di Ridurre à Pace l'inimicitie priuate* (Rome, 1583), pp. 102 and 175; Harold J. Cook, 'The Society of Chemical Physicians, the New Philosophy, and the Restoration Court', *Bulletin of the History of Medicine* 61 (1987), pp. 61–77 and *The Decline of the Old Medical Regime in Stuart London* (Ithaca, 1986), pp. 133–253; George N. Clark, *A History of the Royal College of Physicians*, vol. 2 (Oxford, 1966), pp. 452–5 and 547–73; Bernice Hamilton, 'The Medical Professions in the Eighteenth Century', *Economic History Review*, second series, 4 (1952), pp. 141–69; Ivan Waddington, 'The Struggle to Reform the Royal College of Physicians, 1767–1771: A Sociological Analysis', *Medical History* 17 (1973), pp. 107–26. Hal Cook is currently working on the Groeneveld dispute.

been believed that establishing a lucrative practice was often extremely difficult. Sir John Hawkins contrasted two highly successful London physicians, the elder Schomberg and Fothergill, with twenty failures who lived and died in poverty. In such circumstances, it is hardly surprising that established practitioners attempted to restrict competition by refusing to consult with outsiders. The London physicians fostered a serious dispute when they initially refused to consult with Schomberg, despite his being a licentiate of the College, 'and thereby, for some time, checked his practice'. It has been suggested that the rising income of medical practitioners led to a decline in attacks by physicians on apothecaries. This may be so, but the rewards available for successful practice did not diminish the rivalry between physicians. Greater rewards, and attempts to monopolise them by the construction of micro-hierarchies, led to conflict within groups instead of between them. This, after all, is precisely why highly stratified societies tend to need a complex, institutionalised legal system. The rewards were potentially greater but newcomers posed challenges to existing elite practitioners through the use of novel strategies such as man-midwifery. Poor law contracts and infirmary posts provided new forms of resource control but there was also a perceived need for new styles of controlling existing resources. In a free market, the loyalty of patients was unreliable.[3]

Given the traditional preoccupation of medical history with ideas and institutions, it is perhaps unsurprising that the bitter feuds of provincial practitioners have been given only cursory treatment even though they provide a good picture of the tensions inherent in early modern medical practice. The overwhelming majority of medical practitioners practised far from London and the development of metropolitan institutions, however important for later generations, had only an indirect influence on behaviour outside the seven-mile radius of the College's authority. Although the College was sympathetic to the desire of provincial graduate physicians to control practice in their localities, it was unable to act.[4]

Like panics and epidemics, disputes offer glimpses of rules, beliefs and values which are normally unspoken, despite presenting severe problems of representativeness. Participants talk about the texture of their lives and the ideas that suffuse their ordinary behaviour.

[3] J. Hawkins, *The Life of Dr. Samuel Johnson* (Dublin, 1787), pp. 214–6; Irvine Loudon, 'The Nature of Provincial Medical Practice in Eighteenth-Century England', *Medical History* 29 (1985), pp. 1–32.

[4] Annals of the Royal College of Physicians, 24 March 1709/10; 3 April 1710; 8 Oct. 1713.

Although interesting in themselves, witchcraft accusations are more valuable for the light they shed on the rest of life. To understand the detail and context of any medical dispute, whether predominantly intellectual or professional, requires a great deal of research and patient consideration. The present intention is rather to explore the general outlines of professional disputes through examination of a number of examples, mostly in southern England. For this purpose, it is not necessary to assess the truth of accusations since libel and slander can provide a good indication of the type of behaviour which they are intended to restrict or condemn.[5]

Historians who study disputes in pre-industrial Europe are tempted to turn to legal anthropology for guidance.[6] This is a perilous undertaking for those who are unused to the theoretical underpinnings of other disciplines, since legal anthropology is one of the last bastions of a functionalism that derives from Malinowski and Radcliffe-Brown. The implicit assumptions that inform much research are especially liable to mislead historians working on relatively differentiated societies. There is a danger of assuming the universality of dispute behaviour and filling this category with whatever examples of hostility come to hand. There is a tendency to see a dispute as a temporary disorder, involving individuals rather than interest groups, which requires settlement so that the status quo can be maintained. Influential writers, such as Max Gluckman and Laura Nader, have seen the non-European cultures they studied as dominated by a search for conciliation, which they contrasted with Western adversarial systems of adjudication. They have often underestimated the degree of informal arbitration in European legal systems and the extent of extra-legal disputing but it has also proved necessary to suppress all reference to major aspects of socioeconomic change.[7]

[5] Andrew Cunningham, 'Sydenham Versus Newton: The Edinburgh Fever Dispute of the 1690s Between Andrew Brown and Archibald Pitcairne', *Medical History*, Supplement No. 1 (1981), pp. 71–98; D. N. Harley, 'Disputes in the Career of Henry Bracken of Lancaster' (forthcoming); Peter N. Moogk, '"Thieving Buggers" and "Stupid Sluts": Insults and Popular Culture in New France', *William and Mary Quarterly*, third series 36 (1979), pp. 524–47; Roger Thompson, '"Holy Watchfulness" and Communal Conformism: The Functions of Defamation in Early New England Communities', *New England Quarterly* 56 (1983), pp. 504–22.

[6] John Bossy (ed.), *Disputes and Settlements: Law and Human Relations in the West* (Cambridge, 1983). An attempt to apply anthropology to the development of medical ethics in a very different society has been made by Paul U. Unschuld, *Medical Ethics in Imperial China: A Study in Historical Anthropology* (Berkeley, 1979).

[7] Max Gluckman, *Politics, Law and Ritual in Tribal Society* (Oxford, 1965); Laura Nader(ed.), *Law in Culture and Society* (Chicago, 1969), pp. 69–91; June Starr, *Dispute and Settlement in Rural Turkey: An Ethnography of Law* (Leiden, 1978). Dr Starr omits all reference to the presence of tourists in coastal Turkish villages.

A functionalist perspective is likely to exclude historical change and explanation partly because of its notorious circularity, the institutions' functions being seen as the preservation of the institutions. It ignores the importance of uncertainty and dispute in the historical process, seeing them as entirely dysfunctional despite the stimulating suggestions of Simmel.[8] Like legal theory itself, it sees the parties to a dispute as isolated individuals, and wipes out qualitative differences of ideology and politics between them. There has been a tendency to move from an approval of tribal methods of dispute settlement to an advocacy of their introduction in advanced societies, which unmasks assumptions about cultural universality and the comparability of dispute. Even though the limitations of functionalism have been recognised, in legal anthropology 'established techniques are repeated and consolidated'. Only gradually are efforts being made to break the tradition, notably by Laurence Goldman in his linguistic study of disputing in New Guinea. It is too soon to see where such detailed work will lead since there is still insufficient new material for comparative analysis.[9]

The epistemological difficulties posed by studying disputes are complex and intractable. There is an especial danger of confusing the observer's folk-system of explanation with that of the observed group. In the absence of adequate comparative material, it would be premature to erect an analytical system that attempts to supersede the understanding of the participants, yet some features of contemporary life are not made fully explicit by the disputants and must be partly supplied from other sources. Some assumptions have been made for the sake of the present study: behind the published medical disputes lay tensions between rival groups, to whom participants appealed for support; these tensions were generally the product of political or economic relationships; disputants rarely went to law but sought instead to influence public opinion; affected groups continued to nurse their grievances since general circumstances were not changed by the outcome of any dispute. Even celebrated legal cases such as the College's action against Thomas Bonham can hardly be said to have significantly affected the conflict of interests which they expressed.[10]

The impression that medical arguments were the product of individ-

[8] Georg Simmel, *Soziologie*, 3rd edn (Munich, 1923), pp. 186–255.

[9] Simon Roberts, review article in *Man*, new series, 16 (1981), p. 490; L. Goldman, *Talk Never Dies: The Language of Huli Disputes* (London, 1983).

[10] Harold J. Cook, '"Against Common Right and Reason": The College of Physicians Versus Dr. Thomas Bonham', *American Journal of Legal History* 29 (1985), pp. 301–22.

ual disagreements has been reinforced by frequent reference to the clash between Richard Mead and John Woodward with the comment that 'even physicians were wont to decide their professional altercations at the point of the sword'. This fiasco of a fracas attracted a great deal of attention, being a source of much hilarity. It was remembered long afterwards in the London coffee-houses. Hawkins referred to it in a footnote while describing the irascible character of Akenside; Fothergill alluded to it when he suggested that Myersbach and Lettsom should fight in Warwick Lane.[11] This one case has distorted historical understanding since, although it is true that medical men were occasionally drawn into conflict with military officers or even a colonial judge, they do not appear to have fought duels with one another.[12] There are two documented instances of medical duels in America at a later date, and there is said to have been one in Dublin, but the only medical argument leading to a serious duel that came to public notice in eighteenth-century England occurred in Jamaica. Kirkpatrick, reviewing an account of the fatal dispute, deplored the impolite style of debate and noted that only the death of the two physicians would render the account of interest to English readers. Duelling was not seen as compatible with the Christian morals and healing art of gentlemanly physicians who were seen by themselves as men of sensibility and by others as effete cowards.[13]

Especially after the Restoration, learned physicians affected to abhor quarrels, even when this posture conflicted with their behav-

[11] John Gideon Millingen, *The History of Duelling* (London, 1841), vol. 2, pp. 45–6; Robert A. E. Baldick, *The Duel: A History of Duelling* (London, 1965), p. 70; Joseph M. Levine, *Dr. Woodward's Shield* (Berkeley, 1977), pp. 9–17; Hawkins, *Life of Johnson*, p. 219n.; *Morning Chronicle* 9 Oct. 1776, quoted in W. F. Bynum and Roy Porter (eds.), *Medical Fringe & Medical Orthodoxy, 1750–1850* (London, 1987), p. 74.

[12] Public Record Office, PL 27/3, depositions of 28 April 1760 at inquest on Joseph Jackson; PL 28/2, p. 252; Andrew Steinmetz, *The Romance of Duelling in All Times and Countries* (London, 1868), vol. 2, pp. 243 and 247; Millingen, *History of Duelling*, vol. 2, pp. 327–34; [Simon Ansley Ferrall] *On the Duel* (London, 1838), pp. 25, 27 and 30. The two challenges which Granville Sharp Pattison issued to colleagues were refused and, in a controversy-strewn career, he only fought one actual duel, with a general who was the brother-in-law of one of his professional opponents: F. L. M. Pattison, *Granville Sharp Pattison, Anatomist and Antagonist, 1791–1851* (Edinburgh, 1987), pp. 64, 94–6 and 122–7. I am grateful to Roy Porter for drawing this medical malcontent to my attention.

[13] Millingen, *History of Duelling*, vol. 2, pp. 46 and 319–20; Baldick, *The Duel*, vol. 1, p. 99; Michael T. Ashcroft, 'Publish and Perish: A Fatal Medical Controversy', *Journal of the Royal College of Physicians* 13 (1979), pp. 229–30; *Monthly Review* 7 (1752), pp. 71–4. Scholars and clerics were traditionally seen as able to bestow honour but not to give insult, being as much outside the dispute of honour as women: Geronimo [Ximenez] de Urrea, *Dialogo de la Verdadera Honrra Militar* (Venice, 1566), ff. 102v–103r (in the 1569 Italian translation, ff. 160v–161r).

iour, and carefully defended any entry into controversy.[14] Injured innocence was the only respectable style to adopt, although some writers had difficulty maintaining it. When Robert Wittie of York attacked the chemist William Simpson, he complained that his opponent should have discussed their disagreements privately. He professed to be 'sorry to be put to this unpleasant task of ripping up a weak Brothers Infirmities' but insisted that he was the victim of an aggressive chemist. In a later pamphlet, he suggested 'the most homely of uses' for a book by Simpson and continued to attack the Oxford-educated George Tonstall of Newcastle as a hypocrite while claiming to be himself the injured party and still 'a Friend to Dr Tunstal'. In his reply, Tonstall apologised for descending into Wittie's style of uncivil abuse under provocation, which drew the scorn of Wittie's friend, Nathaniel Johnston, who wrote to Martin Lister: 'If he write long in this manner he will write himself out of repute.' Wittie, Johnston and Lister possessed effective weapons which allowed them to remain aloof from the fray, they employed third parties to prosecute chemists and clerics who practised medicine and they refused to consult with even an extra-licentiate of the College of Physicians because he had not attended Oxford or Cambridge.[15]

Medical controversies of the eighteenth century were ostensibly less charged with political and religious ideology than those of the Interregnum and Restoration. The medical establishment participated in the Whig attempt to achieve the appearance of bland consensus and overtly political attacks on medical practitioners were more often made by religious authors. Joseph Warder, a Dissenting physician at Croydon, was drawn into the theological dispute between Benjamin Hoadly and Andrew Snape when he testified to the sound Anglicanism of a former Jesuit. He was savaged by a Jacobite schoolmaster who accused the Dissenter of deceit, adultery and extreme quarrelsomeness while sarcastically suggesting that the letter printed as written by Warder must be a forgery since it was spelt accurately. Warder

[14] Richard Lower, *Diatribae Thomae Willisii . . . de Febribus Vindicatio adversus Edmundum de Meara* (London, 1665), sig. A3v; 'Alius Medicus', *Animadversions on the Medicinal Observations of . . . Mr. Frederick Loss* (London, 1674), pp. 71–80. This attitude was also adopted by the antiquarian Francis Wise when his work on the White Horse was anonymously savaged, especially for its dedication to Dr Mead: Bodleian Library, Gough Berks. 5, letter to Browne Willis dated 21 Dec. 1740.

[15] R. Wittie, *Pyrologia Mimica* (London, 1669), pp. 3, 8, 115 and 181–8 and *Scarborough's Spagyrical Anatomizer Dissected* (London, 1672), sig. A3v, pp. 14, 15, 101–2 and 127; G. Tonstall, *A New-Year's-Gift for Doctor Witty* (London, 1672), sig. A8r; Bodleian Library, MS Lister 35, f. 17; British Library, Sloane MS 1393, ff. 1[illegible]–17.

complained that his attacker was attempting to destroy a medical practice that was mainly exercised among conformists. The schoolmaster was alleged to be 'ashamed to own the true Spring of his Malice against me, *viz.* my Hatred for *Protestant Popery*, and Zeal for the *Protestant Succession* and for King *GEORGE*'.[16] As the Whig position became increasingly secure, it was not Dissenters but Jacobites who were vulnerable to political attacks. Religious and political opponents attempted to destroy the medical practice of John Burton of York and Thomas Deacon of Manchester in the wake of the 1745 rebellion. It was probably an exaggeration to suggest that Deacon was 'chiefly employ'd by Papists, Jacobites, and Nonjurors' so that alleged disloyalty might well restrict his practice.[17] More effective as a slur was an accusation of dishonesty, since it destroyed a physician's honourable reputation. When Dr Andrew of Exeter was accused of fraudulent intentions in a property transaction, he was so discredited by the mere suggestion that a family which had employed him for twenty years dispensed with his services.[18]

As the experience of John Andrew indicates, medical practitioners depended for success upon their reputation and this was extremely vulnerable to attack by colleagues. The relationship between honour and status, outlined by Max Weber, has been utilised by Waddington to explore physicians' distaste for manual operations and overt trading activity but it has been generally overlooked as a key to the bitter disputes between medical men, despite its evident importance for local office-holders.[19] In any intimate community, honour is easy to lose but difficult to secure. In the absence of any decisive settlement procedure, such as duels or authoritative arbitration, disputes could not die away in a small face-to-face community composed of a county's medical practitioners and their patients. Unless one party conceded defeat and left the area, participants continued to live in the same area and

[16] Francis de la Pilloniere, *A Reply to Dr. Snape's Vindication* . . . (London, 1718), pp. 47–50 and 58; Joseph Warder, *A Vindication of Joseph Warder, Physician at Croyden* (London, 1718), pp. 4 and 6.

[17] George Thompson, *An Account of What Passed Between Mr. George Thompson of York and Doctor John Burton* (London, 1756); Arthur H. Cash, *Lawrence Sterne: The Early and Middle Years* (London, 1975), pp. 91–3, 109–63 and 168–78; *Gentleman's Magazine* 16 (1746), pp. 688–91; 18 (1748), pp. 206–7; Josiah Owen, *Dr. Deacon, Try'd Before his own Tribunal* (Manchester, 1748), pp. 3, 33–7, 45 and 63.

[18] John Andrew, *Remarks on Mr. Tremlett's Letter to Archdeacon Sleech* (Exeter, 1763), p. 28.

[19] *From Max Weber: Essays in Sociology*, ed. H. H. Gerth and C. Wright Mills (London, 1948), pp. 180–95; Waddington, 'Struggle to Reform the Royal College'; A. J. Fletcher, 'Honour, Reputation and Local Officeholding in Elizabethan and Stuart England' in Anthony Fletcher and John Stevenson (eds.), *Order and Disorder in Early Modern England* (Cambridge, 1985), pp. 92–115.

unsettled issues influenced future events. The widening ripples of a dispute shaped attitudes at a considerable distance through critical comment in the London magazines.

One of the most influential disputes was that between Richard Russel of Henley-on-Thames and Anthony Addington of Reading, which has been portrayed as largely concerned with the relative merits of English and foreign degrees. Russel had trained in London and Paris, taken a Rheims MD and accepted an appointment as physician to Christ's Hospital on the testimonial of several eminent physicians. As a licentiate of the Royal College of Physicians, he was astonished when Addington refused to consult with him, claiming that he had entered into an agreement with several colleagues, including Frewin in Oxford, not to consult with those who did not have a degree from Oxford or Cambridge. This was incredible to Russel since he had consulted with two of them and one told him not only that he had not joined any group but 'That he never had heard even that any such Agreement had been entered into in any part of England.' Russel criticised Addington for presuming to 'invalidate all Foreign Degrees, cancel the Licences of the College of Physicians', in favour of those educated at English universities since they were far from being the only source of 'Regular Physicians', the teaching elsewhere being far superior. This was a sore point and many at Oxford would agree with Russel and the London licentiates.[20]

Thus the ostensible ground of the dispute was the familiar conflict between those who had an expensive learned education and those who had a cheaper technical training. According to Russel, however, ungentlemanly behaviour was at the heart of the conflict. When he first came to Henley, Addington had tried to persuade him to move further from Reading and had then spread a rumour that it was unclear whether Russel

> intended to practise as an Apothecary, Surgeon, Man-midwife, or Physician. No Invention could have been more cruel than this, nor more basely calculated to do me mischief; which, by threatening, and seeming to strike at the particular interest of each of the Apothecaries, united them all against me.

Russel accused Addington of being determined to restrict competition in Reading, 'looking upon your Patients as your property, You are

[20] Clark, *History of College of Physicians*, vol. 2, pp. 545–6; Geoffrey Holmes, *Augustan England: Professions, State and Society, 1680–1730* (London, 1982), pp. 209–10 and 226; R. Russel, *A Letter to Dr. Addington of Reading* (London, 1774), pp. 8–9, 11–21 and 33; marginal annotations of the copy of *Remarks on a Pamphlet, Intituled A Letter From a Physician in London to His Friend in the Country* (London, 1735) in the Bodleian Library, Godwin Pamphlets 2902(6).

resolved they shall not be alienated.' He sought to dominate his patients to such an extent that he tried to control their second choice, when he himself was unable to attend them.[21]

A new Whig magazine, the *Monthly Review*, felt that, 'whatever Dr Addington may have to say in his own defence', Russel's criticism 'has entirely the air of veracity, and is expressed in modest and gentleman-like language'. In the same issue, a Cork medical dispute was noted sarcastically as exhibiting 'a like instance of the candid and brotherly regard not unfrequently shewn by the physicians one towards another'. Cork was riven with ecclesiastical contention as well as the medical dispute, in which four physicians attempted to exclude an Edinburgh graduate, Patrick Blair, from consultation, threatening the Cork Infirmary with withdrawal of their services and a campaign to stop subscriptions. Blair endeavoured to vindicate both his practice and his etiquette, and the disputants appealed to Mead in London and Frewin in Oxford for arbitration. Since their opinions appeared to favour Blair's prescription, the dispute remained unresolved.[22]

Russel compared the real cabal formed in Cork with the one which he believed was only in Addington's imagination, when he wrote his second pamphlet on the dispute.[23] Addington, having met only with ridicule when he attempted to answer Russel, had been showing clandestinely a letter from Thomas Bigg, a retired surgeon who had opposed Russel's hospital appointment seven years previously. He had also persuaded his friend, Dr William Lewis of Oxford, to refuse consultations with Russel, even though Lewis was known to consult with distinguished foreign graduates and Addington himself had to break off relations with some practitioners in order to be consistent.[24] Having failed to elicit a satisfactory answer, Russel elaborated on the notion of the public as judge: 'When a person has received injury from another in his character, and cannot procure any redress in a legal way, his only remedy is to accuse the Aggressor, and to bring him before the bar of the Public, as the most proper judge.'[25]

Addington maintained a supposedly dignified silence, at least in print, and concentrated on mustering support among colleagues. He was not entirely fortunate in his choice of allies. He was obliged to deny mentioning Dr Frewin and his close friend, Dr Lewis, became some-

[21] Russel, *Letter to Dr. Addington*, pp. 9–10, 23–4 and 29–31.

[22] *Monthly Review* 1 (Aug. 1749), pp. 277 and 314; *An Account of a Medical Controversy in the City of Cork* (London, 1749), pp. 3 and 38–9; Patrick Blair, *The Case of Mr. Baker Truly Stated* (Cork, 1748).

[23] R. Russel, *A Letter to Mr. Thomas Bigg, Late Surgeon of St. Bartholomew's Hospital* (London, 1751), p. 24n. [24] *Ibid.*, pp. 1–3 and 26–31. [25] *Ibid.*, pp. 19–20.

thing of a liability. They were called in by Mary Blandy, at whose trial for murder they notoriously testified, by which time Lewis was fighting accusations of attempted sodomy with a Christ Church choirboy. A pamphlet attacking him was 'sent Gratis to the Families in his Neighbourhood, obtruded upon Apothecaries, scattered in all Places where it was imagined he might be hurt and injured by it'.[26] This moral blot was stressed by the next participant in the Reading dispute, Francis Pigott, who suggested that Addington and his friends were linked to Lewis by more than mere friendship.[27]

When Addington's close colleague had left Reading, Pigott had been recommended to replace him. He soon realised that Addington's support was double-edged since he had offended so many people, both through his medicine and his politics. Pigott was often advised to oppose Addington, who 'had never made any Friendship he had engaged in, subservient to other than his own Interest'. When Russel moved to Reading, Pigott thought of returning to Oxford but Addington kept offering various baits 'thrown out to keep me here for his Purposes'. There was a secret plan to form a hospital with salaried posts, a secret intention to move to Bath, an offer of Addington's private house and his mad house. Eventually Pigott heard an Oxford rumour that Thomas Bigg's nephew was going to replace Addington, who had not been entirely candid. There appeared to be a deal whereby Bigg's nephew took the Reading practice in return for Addington being helped into a London hospital post. Pigott accused him of not only maligning him but also stealing patients by fraud.[28] 'After having, under the Pretence of Friendship, injur'd and supplanted me in the most disingenuous Manner you have thought proper to refuse as equitable Proposals of Arbitration as ever were made; I am therefore constrain'd to appeal to the Public.' The *Monthly Review* complained that Addington remained silent, failing to 'wipe off the imputation that must remain upon his moral character'.[29]

Addington and his opponents employed notions of honourable behaviour, the senior physician choosing publicly to ignore his critics, relying instead on private conversations. In an attempt to assert his aloof superiority, he engaged in the medical equivalent of cutting a

[26] *Ibid.*, p. 25; *A Genuine and Impartial Account of the Life of Miss Mary Blandy* (London, 1752), pp. 6 and 12–13; *The Genuine Tryal at Large of Mary Blandy, Spinster* . . . (London, 1752), pp. 5–6; William Lewis, *An Answer to the Serious Inquiry into Some Proceedings* (London, n.d.), pp. v and 42–3.

[27] Francis Pigott, *An Appeal to the Public* (Reading, 1754), pp. 1 and 51–2.

[28] *Ibid.*, pp. 2–7, 9–16, 21 and 28–38.

[29] *Ibid.*, p. 1; *Monthly Review* 11 (Nov. 1754), p. 400.

man in the street or blackballing him at the club. Ostracism, excluding a man from cooperative economic activity, was the weapon of first resort for established practitioners. The outsiders were forced into print, thus appearing to be aggressors. Russel, however, had already put himself beyond the pale by combining the attributes of a physician with those of an apothecary and a surgeon, although he only proposed to practise midwifery in conjunction with physic.

The swelling ranks of hospital-trained man-midwives made this increasingly common as a strategy for building a provincial practice, but William Holbrooke found it difficult to compete successfully in his home town in 1737: 'I begin to think I mist it much in not settling in Leicester, instead of Manchester, when I consider you had not a manmidwife within ten miles of Leicester town! nor a Surgeon yt cou'd cut for the Stone!' Nevertheless, fashion and the dissemination of manuals led to much rash practice. Henry Bracken, established as a man-midwife since 1720, recorded a sadly botched delivery performed by 'a Practitioner, who, I suppose, was then like a young Physician, just come from College, with his Head brim-full of the Theory'. Man-midwifery posed severe ethical problems, partly because of its novelty, and one Fellow of the Royal College of Physicians had damages of £1,000 awarded against him in 1741 for criminal conversation with a patient and again in 1754 for negligence. In the latter case, several other man-midwives gave evidence concerning his unethical and mercenary behaviour. Although they rarely achieved more than local notoriety, extremely bitter disputes about malpractice in midwifery could break out in provincial towns. One such was conducted in a Liverpool newspaper by two ecclesiastically licensed man-midwives, John Wareing and Ralph Holt, a pupil of Bracken.[30]

If man-midwifery was a fruitful source of disputes because of its importance in establishing a reputation, another innovation in provincial medicine, the infirmary, posed problems of monopoly because of its importance in consolidating a reputation. As the Cork dispute indicates, physicians could place a great deal of pressure on hospital governors, especially if they had been instrumental in founding the institution. Archibald Cleland was unable to reverse his dismissal from

[30] I. Loudon, *Medical Care and the General Practitioner, 1750–1850* (Oxford, 1986), pp. 85–99; *Notes & Queries*, second series, 10 (1860), p. 144; Henry Bracken, *The Midwife's Companion* (London, 1737), p. 65; Jean Donnison, *Midwives and Medical Men: A History of Inter-Professional Rivalries and Women's Rights* (New York, 1977), pp. 30–1; *The Trial of a Cause Between Richard Maddox, Gent., Plaintiff, and Dr. M—y* (London, 1754), pp. 15–21; *The Lancet*, 10 April 1897, p. 1,047; Cheshire Record Office, Dioc. Misc. bundle 3, nos. 111 and 118 (approximate location in unnumbered bundle).

the hospital of Bath, dominated by William Oliver, despite his success in discrediting evidence against him. He accused David Hartley of 'industriously procuring and spreading those false Reports, where ever he thought they would be credited'. His opponents were 'influencing the Innkeepers of this Place to asperse my Character, to all such Strangers as enquired for me, upon their coming here'. Cleland had no obvious recourse, other than appealing to the public, and he was concerned that his response to anonymous critics might appear acrimonious, which he hoped would be excused as arising from:

> that Warmth, which naturally arises in the Breast of every *innocent Man*, when his *Character* is attack'd, and his very *Bread* and *Being* rendered precarious . . . My ALL is at stake; and the Dispute between me and my *Enemies* is of too serious a Nature to admit of *Compliments*; – it demands *Plainess*; – but nothing, I think can justify *Scurility*; which I hope I have altogether avoided.

Cleland was widely supported and his practice survived the attacks, perhaps because he endorsed Tory virtues of honest individualism and plain speech. Yet he remained an outsider, shunned by the Bath medical establishment, and Smollet noted that Cleland's experience

> justifies the old observation, that an injured person will never be forgiven by those who have done him wrong. Nay, so industrious are his adversaries in the prosecution of their enmity, that all methods, even the lowest arts, are practised to prepossess the minds of strangers against him, by a most malicious misrepresentation of his character . . .[31]

A more substantial assault on the Bath oligarchy was launched by Charles Lucas and William Baylies. In his comparative study of English and European spas, Lucas was not only critical of the squalid bathing facilities at Bath, he ridiculed the previous orthodoxy concerning the supposed constituents of the water. In a dedication to the Earl of Chesterfield, Lucas insisted that arrangements at Bath were badly in need of reform, since 'under an evil or irregular administration, like powerful medicines in the hands of quacks, it can answer few good purposes; unless by accident'. Although the reviewer felt that Lucas was conceited and politically motivated, the newly founded *Critical Review* gave the book extensive coverage. Baylies enthusiastically supported the chemical analysis of Lucas, boasting that they both knew more of chemistry than the Bath establishment because they had trained as apothecaries before becoming physicians. Oxford men might have a polished literary style but they were wholly ignorant of

[31] Archibald Cleland, *A Full Vindication of Mr Cleland's Appeal to the Publick* (Bath, 1744), pp. 27–8n., 29n. and 46–7; Tobias Smollett, *An Essay on the External Use of Water* (London, 1752), p. 43.

the character of the waters, which they 'adulterated with a discordant Jumble of Medicines'. They had no more rational understanding than 'the Quicksilver Doctor and such other Pretenders to Physick'. Baylies looked back to a golden age when there were fewer and better practitioners at Bath. The *Critical Review* found Baylies's work elegant and admirable, especially noting his 'severe, though just animadversions, upon the managers and physicians of the hospital at Bath'. The *Monthly Review* could find nothing good to say about the book, tartly noting that Baylies was an upstart apothecary.[32]

Predictably, the Bath physicians closed ranks. According to Baylies, 'No sooner had Dr Lucas arrived at Bath, than he found that Dr Oliver had been, some time, very assiduous in exclaiming against him, and declaring, before he was asked, that he would hold no consultation with Dr Lucas.' Oliver had previously 'formed a like confederacy, to exclude another gentleman'. Lucas was outraged that his demolition of the soap and sulphur theory of Bath water should lead to

> such an attempt to monopolize, such a destructive association, such a confederacy in iniquity, against the laws of the land, against human benevolence and charity, against the rules and intentions of the healing art, and contrary to the customs and example of all well policied faculties of physic, our great college in particular.

Oliver accused Lucas of having 'abused and misrepresented all the gentlemen of this place, who have had a *regular* education, in the profession of physic'. He refused to consult with Lucas, drawing scorn from the Irishman but sympathy from the *Monthly Review* whose reviewer felt the outsiders were guilty of 'Scandal and Impertinance'.[33]

Lucas had no commitment to Bath practice and went his way, resuming in due course his Dublin political career, but Baylies fought on, publishing a history of Oliver's monopolistic control of the Infirmary. He was scathing in his criticism of Oliver's covert manipulation of the governors, which he depicted as incompatible with medical ethics:

[32] Charles Lucas, *An Essay on Waters* (London, 1756), vol. 3, p.ccxvi; *Critical Review* 1 (1756), pp. 321–45; William Baylies, *Practical Reflections on the Uses and Abuses of Bath Waters* (London, 1757), pp.xx, xxiii–xxv, 6–9, 12–14, 18–20 and 74–5; *Critical Review* 3 (1757), pp. 415–20; *Monthly Review* 17 (1757), pp. 164–9. The policies of these magazines have been frequently discussed, most recently by James G. Basker, *Tobias Smollett, Critic and Journalist* (Newark, 1988). Their impact on the dissemination of medical ideas and the reform of medical attitudes remains to be assessed.

[33] [W. Baylies] *Letters of Doctor Lucas and Doctor Oliver, Occasioned by a Physical Confederacy Discovered in Bath* (London, 1757), sig. A2, pp. 7 and 12; *Monthly Review* 17 (1757), pp. 569–70.

> Honour and humanity are as necessary qualifications for a physician, as knowledge in medicine; and it is impossible for the mercenary, mean, or malicious, to exercise the art of physic in that disinterested and benevolent manner with which it ought always to be practised.

Smollett, writing in the *Critical Review*, approved of Baylies's account but he was pessimistic about the likely outcome, expecting that Oliver and his friends would easily persuade the public 'that the accuser writes from motives of private spleen, and personal interest'. He stressed again the treatment of Cleland as an example 'of most illegal despotism, of the most flagrant iniquity, and cruel oppression'. His expectations were fulfilled. Whigs could see nothing wrong in Oliver's behaviour and suggested that Baylies was angered by the way his opponents ignored both his attacks and his desire for a hospital post. A governor of the Infirmary laid all the blame for the dispute on Baylies:

> If a man appears to be of a litigious, quarrelsome, unsociable temper, who had already done all in his power to disturb the peace of a society, by defaming all the members of it, can such a man, without a most consummate assurance, solicit the members of that society to adopt him into their community?

After an unsuccessful attempt to enter Parliament, Baylies abandoned the unequal struggle and left for a career first in London and then abroad.[34]

Addington and Oliver had no need to answer their critics, being able to employ their authority in informal retaliation, although their silence was differently interpreted by reviewers for political reasons. Their critics appealed to lay and professional opinion to act as passive arbitrators but they did not expect their opponents to concede victory. In more evenly matched disputes, the opposing positions were explicitly stated and the appeal to the reader was direct, as in a controversy at Bury St Edmunds in 1764. A graduate of Cambridge and Leyden joined with a surgeon to complain at the behaviour of an extra-licentiate surgeon-physician. They claimed that rumours of their injudicious treatment of an apothecary, the surgeon's brother-in-law, had been 'with uncommon Industry spread by Mr *Norford*, and his Friends, through this Town and Neighbourhood, (with an Intention to injure our Characters in our Profession)'. The truth of Norford's suggestion, that the treatment was nearly fatal, they left 'to be determined by the

[34] W. Baylies, *An Historical Account of the Rise, Progress, and Management, of the General Hospital, or Infirmary in the City* (London, 1758), pp. 78–9; *Critical Review* 6 (1758), pp. 516–7; *Monthly Review* 20 (1759), p. 85; *A Short Answer to a Set of Queries Annexed to An Historical Account* . . . (Bath, 1759), p. 6.

Suffrage of the Publick in general, and by the Gentlemen of the Faculty in particular' and they apologised for being 'obliged, in this publick Manner, to vindicate our Characters from the Obloquy of our Enemies'. After stating their view of the facts of the case, in which their treatment of the patient's piles was unwarrantably interfered with by Norford, resulting in a potentially dangerous gangrene, they suggested his motive to be resentment. Norford was more concerned with 'his Interest than Reputation' since he was 'determined, at all Events, to revenge himself on Dr *Sharpin*, for refusing to consult with him' on this and a previous occasion. With an air of candour, the authors insisted that they had 'endeavoured to avoid all Heat and Acrimony, which such injurious Treatment is apt to excite'.[35]

Norford's reply began with an air of pained innocence and injured friendship, paying elaborate compliments to the academic education of Sharpin. He was astonished that the suggestion of joint consultation had been met with a complaint of the indignity of consulting with a non-graduate: 'how hard it was to be joined with one who was not regularly educated; and that it had cost you so much more for your education than it had done me'. Stressing the authority of his licence from the College, Norford expressed the familiar belief that 'no person, who had undergone such an examination, was ever before thought unworthy to be admitted into a consultation'. Since they had previously consulted together, when Sharpin had 'behaved like a Gentleman, with great candor, and good nature', Norford suggested that the surgeon, Steward, was responsible for the change. Although he expressed respect for Sharpin, Norford was able to turn the advantages of academic education against a man who admitted being unable to 'stoop so low' as to practise chemistry. Norford claimed to have 'spent whole days and nights in proving the truth of those things, by experiment, which you only have read in books and consider'd in theory'. The physician's gentlemanly upbringing left him unable to diagnose what Norford claimed had been not piles but severe constipation since he had a 'disposition too nice certainly to inspect, much more to touch a business of such a nature'. For all the scorn and invective which he heaped upon his two critics, Norford ended with an expression of concern that he had been 'obliged to a dispute of this kind, with a person I wish'd to live in friendship with – which you are sensible, can't end to the advantage of either of us'. He hoped that partisans would not alter their good opinions of either party but the impartial would

[35] E. Sharpin and T. Steward, *An Appeal to the Public in General, and to the Gentlemen of the Faculty in Particular* (Bury St Edmunds, 1764), pp. 3–4 and 14–15.

consider him 'not the aggressor; but involuntarily drawn into this disagreeable altercation'.[36]

Steward's response flung accusations of 'Malice, Revenge, Falshood, and Ill-nature', insisting that 'Mr *Norford's* Expressions are indecent, and unbecoming a *Gentleman*; his Behaviour insolent to Persons of Education, and regular in their Profession'. He turned back the suggestion of aggression on to Norford, insisting that the original offence lay in his 'imprudent Behaviour, and *calumniating Reports*' which had forced his opponents to publish. This solo contribution by Steward tacitly excluded lay opinion, as the first pamphlet had not. He appealed only to 'the Gentlemen of the Faculty, who are proper Judges where the *Fault* lies; We still rest our Cause upon their Arbitration . . .' He only troubled the public with another pamphlet because 'out of Justice to our Reputations, I ought to clear them from his *slanderous* and *false Asperations*'. Even the patient, despite being an apothecary, 'was not a Judge of his own Case, could know nothing of it, but what Mr *Norford* imposed upon him . . . '.[37]

The non-graduate general practitioner survived to establish a monopoly in due course but Bury seems to have been a contracting medical market-place since the late seventeenth century. The proximity of larger gentry centres and the mobility of patients and physicians led to a decline in Bury's importance as a source of medical services. The three disputants had previously had successful practices in smaller towns but they had been attracted to Bury only to find that there were few pickings to be had, even if it was easier to gain a foothold than it had been for Messenger Monsey. Under such circumstances, relative status was crucial to success and reputations were easily damaged. In Oxford, where competition was especially fierce, one physician accused another of wrong diagnosis, harmful prescription and deceitful behaviour, so a dispute about etiquette and credit for the cure broke out. The accusation was 'of so serious a nature, and has been circulated with such inconceivable industry, all round the country, that I have been called upon from various quarters, to vindicate myself in as public a manner as I possibly can'. Despite being aware of the insignificance of 'the little contentions between a couple of country Doctors about a private case', one of the physicians felt forced 'to rescue myself out of this torment of obloquy' by stating the circumstances and appealing to

[36] W. Norford, *A Letter to Dr. Sharpin* (Bury St Edmunds, 1764), pp. 7–10, 14, 30–1 and 61–2.

[37] T. Steward, *An Appendix to the Appeal, &c* (Bury St Edmunds, 1764), pp. 4–5 and 19–20. I am grateful to Pat Murrell for drawing this dispute to my attention and supplying me with photocopies of the scarce pamphlets.

the reader's 'judgement and candour which of us had the greatest reason to complain'.[38]

Even a distinguished London surgeon could be drawn into an unseemly squabble with country practitioners in order to scotch discreditable rumours. A surgeon-apothecary of Windsor, George Aylett, had urged William Bromfield to let him share in an amputation, contrary to the patient's wishes,

> and mention'd some particulars of the many enemies he had in that place, who would report things greatly to his prejudice if he should not perform a part at least in the operation: particularly that if any accident happened at *Eton* School, the masters might think meanly of a man who was not equal to an operation of that kind; but was obliged to send to *London*.

Following a disagreement about etiquette precipitated by the patient's refusal to see the local surgeon after the operation, Bromfield was induced to sign an apology drafted by Aylett. 'Dr *Lucas* observed it was much the best way, to reconcile matters in an amicable manner, as all dispute of this nature injur'd the profession . . .' Bromfield was startled to find copies of the letter '*with additions* transmitted to every coffee-house and ale-house in town and country, by agents employ'd for that purpose'. The story was also being spread by other country surgeons, 'intending to prejudice me with my brethren'. Thus although publishing first, Bromfield took care to appear hesitant in the extreme, lest he appear the aggressor in a conflict with a mere minnow:

> Application to the publick in matters of private concern, is, I am sensible, in itself extremely wrong, and particularly where few can be supposed judges of the cause of controversy. For this reason, and to prevent scandal to a profession which has always suffer'd by disputes among its members, I would gladly have avoided publishing any thing on the present occasion . . .

Indeed, Bromfield's London colleagues were 'pleased to think I should not have condescended to do it'. The *Monthly Review* deplored his involvement, although sympathetic to his reasons, however unprofessional his actions were.[39]

Aylett's reply was addressed to the Court of Assistants of the Company of Surgeons, whom he suggested might provide an authoritative arbitration, since 'the company of London Surgeons cannot be supposed indifferent to the issue of any dispute, in which the honour of the profession is interested'. He seems to have taken no steps to initiate

[38] J. S. [mith], *A Letter to J. K.[elly], M.D., With an Account of the Case of Mr. T[aunto]n of the City of O[xfor]d* (Oxford, 1765), pp. 4–5 and 18.

[39] William Bromfield, *A Narrative of Certain Particular Facts Which have been Misrepresented . . .* (London, 1759), pp. 5, 9, 22, 32 and 36–7; *Monthly Review* 21 (1759), p. 536.

such a procedure, which would almost certainly have favoured the influential London surgeon. Unusually, the patient entered the fray, publishing a pamphlet which charged Aylett with cruelty and incompetence. He was unimpressed by the professional quarrel:

> *The punctilio's of business* might in many cases raise a warm dispute between you and Mr Bromfield, but they don't affect the present controversy between you and me. They are nothing to the purpose unless you can first prove, that a patient has no right to appoint his own surgeon.

Aylett mocked the amputee as ungrateful and disbelieved his claim not to be fully well: 'He has long been well enough to travel through two or three counties, with a chaise full of his pamphlets, hawking and distributing them about the country, and at horse-races, in order to blacken my reputation . . .'[40]

As might be expected, Kirkpatrick at the *Monthly Review* supported the patient against Aylett, who was seen as tenacious of honour rather than dignity, which was damaged by 'Illiberal sarcasms', although he began to lose patience with the resentfulness of both men. The *Critical Review*, on the other hand, supported Aylett wholeheartedly against Bromfield.[41] The Tory surgeons of the provinces had as good reason to distrust the London surgical grandees as Baylies had to distrust Oliver. They dominated teaching, appointments and hospital admissions, engrossing much of the most lucrative work. When Henry Bracken suggested clinical trials in every county for Joanna Stephens's cure for the stone, he was derided as having a higher regard for the opinion of country practitioners than for the judgement of the learned gentlemen of London. Bracken hinted at London credulity with a reference to Mary Tofts and her rabbits. Dale Ingram, who had practised in Reading, compared London surgeons unfavourably with country surgeons.[42]

The pretensions to gentility and literary prowess of a surgeon like John Ranby could be mercilessly mocked when he tried to combine case-notes, panegyric and self-exculpation.[43] Ranby, Hawkins and

40 George Aylett, *A Genuine State of a Case in Surgery* (London, 1759), pp. 1 and 35; Joseph Benwell, *A Letter to Mr. George Aylett* (London, 1760), p. 38; G. Aylett, *A Full Reply to a Letter Under the name of Joseph Benwell of Eton* (London, 1760), pp. 43 and 50.

41 *Monthly Review* 21 (1759), p. 537; 23, (1760), pp. 329–30; *Critical Review* 8 (1759), pp. 498–9.

42 Henry Bracken, *Lithiasis Anglicana* (London, 1739), pp. 2–3 and 29–30; Omnelio Pitcairne, *The Truth Unvail'd for the Publick Good, or a Treatise of the Stone* (London, 1739), p. 11; Dale Ingram, *Practical Cases and Observations in Surgery* (London, 1731), pp. xxii–xxvi. I am collecting material for a study of the Joanna Stephens controversy.

43 John Ranby, *A Narrative of the Last Illness of the Right Honorable the Earl of Oxford* (London, 1745); 'A Physician', *An Expostulatory Address to John Ranby Esq.* (London, 1745); *Advice to John Ranby, Esq.* (London, 1745).

Bromfield dominated the medical scene only partly through their technical excellence. Their connections at Court gave them considerable patronage, as at Chelsea Hospital. The surgeon from the Royal Hospital at Greenwich, Samuel Lee, complained bitterly at the dealings of Ranby and Hawkins with him. Tangled defamation and perjury cases ensued, but Lee felt his reputation was threatened by 'the Interest and Vanity of some dignified Professors' who had employed both rumour and writing against him. Whatever the truth of the matter, 'finding all private Avenues to Redress closed against him, [Lee] thought it might not be deemed impertinent to submit a fair and candid Account of the whole Proceedings to the Judgement of the Public . . .'.[44] The price that these Court surgeons had to pay for their power was a prostitution of their honour to political necessity, as when Bromfield and Ranby secured a signed statement from John Foot about a man who died following an election riot. Ranby promised on his honour that it should not be shown to anyone other than the Duke of Grafton and Lord Rochford, but it was spread round town, with the interpretation that Foot had changed his mind, in the campaign to reprieve the convicted murderer. Bromfield stated on his honour that a fever, not the blow on the head, was the cause of death. Foot complained that his reputation had been sacrificed for the benefit of a political party. Dale Ingram, criticising Foot, also made use of the rhetoric of 'the tribunal of the public'.[45]

The political divisions of eighteenth-century society affected all aspects of medical theory and practice, to varying degrees, but in most circumstances no resolution of a conflict could be expected before the death or departure of the individuals involved. One of the few contexts in which some kind of settlement seemed necessary was hospital practice. Internecine disputes could fester for years, but a *modus vivendi* had to be found. The surgeons lost their argument with the physicians about admissions to the Bristol Infirmary in the 1770s, but they withdrew cooperation and forced the physicians to concede victory.[46] No hospital organisation was free from political and religious pressures. The ideological divisions tended to reinforce professional divisions, making them virtually intractable, most famously at

[44] Samuel Lee, *A Proper Reply to the Serjeant Surgeons Defence of Their Conduct at Chelsea Hospital* (London, 1754), pp. 3–4.

[45] John Foot, *An Appeal to the Public Touching the Death of Mr. George Clark*, second edition (London, 1769), pp. 7, 30, 38, 49 and 51; [Dale Ingram] *The Blow, or an Inquiry into the Causes of the Late Mr. Clarke's Death* (London, 1769), p. 44.

[46] George Munro Smith, *A History of the British Royal Infirmary* (Bristol, 1917), pp. 107–12. I am grateful to Irvine Loudon for this reference.

Manchester, where the hospital posts were divided between established Tory surgical families and physicians who were reforming Dissenters and Whigs.[47] Out of the conflict at Manchester emerged the *Medical Ethics* of Thomas Percival, first published in 1792 to provide a workable set of rules for infirmary practice. Percival attempted to codify relations in the traditional tripartite division that had always been only a rough guide to actual medical practice, which is why he pays considerable attention to the vexed problems of joint consultation.[48]

Percival's insistence that medical disputes should be referred to arbitration and not made public can best be understood in the context of his stern criticism of duelling and notions of honour.[49] The quasi-legal ideology which Percival sought to establish had many purposes, among them the minimising of party conflict, the establishing of the senior physician's primacy, regardless of what university he had attended, and the paying of due respect to rural general practitioners. Eliminating notions of honour was an essential part of the programme, for political as well as religious reasons. Percival represented the aspirations of moderate non-conformists, seeking to achieve parity of status and respect with graduates of Oxford and Cambridge. Gentry patterns of behaviour could have no place in his system of ethics.

The 'dyadic interaction' of medical disputes was suited to confrontations over honour rather than competition for property, even though the shaming rituals employed, the appeals to a gentlemanly code, were directed at public opinion since the patronage of patients or the control of hospital posts was the property for which the disputants were actually competing. It was always recognised that pamphlet attacks should be written with due decorum – Richard Boulton was cut off from influential patrons for being too intemperate in his criticism of Charles Leigh – but authors found it difficult to restrain their passions.[50] Their reputations and their livelihoods were at stake.

During the eighteenth century, Whig ideologies of dispassionate conduct became increasingly authoritative, building on the Restora-

[47] J. V. Pickstone and S. V. Butler, 'The Politics of Medicine in Manchester, 1788–1792: Hospital Reform and Public Health Services in the Early Industrial City', *Medical History* 28 (1984), pp. 227–49.

[48] Ivan Waddington, *The Medical Profession in the Industrial Revolution* (Dublin, 1984), pp. 153–75, Thomas Percival, *Medical Ethics* (Manchester, 1803), pp. 19–21, 34–7 and 50–1. Charles Webster has reminded me that Percival's work had been gestating for several years prior to the Infirmary dispute but it seems clear to me that its first printing was brought about by the crisis. [49] Percival, *Medical Ethics*, pp. 46 and 87–95.

[50] British Library, Sloane MS 4037, f. 170; Richard Boulton, *A Letter to Dr. Charles Goodall* (London, 1699).

tion attack on 'enthusiasm'. The *Monthly Review* expressed a view of disputes that sprang from the ideology of a dominant group when it criticised the conduct of a quarrel between Giles Watts and Thomas Frewen:

> One great end of science is to enlarge the mind, and remove all contracted views; but this is, in a great measure, defeated, when men of learning descend to personal altercations, and more especially when they stoop so low as to employ means, either to serve their own private interest, or prejudice that of another, which the honest mechanic would be ashamed of.[51]

The medical ethics of the early nineteenth century sought to eliminate the embarrassing public wrangles which had formerly served to define collective attitudes. It explained and defined practice from the viewpoint of dominant groups but it also gave expression to the aspirations of some of the rising groups, which had precipitated eighteenth-century disputes. Neither the individual conflicts nor the ideology which sought to control them can be understood without reference to the relative status and economic strength of the groups involved.

Once stated, such a conclusion acquires the appearance of a truism, yet eighteenth-century medical disputes, especially those concerned with Bath, have been seriously misunderstood over and over again. A good example is provided by the most frequently discussed professional dispute in eighteenth-century English medicine, that between William Withering and the young Robert Darwin. Historians have felt obliged to take the side of one of the protagonists, as if the dispute was primarily about correct clinical judgement. A recent author on Withering's career has at last recognised that the dispute was actually about behaviour and that it is impossible to tell from their letters, 'which are equally vituperative on both sides, which of them, if either, was in the right in this case'. Thanks to the survival of some of Erasmus Darwin's letters touching on the dispute, it has long been clear that the father was at work behind the scenes, gathering anecdotes to support his son's attack on Withering, to whom this activity appears to have been disclosed by Dr Edward Johnstone. Both Darwin and Matthew Boulton were embarrassed by the extent of Withering's information. Although it is true the two luminaries of the Lunar Society had fallen out already, the texture of the dispute is best understood in the context of the other pamphlets discussed in this chapter. Robert Darwin complained that the failure to consult was made more serious by subsequent slander, which he suggested was a regular recourse of Withering,

[51] *Monthly Review* 13 (1755), p. 307.

among the other mean arts by which you attempt to support your business . . . I know that slandering others of the faculty is a cool, deliberate, and determined system which you have adopted . . . A business must be rapidly on the decline which requires such arts to support it.

Withering was critical of the printing of letters, since 'nothing is more foolish or ridiculous, than individuals making their private quarrels the subject of public attention' although it would allow the issue to 'be adjudged by our Peers'. When he published the bulk of the dispute, in the form of an *Appeal to the Faculty*, Robert Darwin was especially infuriated by Withering's self-satisfaction, which he compared to 'the boasting of a stage Charlatan', by his alleged use of rumour, and by his condescension in calling 'the greatest insult it was in your power to offer me, a *breach of ceremony*, and a gross and malignant slander, a *difference of opinion*'. Even if the roots of the quarrel lay elsewhere, a young practitioner such as Robert Darwin had no recourse except to the familiar rhetoric of the dispute of honour as practised by medical men throughout provincial England.[52]

This brief study has broken little new ground, implicitly relying on such familiar parameters as relationship between disputants, grievance type, dispute process and sanction. Future studies of this material might usefully consider dispute pamphlets as a literary genre, directed to a specific audience of patrons. Provincial newspapers contain examples of similar disputes, although it is often difficult to follow their progress. One might also compare medical quarrels with those conducted by clergy or with the formal disputes conducted by medical men in more highly regulated countries.[53] The context and language of insult is beginning to be explored by historians and should provide a new foundation for considering the importance of reputation outside

[52] J. K. Aronson, *An Account of the Foxglove and its Medical Uses, 1785–1985* (Oxford, 1985), p. 260; *The Letters of Erasmus Darwin*, ed. Desmond King-Hele (Cambridge, 1981), pp. 182–9; T. Whitmore Peck and K. Douglas Wilkinson, *William Withering of Birmingham* (Bristol, 1950), pp. 97–122; R. W. Darwin, *Appeal to the Faculty Concerning the Case of Mrs. Houlston* (Shrewsbury, 1789), pp. 4–5, 10, 26–7 and 43–5; E. Posner, 'William Withering Versus the Darwins'. *History of Medicine* 6 (1975), pp. 51–7. I am grateful to Dorothy Porter for sending this article to me.

[53] *A Letter to the Reverend Dr. Lowth* (London, 1768); Neast Havard, *A Narrative of the Origin and Progress of the Prosecution against the Rev. Edward Evanson* (London, 1778); *The Defence of the Rev. Reginald Bligh* (London, 1780); Alvar Martinez Vidal, 'La vinculación de Andrés Piquer al Hospital General de Valencia', *Medicina & Historia* 20 (1987), pp. 1–16. I am grateful to the author for sending me this article and to Johanna Geyer-Kordesch and Larry Brockliss for comments on the methods of resolving disputes employed by German and French practitioners.

the duelling classes.[54] Although such approaches have scarcely been touched upon in the present study, it is possible to make some tentative observations on the structure of conflict between medical practitioners in eighteenth-century England.

Precipitating factors often involved unfamiliar issues, such as hospital practice or man-midwifery or general practice, which posed a threat to the status and power of elite groups accustomed to maintaining an appearance of non-competitive activity. In the absence of any likelihood of actual violence, there was no restraint on the level of hostility and dispute behaviour did not exorcise the grievances, which were apt to be remembered for many years. Bromfield's critics reminded the public of his behaviour towards Aylett, ten years after the dispute had taken place. Moreover, the unrestrained hostility of medical practitioners was satisfied only by the death or departure of an opponent. It was silenced only by the disapproval of peers, although there was an abiding tension for practitioners of higher status between the shame of silence and the shame of disputing with inferiors. Despite having roots in economic rationality, the disputes were couched in the language of honour and conflicting notions of professional integrity. The development of new economic relationships and new strategies of practice, the wider distribution of a variety of credible qualifications and the desire of a widening circle of consumers to receive cures from a reputable source were all factors which increased uncertainties about the value of hierarchies of social stratification within medicine.

[54] Peter Burke, *The Historical Anthropology of Early Modern Italy* (Cambridge, 1987), pp. 95–109; David Garrioch, 'Verbal Insults in Eighteenth-Century Paris' in P. Burke and R. Porter (eds.), *The Social History of Language* (Cambridge, 1987), pp. 104–19; Thomas Brennan, *Public Drinking and Popular Culture in Eighteenth-Century Paris* (Princeton, 1988), pp. 20–75.

Appendix: Henry Bracken's dispute in 1747–8

In this chapter, disputes have been given cursory treatment since the pamphlets involved are fairly lengthy. The example reproduced below is representative but relatively concise, and it is only known from the slightly abbreviated transcript printed by an antiquarian in the *Preston Guardian* of 4 September 1880.

Henry Bracken was a physician, surgeon and man-midwife in Lancaster. His career is outlined in the *Dictionary of National Biography*, although he is mistakenly credited with an MD. Apart from his non-graduate status, his most important characteristic was his staunch Toryism, which had led to his being imprisoned during the investigation of the 1745 rebellion. His interrogators were a Whig clergyman and a Whig physician. Although his son died of gaol fever, Bracken recovered his standing and was made mayor in 1748.

Bracken's opponent, Preston Christopherson, was a young man, aged about thirty-five at the time. The son of a Cumberland vicar, he had been educated at St John's College, Cambridge, before becoming a Fellow of Pembroke. Whereas Bracken was a Tory alderman, Christopherson was a Whig common councillor. The main patient mentioned, Thomas Butterfield, was a wealthy Whig merchant and apothecary whose family had been prominent in Lancaster non-conformist circles for many years. He is mentioned in Stout's diary and his father, twice mayor, is mentioned in Tyldesley's diary. Christopherson's colleague, George Carlisle, was a graduate of Leyden who practised at Kendal. The only MD here mentioned, he was probably a non-conformist.

The Dr White of Manchester recommended by Bracken was Thomas White, father of the more famous Charles White. He had trained as a surgeon in London, was an extra-licentiate of the College of Physicians, and practised as a physician-surgeon. He was a Tory. Mrs Sarah Haresnape was a Lancaster midwife whose evidence was called by Bracken when he acted as coroner in a case of infanticide in August 1748. She thought the child had been born alive at full term. Thomas Worthington was a member of the Catholic family of medical practitioners who dominated the Wigan area after the Restoration. His father and brother are mentioned in Nicholas Blundell's Diurnal.

This dispute contains two important strands, the political division between Whigs and Tories, commonly reinforced by religious differences, and the professional division between the older surgeon-physicians and the swelling ranks of graduates. Bracken was a well-known author who had been persecuted by his Whig opponents. Christopherson was precisely the sort of practitioner he had always detested, although historians have generally focused only on his remarks about incompetent midwives. Here he expresses the widespread contempt of practical medical men for mere theoreticians as well as the concomitant anxiety about paper qualifications.

Men like Bracken were being supplanted as general practitioners by surgeon-apothecaries but his account of his own training gives an idealised view of this type of medical man. It has not proved possible to corroborate the autobiographical details as yet. Bracken's papers seem to have disappeared since the late eighteenth century.

TO PRESTON CHRISTOPHERSON, M.B., A.P.S., IN LANCASTER.

Sir, – I received your printed letter to me, wherein you complain of injuries, aspersions, and what not, offered (in a clandestine manner) by me against your character; I suppose you mean your character as a physician; and if this is the case, I might undertake to make out everything that I at any time might express relating to your practice. And for you, such a junior, to pretend to call me to account, is very odd, for I am ready to shew that, although you may be a Fellow of Pembroke Hall, yet you are but a silly Fellow, by reason your letter is full of little else besides vain boasting and self-conceited ignorance. It is not the number of mystical letters following your Name, and thrown after you by the College, that can make you a true Physician. No, no, Sir, I have been at the proper schools for such purpose, and where many young gentlemen, as really wise as you pretend to, from Oxford and Cambridge, thought it necessary to come to finish their studies, well knowing that no such opportunities offered in England, Wales, or Berwick-on-Tweed; no, not even in Scotland itself. But to the point.

Mr. *Kirkby* was killed by a fall from his Horse, it is plain; but how you and Dr. Carlisle could be well assured his Skull was perfectly safe, is something extraordinary, because there are *fissures* as well as *fractures* and contusions, you should know; and therefore you are only a Novice in cases of surgery; and I cannot help thinking but that the operation of the trepan might have prolonged his life, notwithstanding you may be a stranger to the reason why it might be so.

Secondly, as to the paragraph in the St. James's Evening Post, which you hint at as false, scandalous and malicious, I believe it is false in respect to that part you mention, of the Surgeons giving their opinion, &c., but the true MSS. I now tell you ran thus, viz., 'but the Surgeons are of opinion', &c., so you should have first inquired whether the Author or the Printer was wrong, before you vented your invective. In fine, I am well satisfied that Mr. Kirkby's case was more a case of surgery than physick, and that it was a piece of pride and presumption in you not to hear a better opinion than your own.

The next thing you mention is the case of the late Mr. *Thomas Butterfield*, a person whom I had a great esteem for, notwithstanding Party divisions, and disputes about Elections, had prevented that intimacy that otherwise might have subsisted between us; and it is my opinion you had much better have let that affair been buried in oblivion; for when I was applied to, he was in the very last stage of a dropsy, and by your directions had drunk such large quantities of cold water, along with a course of soapy medicines, that it was not possible to set him to rights; and therefore, you saying my myrmidons spread it abroad that I had performed a cure, must be a victim of your own brain . . . You say farther relating to Mr. Butterfield, that four physicians were employed, amongst whom you had the honour to be one, and that I disregarded everything that had been done by men much better than myself; but this is only one Doctor's opinion, and I take that doctor to be no judge of the matter, so shall rest it here, and pass to what you insinuate about Mrs. G—, the plain truth of which is as follows:

Mrs. G—t had been your patient many months, but as to a fever, I never heard she had any whilst under your care: therefore am apt to believe you often fancy strange things, and prescribe accordingly . . . Mrs. G—t only asked my opinion the morning she left Lancaster, and I told her she had the dropsy. Accordingly I writ to Mr. Walmsley, of Wigan, where she was going, that Dr. White of Manchester was a proper person to be employed; and that as to the course of medicines she had been under at Lancaster, I was an entire stranger to; so pray, why are you displeased at my recommending a person more likely to do her service than you, that never told her the true cause of her illness, nor ever found a name for her distemper?. . I must now answer your charge relating Mrs. R—n, and tell you in plain terms you are the author of falsehood; for I never uttered anything like the substance of what you say, nor do I take it for granted that Mrs. Haresnape, or any other midwife, is able to state a case sufficient to ground prescription upon, notwithstanding I dare venture to affirm that Mrs. Haresnape knew Mrs. R—'s case much better than yourself, who compared the swelling of the stomach to a swelled face in the tooth-ache; – fy, fy, Doctor, burn your books and begin *de novo*.

Thirdly and lastly, I must be obliged to tell you that you are only a mere Harlequin in physics, and that, although you may be dubbed Bachelor of Physic at Cambridge, yet you may return thither *re infecta*, and therefore the best judges in the Kingdom, according to your own words, must have turned you out too soon of your Dadling strings, and that you entertain a better opinion of yourself than others do, that have experienced your prescriptions, excepting a few fiddle-faddle folks, who stand in no more need of a physician than I do of your instruction or recommendation, because *exigi monumentum* – but where yours is, the Lord above knows; however, lest I should be thought behind you in education, let me acquaint you with mine, as you have done me the favour to tell me yours, for it is irksome to me to dispute with you about people yet living.

First, then, I began my Education under Mr. *Bordley*, Schoolmaster at Lancaster (who, I fancy, was as good a scholar as your Mr. *Yates* of Appleby, excepting the French Language), and finished my School-Learning under the late Rev. Mr. *Thomas Holmes*, a very ingenious and good man. After this, I was six years with the late Dr. *Thomas Worthington* (commonly called Worton) of Wigan, a Man known through the kingdom, for his Physical and other performances in the art of healing; under him, I had the opportunity of seeing a very extensive practice, and a great variety of cases, and courses of chemistry were frequently performed by good hands in a Laboratory he built for the purpose; to these were added the advantage of an excellent Library, that contained the works of most of the learned men in all ages of the Profession; so that Dr. Worthington's pupils had the advantage of studying the history of Diseases, and seeing the operation of Medicines upon human bodies, at one and the same time, while you young Cantabs only run over the theory, and fancy you can turn the Moon with your heels. From Dr. Worthington I went to London, with design to perfect myself in the knowledge of Anatomy, &c.; but when I came to inquire at St. Thomas's Hospital and other places, I found there were few dead subjects allowed for dissection this was about thirty years ago, so I contented myself for three months with looking on at the said Hospital, and attending to the practice of Dr. *Wadsworth* and Dr. Plumtree, to whom I was recommended by my very sincere and good friend Roger Braddyll, Esq., an East India Merchant; after this I went over to Paris and attended the hospitals there, but more particularly the Hospital called the Hotel de Dieu, which place you must be a stranger to, or you would not vaunt yourself on that Hospital in miniature which you have mentioned; because in the Hotel de Dieu there are seldom less than 3,000 sick Patients, whereas 400 is higher than you ever saw at the other, not to mention the opportunities of attending many more in Paris, much superior to Bartholomew's Guy's, the London Infirmary, &c., where you was a-dabbling.

The dissection of diseased dead bodies must give the greatest insight into the cure of distempers, provided a man makes good use of his time, and has a well-turned head; and, where I attended, we had fifteen or twenty bodies every day during the cooler months, that is, from September till March inclusive; and lectures many times a day upon different parts of human bodies; so that we abroad are not put to the pitiful shifts of stealing half-rotten bodies out of their graves, or begging an executed Malefactor, now and then, from a Sheriff. No, no, 'tis better, when the war is over, for you to go and see things as I have, and you'll then own the folly of your expressions, and ingenuously acknowledge that before such time you knew nothing, which is what I have several times heard owned by gentlemen from Oxford and Cambridge that I saw at Paris, pursuing the like study with myself. It would be too tedious for me to relate to you the superior advantages we have at Paris, with respect to many branches of the profession, though their Physic Schools are the least worth attending; however, a Bee will gather honey from a— —, and therefore we ought to try all, and stick to that which is best.

From Paris I travelled to that ever-memorable Man, Professor *Boerhaave* of Leyden, and attended his lectures eighteen months, and saw much of his private Practice, and have had the honour to prescribe in his presence to some of his patients, and he dictated to me when he found necessary. From this great Physician and true philosopher, I came back to London, and was a second time, several months attending the practice of two Ingenious Men I have mentioned before, in order to form a judgement between our Home-way of prescribing, and that which I have seen abroad; wherefore, thus qualified (most magnificent Doctor) I entered into the Profession, tho' I will not say perfectly qualified, as you do because I should not run counter to the first aphorism of Hippocrates; however, I wish you would read, mark, learn, and inwardly digest this my Admonition, and you'll see what time you have lost in travelling much at home to no purpose, as well as the necessity there is of you taking upon you such a journey as I did, and of creating the like acquaintance; for you make the noble Art of Healing more a Trade than a Science, and consequently you prescribe more for your own and the Apothecary's gain, than the Patients' health, otherwise you have no occasion to dangle so much after people in imaginary illnesses.

P.S. – Your Postscript is so low and mean that it is scarce worth any notice, and your dispersing your printed Letter among your own set of creatures cannot at all affect me; for when any of your patients are at a dead Lift, I am almost sure of a good Fee, though, indeed, some of them die hard I must own; therefore, finally, take this from me, viz., You resemble the Scholar in the fable that threw away his corks before he had sufficiently learned to swim. – HENRY BRACKEN.

Lancaster, Feb. 10, 1747–8

7

Medicine, morality and the politics of Berkeley's tar-water

MARINA BENJAMIN

You see, Hylas, the water of yonder fountain, how it is forced upwards, in a round column, to a certain height; at which it breaks and falls back into the basin from whence it rose: its ascent as well as descent, proceeding from the same uniform law or principle of gravitation. Just so, the same principles which at first view lead to scepticism, pursued to a certain point, bring men back to common sense.

Berkeley, *Three Dialogues Between Hylas and Philonous* (1713), the third dialogue.

In 1744 Bishop Berkeley (1685–1753) published *Siris: A Chain of Philosophical Reflections and Inquiries Concerning the Virtues of Tar-Water and Divers Other Subjects Connected Together and Arising One from Another*, his last and most sophisticated major composition. While *Siris* deals with medicine, philosophy, natural philosophy and theology, it is most often celebrated for its introduction of tar-water – an unlikely cordial of water impregnated with pine rosin – as a universal remedy. Not only did Berkeley suspect that tar-water was a panacea, but he also believed that its 'virtues are divine'.[1] The term 'divine' offers a key to the interpretation of *Siris* as a coherent and mature text, for *Siris* represents Berkeley's attempt to provide the High Church with a Trinitarian natural philosophy. We will see that what has been described as 'an old man's ramble through quack remedies to Elysian fields'[2] was a text deliberately designed to undermine the version of natural philosophy which Berkeley ascribed to Newton's followers. This version, based on Newton's statements about an aether published in the 1717 *Opticks*, involved an account of God's role in the

Acknowledgement: My thanks to Simon Schaffer, Geoffrey Cantor and Michael Barfoot for their advice and comments on this chapter.

[1] *The Works of George Berkeley, Bishop of Cloyne*, ed. A. A. Luce and T. E. Jessop, for the *Bibliotheca Britannica Philosophica*, 9 vols. (London/Edinburgh, 1948–57); hereafter *Works*. From the poem 'On Tar' in vol. 5, p. 225.

[2] T. E. Jessop, 'Is there a Berkeleian Philosophy?', *Hermathena* 1 (1936), p. 197. A more sympathetic treatment of *Siris* can be found in the Introduction to *Works*, vol. 5.

natural world, which according to Berkeley was a direct invitation to atheist materialism.

A cursory glance at the secondary literature reveals that traditional interpretations of Berkeley's writings classically demonstrate the stranglehold of today's anachronistic disciplinary boundaries. Berkeley is almost exclusively read as a philosopher, according to modern-day usage of the term, and his later works are usually seen through the lenses of his early idealist theories.[3] While philosophers intent on separating text from context have paid little attention to history, historians in turn have radically underestimated the hostility which a possible materialism could engender. Berkeley's antipathy towards Newtonian materialism has persistently been dismissed or ignored, most significantly by historians of matter theory.[4]

I would like to offer a reading of *Siris* as Berkeley's ultimate stand in response to the High Anglican cry of 'Church in danger',[5] seeking not to privilege the Bishop's theological commitments over his philosophical ideas, but rather to suggest that these two categories were inseparable. Such a reading provides a framework within which to interpret all Berkeley's work, recommends a revaluation of his juvenilia composed before 1713, and serves as a means of understanding the way in which the various themes in *Siris* are connected. Taking *Siris* seriously as a medical text goes hand in hand with recognising that the medical men were generally perceived to be in the vanguard of atheism and materialism; men like Porterfield, Whytt, Cullen and Monro, for example, had continually to rebut this accusation. And taking tar-water seriously as a medicine entails acknowledging that its significance far exceeded that of a simple remedy or fashionable drink, for in the natural-philosophical basis of tar-water's effectiveness, Berkeley saw a means of combating materialist irreligion.

THE RELATION OF 'SIRIS' TO BERKELEY'S EARLIER WORK

As a High Churchman and Tory, Berkeley was deeply opposed to what he saw as the natural-theological consequences of a Newtonian ma-

[3] *Essays on the Philosophy of George Berkeley*, ed. Ernest Sosa (Dordrecht; Lancaster, 1987); A. C. Grayling, *Berkeley: the Central Arguments* (London, 1986); *Essays on Berkeley, A Tercentennial Celebration*, ed. John Foster and Howard Robinson (Oxford, 1985); John T. Richetti, *Philosophical Writing: Locke, Berkeley, Hume* (Cambridge, MA, 1983). An exception is *George Berkeley: Essays and Replies*, ed. David Berman (Dublin, 1986).

[4] For example, Arnold Thackray, in tracing the development of matter theory in the eighteenth century maintains, 'Berkeley's own radical idealist theories cannot concern us here, except to note their Newtonian filiations', *Atoms and Powers* (Oxford, 1970), p. 245.

[5] Steven Shapin, 'Of Gods and Kings', *Isis* 72 (1981), pp. 187–215. See pp. 202–5.

terialism, which had become allied to the Whiggery and, in his opinion infidelity, of the Latitudinarian Low Church.[6] We will see later that such natural philosophy could be used to deny the existence of the Trinity. For Berkeley, deists and freethinkers like John Toland, Matthew Tindal and Anthony Collins, who favoured the use of reason over revelation in Biblical exegesis, exemplified the political threat of Newtonian natural philosophy at its most base level. The Whig radical John Toland, who looked upon Newton's discoveries achieved independently of revelation and tradition as being paramount exemplars of Lockean rationalism, frequently cited Newton in his *Letters to Serena* (1704) to lend support to his claim that 'Motion is essential to matter no less than extension.'[7] By attributing activity to matter, Toland defied Newton's insistence on the primacy of force and dispensed with the need to invoke God's intervention in the maintenance of the natural world. He argued by analogy that the social order was no more God-given than the natural order: 'none is born a Divine, Philosopher, or Politician, therefore every man at the beginning stands on the same ground as the vulgar'[8]. Thus Toland saw in immanentism, the doctrine that motion is inherent in matter, a natural-philosophical justification for his deism and republican politics.

Berkeley initiated his challenge to the deists in *A Treatise Concerning the Principles of Human Knowledge* (1710) where he argued that matter was simply an idea and consequently passive, claiming triumphantly: 'Atheists are forever silenced upon supposing only spirits and ideas.'[9] This optimistic conclusion is not unconnected to the fact that the Tories, who were concerned to preserve the sanctity of the Church of England, enjoyed considerable power during Anne's reign which enabled them to legislate against Dissent. In 1711 they managed to implement the Occasional Conformity Bill, and in 1714 the Schism Act

[6] For alliance between Newtonians and Low Church see Larry Stewart, 'Samuel Clarke, Newtonianism and the Factions of Post-Revolutionary England', *Journal of the History of Ideas* 32 (1981), pp. 53–73; Shapin, 'Of Gods and Kings'; J. R. Jacob and M. Jacob 'The Anglican Origins of Modern Science: The Metaphysical Foundations of the Whig Constitution', *Isis* 71 (1980), pp. 251–67; M. Jacob, *The Newtonians and the English Revolution 1687–1720* (Cornell, 1976).

[7] John Toland, *Letters to Serena* (New York, 1704), reprinted in facsimile for Garland Publishing Inc., 1976, Preface, Sect. 14. See also R. E. Sullivan, *John Toland and the Deist Controversy* (Cambridge, MA, 1982); H. F. Nicholl, 'John Toland, Religion Without Mystery', *Hermathena* 100 (1965), pp. 54–65; David Berman, 'Anthony Collins; Aspects of His Thought and Writings', *Hermathena* 120 (1975), pp. 49–71.

[8] Toland, *Letters to Serena*, p. 173.

[9] Berkeley, *Principles*, (London, 1710), reprinted in *Berkeley's Philosophical Works*, notes and introduction by M. R. Ayers (London, 1980), section. 133, p. 119.

came into effect.[10] Men of Latitude had difficulty in divesting themselves of all association with the deists and thereby exonerating themselves from the charge of infidelity; their support of natural over revealed religion, and their implied reliance on a Lockean philosophy upon which Whig advocacy of the contract theory and doctrine of resistance rested, meant that the High Church could look upon Latitudinarianism and deism with the same disdain.[11] In 1711 the Low Church Newtonians Samuel Clarke and William Whiston failed in their attempts to convince Tindal and Collins of the truth of established Christianity, and the High Church, who remained convinced that atheism infected the Whig party, extended their charge of atheism to embrace the Newtonian divines. Yet such religious persecution was short-lived, since the Hanoverian succession in 1714 and the failure of the Jacobite rebellion in 1715, placed the Whigs firmly in power. And in the following years, as Chris Wilde has indicated,

> The alliance of Whigs and Latitudinarians continually thwarted the attempts of the High Church party to take effective political action against Deism, Socinianism and anticlericalism and to strengthen the Church against intrusion by dissenters. Because of this Newtonianism could be seen to be implicated in a plot to undermine the true religion of the Church of England.[12]

From Berkeley's viewpoint Latitudinarian Whigs were irredeemably tarred with the brush of Dissent.

Newton's introduction of the 1717 aether, which is widely acknowledged as embodying his bid to extricate himself from Leibniz's charge that gravity was occult, can also be seen as an attempt to deny any similarities between his own natural philosophy and that expounded by the deists. But the materialist treatment of the *Opticks* by Newton's Low Church disciples only compounded Berkeley's belief that the unholy alliance between Whigs and Latitudinarians was responsible for the irreligion and moral corruption of the nation. Berkeley held the materialism and atheism of the Walpole administration to blame for the social turmoil and financial chaos resulting from the failure of the South Sea Scheme. Giving vent to his grievances in *An Essay Towards*

[10] G. M. Trevelyan, *England Under the Stuarts* (London, 1965), see chapter 15. The Occasional Conformity Bill prohibited Dissenters gaining government office. The Schism Act prevented Dissenters from educating their own children. See also, J. P. Kenyon, *Revolution Principles* (Cambridge, 1977).

[11] J. E. Force, *William, Whiston, Honest Newtonian* (Cambridge, 1985); H. T. Dickinson, *Liberty and Property: Political Ideology in Eighteenth Century Britain* (London, 1977); J. Redwood, *Reason, Ridicule and Religion: the Age of Enlightenment in England 1660–1750* (London, 1976).

[12] C. B. Wilde, 'Hutchinsonian Natural Philosophy and Religious Controversy in Eighteenth Century Britain', *History of Science* 18 (1980), pp. 1–24.

Preventing the Ruine of Great Britain (1721) he lamented the fact that the island's inhabitants, once 'a religious, brave, sincere people, of plain uncorrupt manners', had fallen. He complained that

> they degenerated, grew servile flatterers of men in power, adopted Epicurean notions, became venal, corrupt, injurious, which drew upon them the hatred of God and man, and occasioned their final ruin.[13]

Berkeley's religiously inspired philanthropic commitments, evident in the *Essay* and in his later foray into medicine, became the essential motivation behind his ill-fated Bermuda project which involved building a college or seminary dedicated to converting the natives to Protestant Christianity. Berkeley hoped that,

> Rivulets perpetually issuing forth from a Fountain or Reservoir of Learning and Religion, and streaming through all parts of America, must in due time have a great Effect in purging away the ill Manners and Irreligion of our Colonies.[14]

Berkeley may have intended to undo some of the wrongs inflicted on the colonies by the South Sea Company, by heroically rescuing historic Christianity, but his project was not to be realised. Walpole refused to forward a £20,000 grant promised by Parliament for the scheme, thus obliging Berkeley, who had set sail for America three years earlier, to return embittered to London in 1731. In a furious onslaught on Newtonian materialists, now irremediably linked with Walpole in his demonology, *Alciphron* (1732), *The Theory of Vision* (1733) and *The Analyst* (1734) were published by Berkeley in rapid succession.

In 1734 Berkeley returned to his native Ireland upon being appointed Bishop of Cloyne. And although he had not been able to achieve the spiritual, moral and bodily cleansing of the New World, by the 1740s he became aware of the need to institute such a purifying project at home. *Siris* was the culmination of the critical project Berkeley embarked on in 1710 and the reincarnation of the Bermuda project, and tar-water was the redeeming spiritual agent. Berkeley enthused that tar-water 'cheers but not enebriates', producing a 'calm and steady joy like the effect of good news' (p. 217). Tar-water could bring wandering souls back to true religion.

Throughout Berkeley's writings there was a close link between his

[13] Berkeley, *Essay*, in *Works*, vol. 6, pp. 84–5.

[14] Berkeley, *A Proposal for the Better Supplying of Churches in our Foreign Plantations and for Converting the Savage Americans to Christianity* (London, 1724). This work is listed for 1724 in Jessop, *A Bibliography of George Berkeley* (London, 1973); it was included in Berkeley's *Miscellany* (London, 1752). See also Edwin G. Gaustad, *George Berkeley in America* (New Haven, 1979), pp. 49–50; Benjamin Rand, *Berkeley's American Sojourn* (Cambridge, MA, 1932).

religious and political polemic against deist free-thought and its allies, and his epistemological and natural-philosophical attack on materialism. *Siris* was no exception. In 1744 as in 1721, the political climate in Britain was characterised by crises; Tory frustration was at its apogee, for the Whig oligarchy did not fall with Walpole's resignation in 1742, although its leadership still hung in the balance. Furthermore, Jacobite unrest, which was to culminate in the 1745 rebellion, posed an unprecedented threat to Whig hopes of achieving stability.[15] While it is worth pointing to certain continuities in the political scene, it is arguable that Berkeley continued to read the political dramas of the 1740s in terms of an older debate – such historical entrenchment seems a feature of Tory ideology generally. Berkeley's timing did not go unnoticed by one of *Siris's* critics who warned his readers:

> Judge then how dangerous a Commonwealth's-Man this insinuating Writer may prove in a Reform'd Nation; and particularly, at a Time that we are at War with France, and that the Pretender's Son is within Call? It is pretty extraordinary too, that he should chose to publish this his latent Poison, in so very critical a Conjuncture of the present.[16]

The accusation of 'Jacobite', here implied, was the standard Whig term of abuse hurled at Tories and High Church ministers as indiscriminately as the High Church faction branded their enemies 'atheist'. It is in this context of political and theological controversy and polemicism that our discussion of *Siris* must take place, for by the 1740s it was possible for Berkeley to display the Newtonian materialism based on the 1717 *Opticks* as akin to the materialism of the deists and as carrying with it an equivalent threat to revealed religion and Tory politics.

THE MEDICAL TARGET

Siris represents a dark cloud on the Newtonian medical landscape. The starting point from which such a claim gains support lies in a provocative comment Berkeley made in a published letter to his life-long friend and compatriot, Thomas Prior: 'If physicians think they have a right to treat of religious matters, I think I have an equal right to treat of

[15] For a brief account of the political tension in the 1740s see J. H. Plumb, *England in the Eighteenth Century* (Harmondsworth, 1950; 1985), pp. 105–15 and Dickinson, *Liberty and Property*. For a history of Jacobite activity in Britain, Bruce Lenman, *The Jacobite Rising in Britain, 1689–1746* (London, 1980).

[16] *Anti-Siris or English Wisdom Exemplify'd by Various Examples, But Particularly the Present General Demand for Tar-Water, on so Unexceptional Authority as that of a R—t R—d Itinerant Schemist, and Graduate in Divinity and Metaphysics*, anonymous (London 1744), p. 34. '*Anti-Siris*' accused Berkeley of Popery several times, e.g., pp. 12, 34 and 38.

medicine.'[17] This is a highly significant indication of the kind of programme Berkeley set out in *Siris*. Just as in *The Analyst* Berkeley had shown that Newtonians and deists were incompetent mathematicians,[18] so in *Siris* he would challenge the authority of Newtonian physicians. While Berkeley evidently sought to circumscribe the physician's role, we should not be led into thinking that interactions between medical men and clergy were typically competitive or adversarial. Indeed, recent scholarship, contrary to convention, supports the view that medicine and religion were characteristically compatible if not symbiotic. Afflictions of the soul carried equal weight with those of the body in the eighteenth century's symptom-based nosology. If the faculty and the cloth, usually because of divergent natural-theological convictions, fell out over theory, they generally saw eye to eye in practice; the purveying of medicines and the attendance on the sick and dying being instances of appropriate duties for both.[19] It is therefore necessary to look behind Berkeley's polemic, and define his theological and medical target more precisely.

Newton's natural philosophy formed the theoretical basis of much eighteenth-century medical thought. The physiology of those physicians belonging to the Pitcairne–Gregory circle, drawing its inspiration from the *Principia*, explained the operations of the body through the actions of short-range forces which were seen to be analogous to gravity. Anita Guerrini has pointed to the demise of this essentially mechanistic physiology after the publication of James Keill's *Account of Animal Secretion* in 1708.[20] We have seen that this was a time when the High Church exploited the theological, not to say political, implications of Newtonian matter theory, linking it to the immanentist natural philosophy of Toland, Tindal and their deist followers. Their symbolic ritual sacrifice, the withdrawal from William Whiston of his Lucasian professorship, demonstrated that even the protective cover of

[17] Berkeley, 'First Letter to Prior' dated 19 June 1744, *Works*, vol. 5, section. 6, p. 173.

[18] Geoffrey Cantor, 'The Analyst Revisited', *Isis* 76 (1984), pp. 668–83. For Berkeley's inspiring Smart and Blake see D. J. Greene, 'Smart, Berkeley, the Scientists and the Poets', *Journal of the History of Ideas* 14 (1985), pp. 327–52.

[19] Roy Porter, 'Medicine and Religion in Eighteenth Century England: A Case of Conflict?', *Ideas and Production*, Issue 7 (1987), pp. 4–17. See also the essays by Andrew Wear and Jonathan Barry in *Patients and Practitioners*, ed. Roy Porter (Cambridge, 1985) and the essays by Michael Macdonald and Henry D. Rack in *The Church and Healing*, ed. W. J. Sheils (Oxford, 1982).

[20] Anita Guerrini, 'James Keill, George Cheyne, and Newtonian Physiology', *Journal of the History of Biology* 18 (1985), pp. 247–66; see also Roger French, 'Ether and Physiology', in *Conceptions of Ether: Studies in the History of Ether Theories*, ed. G. N. Cantor and M. J. S. Hodge (Cambridge, 1981) and Geoffrey Bowles, 'Physical, Human and Divine Attraction in the Life of George Cheyne', *Annals of Science* 31 (1974), pp. 473–88.

Newton's patronage could be penetrated. However, the spectre of materialism was not so easily exorcised; Whig stability provided the Latitudinarians with a firmer social footing and curbed High Church lust for religious persecution, thus ensuring that after the publication of the 1717 *Opticks* Newtonian medicine could be revitalised without challenge.

This second school of physiological thought received its impetus from Newton's revival of the aether hypothesis, briefly alluded to in the 'General Scholium' of the 1713 *Principia* but developed more coherently in the *Opticks*. In the 1717 queries, Newton described the aether as 'rare', 'subtle' and 'elastick'; he referred to the 'exceeding smallness of its particles' and claimed that it 'dilates', 'contracts', 'condenses' and 'vibrates'.[21] To his disciples this aether was for all intents and purposes material, but more importantly, as Peter Heimann has indicated,

> Newton's theory of the micro-structure of the aether as the embodiment of repulsive forces . . . was to enable eighteenth-century thinkers to transform his concept of the aether into that of 'active substances' by conflating his concepts of the aether and active principles.[22]

Newton always maintained that God worked through secondary causes, and active principles, as manifestations of such causes, were defined in relation to God's omnipotence. Active principles are not to be equated with force: they cause forces. But since in 1717 Newton proposed the aether as the cause of both gravity and the short-range attractive and repulsive forces underlying chemical phenomena, his followers were able to identify the aether with active principles, and so treat force as an intrinsic property of matter.[23] The activity of nature was thus explained in terms of the material operations of an aethereal medium, and Providential intervention became redundant. In medical terms, the body represented a microcosm of the Newtonian universe and the actions of an aethereal fluid were taken as the basis of physiological explanation.

While most of the physicians who flocked round Newton at the start

[21] Newton, *Opticks* (London, 1717), reprinted for Dover Publications, based on the 1730 edition, 1952. Queries 17–22, pp. 347–54.

[22] Peter Heimann, 'Nature is a Perpetual Worker, Newton's Aether and Eighteenth Century Natural Philosophy', *Ambix* 20 (1973), pp. 1–25, see p. 5.

[23] *Ibid.*; Eric Forbes, 'Newton's Science and the Newtonian Philosophy', *Vistas in Astronomy* 22 (1978), pp. 413–18. P. M. Heimann and J. E. McGuire, 'Newtonian Forces and Lockean Powers: Concepts of Matter Theory in Eighteenth Century Thought', *Historical Studies in the Physical Sciences* 3 (1971), pp. 233–306, see pp. 237–8. Joan L. Hawes, 'Newton's Revival of the Aether Hypothesis and the Explanation of Gravitational Attraction', *Notes and Records of the Royal Society* 23 (1986), pp. 200–12.

of the century had High Church sympathies, among them Pitcairne, John and James Keill and George Cheyne, those who worked closely alongside him in the 1720s were mainly of Broad Church persuasion. James Jurin, educated at Trinity College, Cambridge and Leiden, and later President of the Royal College of Physicians, which by the 1720s had become something of a Whig bastion,[24] was from 1721 to 1727 Secretary of the Royal Society. In this capacity he is reputed to have 'imbibed the Newtonian philosophy from Newton himself',[25] putting it to use both in his attempts to determine, quantitatively, the impulsive force of the heart,[26] and in his lesser known pamphlet attacks on Berkeley. Jurin also edited the third edition of the *Principia*, working closely with fellow physician Henry Pemberton, who had been entrusted with writing the introduction. Pemberton, later Gresham professor of physic, first brought himself to Newton's attention in 1722 with a paper refuting Leibniz's measure of the force of moving bodies,[27] and the following year Jurin, presumably convinced of Pemberton's Newtonian loyalties, invited him to produce an introduction on muscular motion for an edition of William Cowper's *Myotomia Reformata*.[28]

Perhaps most menacing to Berkeley was the fact that Newtonian physiology was thought to be capable of resolving the mind–body problem. The implications for Trinitarianism of the breakdown of mind–body duality, were as pernicious as the blurring of boundaries between the spiritual and material, the sacred and the profane. Ironically, it was Newton himself who, though never wavering in his commitment to a belief in the sluggishness of matter, raised the question:

> How do the Motions of the Body follow from the Will, and whence is the Instinct in Animals? Is not the Sensory of Animals that place . . . into which the sensible Species of Things are carried through the Nerves and Brain, that there they may be perceived by their immediate presence to that Substance?[29]

[24] This had not always been the case, see R. J. J. Martin, 'Explaining John Freind's *History of Physick*', *Studies in History and Philosophy of Science* 19 (1988), pp. 399–418.

[25] *Dictionary of National Biography* (Oxford, 1909 edn), vol. 10, p. 1,117.

[26] James Jurin, 'De Potentia Cordis . . .', *Philosophical Transactions* 30 (1718), pp. 863–72; see pp. 867–70.

[27] Henry Pemberton, 'A Letter to Dr. Mead, Coll. Med. Lond. & Soc. Reg. S. Concerning an Experiment, Whereby it has been Attempted to Shew the Falsity of the Common Opinion, in Relation to the Force of Bodies in Motion', *Philosophical Transactions* 32 (1722), pp. 57–68; *Dictionary of National Biography* (Oxford, 1909 edn), vol. 15, pp. 725–6.

[28] Theodore M. Brown, 'Medicine in the Shadow of the Principia', *Journal of the History of Ideas* 48 (1987), pp. 629–48.

[29] Newton, *Opticks*, Query 28, p. 370 and Query 24, pp. 353–4. See also Philip C. Ritterbush, *Overtures to Biology, the Speculations of Eighteenth Century Naturalists* (New Haven, 1964).

Taking Newton's cue further than had been intended by him, John Cook in his *Anatomical and Mechanical Essay on the Whole Animal Economy* (1730) suggested that the mind was 'clothed with a material vehicle' and proposed the aether as such an 'intermediate vehicle'. The Dublin physician Bryan Robinson, who in 1745 was to become professor of physic at Trinity College, built upon a similar distortion of the queries in *A Dissertation on the Aether of Sir Isaac Newton* (1742). Here he relied on the crude mechanics of contact action to explain the phenomena of light, heat, gravity, muscular motion and the transmission of nervous impulses in terms of the sizes and motions of aether particles. This dissertation was a more focused reiteration of an earlier work, *A Treatise of the Animal Oeconomy* (1732), where Robinson first claimed that 'Muscular Motion is Performed by the vibrations of a very Elastick Aether.'[30] Berkeley owned a copy of this work and was therefore aware of materialist irreligion having become a threat on Irish soil.

Physicians, however, were not the only group on whom Berkeley took revenge in *Siris*, for health was the locus where medicine met with chemistry, pneumatics and electricity – areas which after publication of the 1717 *Opticks* had one by one become infected with materialism. With *Siris* located precisely where these central strands of Newtonian thinking converged, natural philosophers as well as physicians were objects of Berkeley's attack.

The predominantly chemical context in which Newton presented his statements about an aether led his disciples to look to pneumatics and electricity for experimentally verifiable evidence of a 'repulsive virtue'. Such research paved the way towards an immanentist cosmology, since Newtonians had simply to show the existence of repulsive force to confirm that a material aether was the source of activity in nature. The Revd Stephen Hales's *Vegetable Staticks* (1727) represents a landmark in this programme. Hales accepted that matter was 'endued with a strongly attracting power' but stipulated that it was absolutely necessary 'that there should be every where intermixed with it a due proportion of strongly repelling elastick particles, which might enliven the whole mass'.[31] His argument was that heat or fermentation were able to put air particles into such a 'vigorously elastick and permanently repelling state'.[32] Yet only air was amphibious, that is,

[30] Bryan Robinson, *A Treatise on the Animal Oeconomy*, second edition (Dublin, 1734), p. 87.

[31] Stephen Hales, *Vegetable Staticks* (London, 1727; reprinted London, 1961), p. 178, as cited in D. E. G. Allan and R. E. Schofield, *Stephen Hales: Scientist and Philanthropist* (London, 1980), pp. 30–48; see p. 41.

[32] *Ibid.*, p. 40, citing Hales, *Vegetable Staticks*, p. xxvii.

capable of being changed from a strongly repelling state to as strongly an attracting state and back again. Thus the physical world for Hales consisted of two fundamentally different types of matter: ordinary matter, composed of permanently inelastic particles, and air, composed of possibly elastic ones. Although Hales rejected Newton's central doctrine of inertial homogeneity – the notion that any two units of matter of the same volume were of the same inertial mass – he frequently cited the *Opticks* in support of his claims. Jean Theophilus Desaguliers, who had studied under John Keill at Oxford before following Hauksbee as curator of experiments for the Royal Society, and who publicised both his poetic inclinations and Whig allegiance in *The Newtonian System of the World, the Best Model of Government* (1728), was influenced by Hales's work in his own search for repulsive force. As early as 1729, he confidently announced 'We have too many Observations and Experiments to leave any doubt of the Existence of the repellent Force.'[33] For Desaguliers, as for William Whiston and Stephen Gray, this experimental evidence came principally from electrical phenomena, which were represented as manifestations of active powers in matter, since electricity was itself identified with an aethereal principle. Desaguliers saw in the electrical properties of bodies, to which he reduced explanations of elasticity, combustion and evaporation, the key to the causation of force; he elaborated this conceptual scheme, which defied Newton's dichotomy between attractive and repulsive states of force, in his *Dissertation Concerning Electricity* (1742) where he claimed 'Electricity is a property of some bodies whereby they alternately attract and repel small bodies when brought near them.'[34]

By the 1740s natural philosophers like Desaguliers, by appealing to an aethereal agent, were attempting to provide chemical and electrical phenomena with a common theoretical basis. Novel sources were incorporated into this burgeoning school of natural philosophy to extend its explanatory value. Boerhaave's chemical writings were of prime importance in this development. For Boerhaave, fire was 'the cause of almost all the effects cognizable by our senses', it was 'the

[33] J. T. Desaguliers, 'An Attempt to Solve the Phenomenon of the Rise of Vapours and Formation of Clouds and Descent of Rain', *Philosophical Transactions* 407 (1729), p. 18.

[34] J. T. Desaguliers, *A Dissertation Concerning Electricity* (London, 1742), p. 1. For Hales and Desaguliers contradicting Newton see A. Quinn, 'Repulsive Force in England, 1706–1744', *Historical Studies in the Physical Sciences* 13 (1982), pp. 109–28. For electricity as political and theological and moral instruction, see S. Schaffer, 'Natural Philosophy and Public Spectacle', *History of Science* 21 (1983), pp. 1–44.

great changer of all things, in the universe'.[35] The similarity of this fire to Newton's 1717 aether is clear; moreover it appealed to many eighteenth-century natural philosophers because it was material yet non-gravitational. Chiefly responsible for the introduction of Boerhaave into English natural philosophy was the self-taught physician, Peter Shaw, who had studied under Boerhaave at Leiden. Shaw's translation of the *Elementa Chemiae* in 1741 was a Newtonian rendition of Boerhaave's writings, replete with extensive footnotes linking his chemical theory to ideas derived from the 1717 *Opticks*. In a footnote to Boerhaave's comments on motion as the universal cause of chemical change, Shaw, drawing from query 31 stated:

> all the phaenomena, all the changes in the universe are the effects of motion. Accordingly to have a succession of such changes, the author of nature has added to bodies certain active principles to be sources of motion.[36]

Boerhaave's writings were seen by Shaw's contemporaries to be consistent with the Newtonian programme of developing a quantitative science of interparticulate forces based on the operations of an aethereal medium.

From Berkeley's perspective, health had become an area of materialist thought; the immanentism, which at the start of the century had been confined to wayward radicals, and denounced by High and Low Church alike, had by the 1740s been embraced by respected establishment natural philosophers and physicians. In 1734, Berkeley had illustrated how easy it was for materialists to sink from religious scepticism to immanentism and atheism, for this was the slippery slope down which Alciphron slid. But those materialist thinkers loyal to a politics of Broad Church Whiggery, who between 1704 and 1744 sought to establish a coherent picture of the universe which faithfully followed the tenets of Newton's programme, shunned the warning contained in Alciphron's fate, and therefore stood in need of further rebuke.

THE RECEPTION OF TAR-WATER

The 1720s to 1740s witnessed the growth of a Patrician culture obsessed with morality, manners and clean living. A healthy life-style was

[35] Herman Boerhaave, *A New Method Of Chemistry: Including the History, Theory and Practice of the Art*, translated by Peter Shaw from the original Latin of Dr Boerhaave, *Elementa Chemiae* (London, 1741), p. 206 and p. 362.

[36] *Ibid.*, p. 157. See Jan Golinski, 'Peter Shaw: Chemistry and Communication in Augustan England', *Ambix* 30 (1983), pp. 19–29.

seen to be commensurate with politeness and civilisation, and a sound physical constitution became consistent with an enlightened mind. Health was therefore more than an arena in which natural philosophers and physicians vied for the definitive word, it was also a concern which had captured public interest. As a subject for scrutiny, health had been swept along by the tide of improvement beyond the domain of the professional medical elite and into Enlightenment culture generally. As Roy Porter concludes from his survey of lay involvement with medicine based on evidence from the *Gentleman's Magazine*, 'being familiar with medicine was not an individual and private matter, but integral to the public role of the well-informed, public-spirited and responsible layman'.[37] *Siris* must therefore be located in the broad context of public concern with health for it was here that Berkeley found a wide and receptive audience.

The Georgians were noteworthy medicine takers, in sickness and in health, so that the prescribing of medicines, properly the province of physicians but in practice an open market, became a lucrative enterprise.[38] This did not go unnoticed by the Revd John Wesley who, to add to his other achievements, was the century's best-selling medical author:

> Physicians now began to be had in Admiration, as Persons who were something more than Human. And Profit attended their employ as well as Honour; so that they now had Two Weighty Reasons, for keeping the bulk of Mankind at a distance, that they might not pry into the Mysteries of the Profession.[39]

Yet however hard some physicians sought to defend their territorial rights, denouncing all trespassers as empirics or quacks, their authority could always be undermined by those among their rank who proffered some or other medical fad. In this context of the competitive offering of health treatments, medical orthodoxy merged with heterodoxy; Dr John Arbuthnot's diet of 'asses milk', Dr Joshua Ward's 'Pill and Drop', Dr Thomas Dover's 'Mercury Powders' and Dr Robert James's 'Fever Powders' all defeat conventional categorisation. The status of

[37] Roy Porter, 'Lay Medical Knowledge in the Eighteenth Century: The Evidence of the *Gentleman's Magazine*', *Medical History* 29 (1985), pp. 138–68; Virginia Smith, 'Cleanliness: The Development of the Idea and Practice in Britain 1770–1850', unpublished Ph.D. thesis (LSE, 1985) and Chris Lawrence, 'William Buchan: Medicine Laid Open', *Medical History* 19 (1975), pp. 20–35.

[38] Irvine Loudon, 'The Nature of Provincial Medical Practice in Eighteenth-Century England', *Medical History* 29 (1985), pp. 1–32 and Joseph Kett, 'Provincial Medical Practice in England', *Journal of the History of Medicine* 19 (1964), pp. 17–29.

[39] John Wesley, *Primitive Physick: OR AN Easy and Natural METHOD OF CURING most Diseases* (London, 1747), Preface, pp. x–xi. See G. S. Rousseau, 'John Wesley's *Primitive Physic* (1747)', *Harvard Library Bulletin* 16 (1968), pp. 242–56.

physician was barely distinguishable from that of quack. Strategically, medical orthodoxy was increasingly defined in social terms serving the interests of those members of the profession with a university training and those belonging to the Royal College of Physicians, thus creating a medical hierarchy based on educational and institutional elitism.[40] Ultimately in medicine, as in commerce, the discriminating consumer sat in judgement of what was on offer, and in the consultative relationship the patient, with potential to bestow patronage and celebrity on the physician, took the dominant role.[41] The public success of Berkeley and Wesley, set against this background of intense rivalry between physicians, lay in their recognition that the patient was the final medical arbiter, as the end of a verse which Berkeley intended as a reply to Jurin bears out:

What agrees with his stomach, and what with his head,
The drinker may feel, though he can't write or read.
Then authority's nothing: the doctors are men:
And who drinks tar-water will drink it again.[42]

The public impact of *Siris* was enormous, and probably warmed Berkeley's heart more than his pocket, for unlike some of its more exotic rivals, tar was both readily available and cheap. Tar-water flooded the medicine market, and the Bishop rapidly became a household name. As Marjorie Nicolson and G.S. Rousseau remark, 'The effect of Siris was almost instantaneous. Tar-water ware-houses were established in London and elsewhere. Advertisements for tar and tar-water appeared widely in periodicals.'[43] The 'Proprietors of the Tar Water warehouse' which opened in St James's Street in 1744, published an abstract of *Siris, The Medicinal Virtues of Tar-Water Fully Explained*. To this was added 'The Receipt for making it' together with 'A Plain Explanation of the Bishop's physical terms'. Presumably this spare handout catered for the many drinkers of the salubrious fluid

[40] N. D. Jewson, 'Medical Knowledge and the Patronage System in Eighteenth-Century England', *Sociology* 8 (1974), pp. 369–85; esp. pp. 374–77; Geoffrey Holmes, *Augustan England: Professions, State and Society, 1680–1730* (London, 1982) and G. N. Clark, *A History of the Royal College of Physicians of London* (Oxford, 1966), vol. 2.

[41] Jewson, 'Medical Knowledge' and N. D. Jewson 'The Disappearance of the Sick-Man from Medical Cosmology 1770–1870', *Sociology* 10 (1976), pp. 225–44.

[42] Berkeley, from a verse 'On the Disputes about Tar-Water' enclosed with Berkeley's 'First Letter to Prior', dated 19 June 1744, *Works*, vol. 8, p. 225. In another letter to Prior dated 3 September 1744, Berkeley enclosed another verse intended for publication complaining, 'The doctors, it seems, are grown very abusive', *Works*, vol. 8, p. 274.

[43] Marjorie Nicolson and G. S. Rousseau, 'Bishop Berkeley and Tar-Water' in *The Augustan Milieu*, ed. Henry Knight Miller, Eric Rothstein and G. S. Rousseau (Oxford, 1970), pp. 102–37. For the reception of Ward's 'Drop' see M. H. Nicolson, 'Ward's Pill and Drop and Men of Letters', *Journal of the History of Ideas*, 29 (1968), pp. 173–96.

who had little interest in Berkeley's natural-philosophical gymnastics, for tar-water became something of a vogue. On 10 June 1744, William Duncombe wrote to Archbishop Herring that tar-water 'is the common discourse both among the rich and poor, high and low; and the Bishop of Cloyne has made it as fashionable as going to Vauxhall or Ranelagh'.[44]

Supporters of tar-water spanned the political spectrum, Prior, Percival and Faulkner were all in favour of tar-water. Among those who drank it were Lady Egmont, Princess Caroline, Thomas Grey, William Trollope, Elizabeth Carter and Berkeley himself. Horace Walpole confessed to Sir Horace Mann on 29 May 1744 'We are now mad about tar-water.' Testifying with jocularity to the success of tar-water, he wrote 'A man came into an apothecary's shop t'other day, "Do you sell tar water?" "Tar-water!" replied the apothecary "why I sell nothing else!"'[45] Letters and testimonials praising the medicinal virtues of tar-water appeared frequently in the *Gentleman's Magazine* and Prior began collecting these for his *Authentic Narrative of the Success of Tar-Water, in Curing a Great Number and Variety of Distempers* (1746). The book, which is devoted to brief case-histories of cure or relief by tar-water, contains 120 testimonials, many of which were used for advertising by the tar-water warehouse in St James's Street. Prior enthused:

> Thousands have received benefit, and daily do receive benefit in Ireland, England, Holland, Portugal, and Germany, by the use of tar-water. The letters sent to me signify the same and the least enquiry may satisfy others of the truth thereof . . .[46]

At face value it would appear that the popularity of tar-water met with no political objections. Yet a gentle probe beneath the public craze for tar-water reveals that Berkeley provoked the wrath of several Whig physicians, including one Thomas Knight MD who boasted, 'Every body takes Tar-Water but that is not sufficient reason for me to take it.' Knight attacked Berkeley's theory of the virtue of tar-water, claiming in Newtonian tones that it 'is no more than a bare Hypothesis being not founded upon real but imaginary principles'.[47]

[44] Quoted in A. A. Luce, *The Life of George Berkeley* (London, 1949), p. 201.

[45] *Horace Walpole's Correspondence with Sir Horace Mann*, vol. 2, ed. W. S. Lewis, Warren Hunting Smith and George L. Lamb (= vol. 18 of *The Yale Edition of Horace Walpole's Correspondence*, ed. W. S. Lewis (New Haven, 1955)), p. 452: 'We are now mad about tar-water, on the publication of a book that I will send you, written by Dr Berkeley Bishop of Cloyne. The book contains every subject from tar-water to the Trinity: however all the women read it, and understand it no more than they would if it were intelligible.'

[46] Thomas Prior, *Authentic Narrative* (London, 1746), section 294.

[47] Thomas Knight, MD, *Reflections on Catholicons* (London, 1749), pp. 106–7 and pp. 34–5. See also Dr Thomas Reeve, *A Cure for the Epidemical Madness of Drinking Tar-Water* (London, 1744). Reeve followed Jurin as President of the Royal College of Physicians.

Siris was in fact the cause of a veritable pamphlet war, at least nine replies and defences appearing within the first year, 1744.[48] Among these was James Jurin's *Letter to the Right Reverend the Bishop of Cloyne*. Jurin, an established opponent of Berkeley's, had already written him two replies in 1734, one against *The Analyst* and the other against *Alciphron*. Both *Geometry no Friend to Infidelity* and *The Minute Mathematician* were defences of Newtonian calculus. In 1744, Jurin accused Berkeley of employing 'Occult Qualities' to bring 'Primitive Darkness' to medical knowledge. The tone of his conclusion was bitter: 'as Bishop of Cloyne I honour and respect you, but as a physician I pity and despise you'.[49] These were loaded criticisms and in order to appreciate their theological and political significance, it is necessary to provide some account of the context in which Berkeley was introduced to tar-water, and of how he was led subsequently to admit, 'I freely own that I suspect that tar-water is a panacea',[50] thus opening himself to Jurin's charge of occultism.

The likeliest source for Berkeley's information concerning tar-water is a piece in the *Gentleman's Magazine* for 1739. The claim was that 'By this remedy several persons in Charles Town South-Carolina, where the smallpox was lately very much mortal, escaped the infection.'[51] His first mention of tar-water in the extant correspondence is in a letter to Prior dated 8 February 1740/41. Here, Berkeley, referring to the 'epidemical bloody flux' maintained 'I believe tar-water might be useful to prevent (or to perfect the cure of) such an evil.'[52] The winter of 1739/40 had been a particularly harsh one causing a famine, and a severe smallpox epidemic followed in its wake. One witness to the devastation of Ireland's populace wrought by these circumstances described the

> Want and misery in every face; the rich unable to relieve the poor; the road spread with dead and dying bodies; Mankind the colour of the Docks and Nettles which they fed on; two or three sometimes more going to the grave for want of bearers to carry them, and many buried only in the fields and ditches where they perished.[53]

[48] Nicolson and Rousseau, 'Bishop Berkeley and Tar-Water', p. 116.

[49] James Jurin, *Letter to the Right Reverend the Bishop of Cloyne, Occasioned by his Lordship's Treatise on the Virtues of Tar-Water. Impartially Examining how far that Medicine Deserves the Character his Lordship has Given it* (London, 1744), pp. 8–11.

[50] Berkeley, 'First Letter to Prior' section 2, p. 171.

[51] *Gentleman's Magazine* 9 (1739), p. 36. The author claimed that tar-water 'is not only a Preservative but an Antidote, and consequently far preferable to Inoculation itself'. That this was indeed Berkeley's source of information concerning tar-water has been well argued by Ian Tipton, 'Two Questions on Berkeley's Panacea', *Journal of the History of Ideas* 30 (1969), pp. 203–44.

[52] Berkeley, letter to Prior dated 8 February 1740/41, *Works*, vol. 8, pp. 248–9.

[53] From a pamphlet entitled *The Groans Of Ireland*, see *The Gentleman's Magazine* 11 (1741), pp. 638–41.

It was during this smallpox epidemic that Berkeley wrote to Prior first on 8 February then again on the 15 February; in this second letter he announced, 'By new trials, I am confirmed in the use of the rosin.'[54] Presumably then, Berkeley had some success in his attempt to curb the spread of the disease among his parishioners. Yet his interest in matters medical does not sufficiently account for his transition from observer and critic to practitioner; there is an additional consideration, for as Berkeley explained in *Siris*, 'I live in a remote corner, among poor neighbours, who for want of a regular physician have often recourse to me, I have had frequent opportunities of trial.' (72)[55] Smallpox was a scourge throughout the early eighteenth century and many Whig physicians and natural philosophers had concentrated their efforts on attempting to thwart it, notably through the practice of inoculation in London society. It was Berkeley's claim for tar-water's success in the treatment of smallpox which unleashed Jurin's enmity, for the physician was the leading proponent of inoculation.

The introduction of inoculation earlier in the century had sparked a furious controversy which divided the medical community in two, largely on the basis of religious sensibility. Many representatives of the High Church saw the finger of God behind all affliction; disease was represented as God's revenge, trial or punishment of man, whose right to employ interventionist medical treatments was thus highly questionable.[56] On the other side of the fence Broad Church physicians sought to establish, quantitatively, the practical value of inoculation, and Jurin undertook the central research programme in their campaign. His *Account of the Success of Inoculating the Small-pox in Great Britain* (1724) presented the results of a major statistical survey which was repeated for the following four years. Larry Stewart has recently shown that physicians like Jurin appealed to Newtonian rather than Scriptural authority in their attempts to counter High Church antagonism, turning to the 1717 *Opticks* 'for notions of air as an elastic fluid which might help explain the phenomenon of contagion of epidemic diseases as well as legitimize intervention in their prevention'.[57] Initially, and in spite of angry protest from Providentialists, inoculation enjoyed a warm public reception aided by the patronage of

[54] Berkeley, letter to Prior dated 15 February 1740/41, *Works*, vol. 8, pp. 250–1.

[55] Berkeley, *Siris*, *Works*, vol. 5, section 72. Hereafter only the section references will be given.

[56] Porter, 'Medicine and Religion'; Larry Stewart, 'The Edge of Utility: Slaves and Smallpox in the Early Eighteenth Century', *Medical History* 29 (1985), pp. 54–70; A. D. Farr, 'Medical Developments and Religious Belief: With Special Reference to Europe in the Eighteenth and Nineteenth centuries', unpublished Ph.D. thesis (Open University, 1977), pp. 30–45; Genevieve Miller, *The Adoption of Inoculation for Smallpox in England and France* (Philadelphia 1957).

[57] Stewart, 'The Edge of Utility', p. 59.

the aristocracy which peaked with the Princess of Wales having two of her children inoculated. However, the deaths of several distinguished persons in the 1720s swung public favour over to non-interventionist methods of treatment, and it was not until the end of the 1730s amidst new outbreaks of smallpox that interest in inoculation was rekindled.

But the long fallow period of disfavour had made proponents of the practice increasingly intolerant of the persistent competition from wonder-drugs and catholicons. Unlike the inoculators, who relied on sophisticated theories of contagion to advance their cause, dealers in panaceas had little regard for theoretical speculation; they relied instead on testimony, and the faith of a credulous public. It is little wonder then, that Jurin damned tar-water's virtues as occult. Although the eighteenth century had already seen the rise and fall of Ward's 'Pill and Drop', 'Mill-flower water' and 'Quick-silver and Lime-water', all put forward as catholicons, the popularity of tar-water indicates that public enthusiasm for panaceas was unabated, and that tar-water became a viable alternative to the practice of inoculation. It is arguable that a medical Providentialism set Berkeley against interventionist treatments, and moreover that his belief in a panacea was a reflection of his belief in miracles. Indeed, Lady Mary Wortley Montagu, a Whig and most celebrated backer of inoculation, denounced tar-water, linking it with religious mystery. She said, 'I find tar-water succeeded to Ward's drop', admitting, 'we have no longer faith in miracles and reliques, and therefore with the same fury run after receipts and physicians'.[58]

The promotion of inoculation was not the only Newtonian research programme which tar-water managed to encroach upon. This nostrum was in direct competition with another medical vogue, namely mineral waters, which had, through the patronage of the upper and moneyed classes, become associated with improvement. Spas were a product of this cultural preoccupation, and the towns of Bath and Scarborough, which boasted mineral springs, became centres of activity.[59] The study of the medicinal virtues of mineral waters became an important branch of pneumatics and attracted the attention of Newtonians. Peter Shaw, who later commentated on Boerhaave, was in the 1730s engaged in the investigation of the chemical and medicinal

[58] *The Complete Letters of Lady Mary Wortley Montagu*, ed. Halsband, 3 vols. (Oxford, 1967): Letter to Wortley, 24 April 1748, vol. 2, p. 397. For Lady Mary's role in the introduction of inoculation see Genevieve Miller, 'Putting Lady Mary in her Place: A Discussion of Historical Causation', *Bulletin of the History of Medicine* 55 (1981), pp. 2–16.

[59] Barbara Brandon Siebenschuh, 'Medical Men of Bath', *Studies in Eighteenth Century Culture* 13 (1984), pp. 189–203.

properties of mineral waters, a study which came to fruition in 1734 as *An Enquiry into the Contents, Virtues and Uses of Scarborough Spa Waters with the Method of Examining any Other Mineral Water.* Jon Eklund has argued that what is important about Shaw's work and that of some of his contemporaries is that they believed that

> certain elusive substances were responsible for one or more striking chemical and medicinal properties of mineral waters. In attempting to describe and comprehend these elusive substances they understandably tried to anchor their conceptions in analogies with air and thus adopted such adjectives as 'aerial'.[60]

Shaw proposed that mineral waters were somehow able to 'fix' such aerial substances, and he attempted to isolate this active, material 'mineral spirit' by collecting evaporated spirit in a bladder, in a manner reminiscent of Hales's experiments on combustion in the 1720s.

It is in the context of balneotherapy and pneumatics that *An Account of some Experiments and Observations on Tar-Water* (1745) must be seen. The author of the pamphlet, the Low Church minister, Stephen Hales, was primarily concerned 'to inquire whether any, or what quantity of Tar, there was in Tar-Water, made with different kinds of Tar, different Degrees of stirring, and in different ways of making it'.[61] Hales grounded his interpretation of this quantitative analysis in ideas imported from the 1717 *Opticks*; he claimed, drawing from query 31, that the medicinal virtue of tar-water was due to its being impregnated with 'the volatile acid spirit', which was conveyed to the remoter vessels of the body 'in the same manner that Mineral waters are conveyed'.[62] He admitted that 'were it possible in the Nature of Things, that there could be such a thing as a Panacea', it was never more needed than to counter the ill-effects of alcohol, 'that great bane of mankind'.[63] Hales suggested enthusiastically that instead of searching for catholicons, man should look to Christ for salvation:

> Yet how eagerly do mankind catch at every semblance of a Panacea, in hopes to prolong the present life; tho' but too neglectful of that truly salvatory Water of Life, which kind Providence renders us in order to extend life thro' a happy eternity.[64]

Hales, ever loyal to Low Church rationality, was no believer in panaceas and therefore refused to award to tar-water a value superior

[60] Jon Eklund, 'Of a Spirit in the Water', *Isis* 67 (1967), pp. 527–50, p. 529. See also Golinski, 'Peter Shaw'; Noel Coley, 'Physicians and the Chemical Analysis of Mineral Waters in Eighteenth Century England', *Medical History* 26 (1982), pp. 123–44.

[61] Stephen Hales, *An Account of Some Experiments and Observations on Tar-Water; Wherein is Shown the Quantity of Tar That is Therein; And Also a Method Proposed Both to Abate That Quantity and to Ascertain the Strength of the Tar-Water*, read before the Royal Society (London, 1745), p. 1. [62] *Ibid.*, p. 10. [63] *Ibid.*, pp. 16–17. [64] *Ibid.*, pp. 25–6.

to that of mineral waters. While he may not have extolled the virtues of tar-water to the extent characteristic of the Irish divine, he nevertheless was sufficiently persuaded of its benefit to take it himself. In a letter to Bishop Hindesley dated October 1760, Hales recommended a dose of 'one fourth of a pint, at four several times' adding, 'I took it thus in the early spring, with good effects and intend to begin again in fourteen days.'[65]

One of the most incisive rebuttals of the effectiveness of tar-water is to be found in an anonymous pamphlet entitled *Anti-Siris*. Here, tar-water is associated with Dr Slayer's advocacy of sugar, Ward's 'Pill and Drop', and Mr Hancock's praise of cold water as a universal remedy – in other words with panegyric not panacea. *Anti-Siris*, noting professional opposition to this new medical fad, remarked:

> Tis already advertised in every News Paper, is to be had at every Public House and already drank by every creature in this great Metropolis except slow unbelieving Foreigners, Physicians, and all their Under Rags of the profession.[66]

This adversary, getting to the core of the issue, exposed deism as the target of Berkeley's learned 'Medley of Politics and Metaphysics'. He implicitly linked Newton with the deists by conceding that Newton was as wrong to dabble in theology as Berkeley was to dabble in physic; none the less he reproached the Bishop's reluctance to attack deism directly. Instead, 'He begins with Tar, the thing in the world farthest from his heart, to be able the more imperceptibly to come at *Ministers and Deists*.'[67] While tar-water was by no means far from Berkeley's heart, *Anti-Siris* was correct in supposing that 'The cure of the natural world was not the only view of this universal physician; he had the Body Politic likewise in view; and probably that of the soul too'.[68]

This survey shows how enormous was the effect of *Siris*. The hostility from Whig physicians, the public craze for tar-water, and the persistent religious tone to the controversy, demonstrate how important the text was in its eighteenth-century setting, and how crucial the moral of the text was for Berkeley's argument.

'SIRIS' AS MATURE PHILOSOPHY

Berkeley is unrepresentative of the century's dealers in panaceas in that his advocacy of tar-water not only rested on sophisticated natural-philosophical arguments, but on a critique which was designed to demolish the theoretical resources relied upon by those establishment

[65] Hales, letter to Bishop Hindesley, quoted in Allan and Schofield, *Stephen Hales*, p. 117.
[66] *Anti-Siris*, p. 52. [67] *Ibid.*, p. 56. [68] *Ibid.*, p. 33.

physicians and natural philosophers who had brought irreligion to medicine. *Siris* is a masterly attack on the programme of natural philosophy which centred on the problem of the causation of force, and which therefore drew on Newton's statements about an aether. Berkeley was unaware of Newton's early aethereal speculations, those which arose from his unpublished alchemical explorations, and those revealed in his letters to Oldenburg (1676) and Boyle (1697), both of which were only published in 1744.[69] It must therefore be the case that *Siris* was directed principally against eighteenth-century Newtonians whose knowledge of Newton's aether was confined to the 1713 'General Scholium' and the 1717 *Opticks*. In 1717 Newton had made the epistemological status of his aether quite clear. Referring to the fact that he had added 'some Questions' to the end of the *Opticks*, he explained:

> And to show that I do not take Gravity for an essential Property of Bodies, I have added one Question concerning its Cause, chusing to propose it by way of a Question, because I am not yet satisfied about it for want of Experiments.[70]

Subsequent thinkers, however, not only materialised this aether, but awarded it the epistemological status of natural fact. Desaguliers commented that Newton's queries 'contain a vast fund of philosophy: which (tho' he has modestly delivered under the name of Queries, as if they were only conjectures) daily experiments and observations confirm'.[71] And in the words of Bryan Robinson: 'This aether being a very general material Cause, without any Objection appearing against it from the phaenomena, no doubt can be made of its Existence.'[72] By identifying a material aether with active principles, these natural philosophers and their many allies were able to attribute activity to matter. Such a manoeuvre implied that the natural world was self-activating and self-sufficient and thereby contradicted Berkeley's voluntarist belief that all activity in the natural world was the result of God's direct and continual intervention.[73]

Berkeley was not alone in his antipathy to Newtonian cosmology. A.J. Kuhn has pointed out that William Law, John Freke, John

[69] *Isaac Newton's Papers and Letters on Natural Philosophy (and related documents)*, ed. I. B. Cohen and R. E. Schofield, (Cambridge, MA and London, England, second edition, 1978): Letters to Boyle and Oldenburg, pp. 70–4. Newton expressed similar views in his letters to Bentley, not published until 1756.

[70] Newton, *Opticks*, second advertisement, p. cxxiii.

[71] J. T. Desaguliers, *A Course of Experimental Philosophy*, 2 vols. (London, 1734–44), vol. 1, Preface.

[72] Bryan Robinson, *A Dissertation on the Aether of Sir Isaac Newton* (London, 1742), 1747 edition, Preface.

[73] For Berkeley's voluntarism see *Principles*, sections 27 and 59–65. A. A. Luce, *Berkeley and Malebranche* (Oxford, 1934; 1961), chapters 2–4.

Hutchinson, Johnathan Edwards and John Wesley, to name but a few, all shared Berkeley's hostility to the dominant world view.[74] Moreover, *Siris* was recognised as an anti-Newtonian work by many of Berkeley's contemporaries; in addition to the replies discussed earlier, *Siris-Theologica-Metaphysica* appeared anonymously in 1747. This book, which contains a sharp attack on immanentism directed against Broad Church natural philosophers and clerics such as Halley, Warburton, Cadwallader Colden and Benjamin Martin, is very Berkeleian in character and shows that *Siris* had become a label for anti-Newtonian attacks.

Berkeley's elaborate arguments against materialism consist in undermining the very basis of eighteenth-century Newtonianism, the 1717 *Opticks*. By stressing the tentative nature of Newton's queries, he accused those Newtonians who had treated the existence of the aether as fact, of founding their natural philosophy on hypotheses. The structural core of Berkeley's argument can be characterised by what Geoffrey Cantor calls the 'Matthew strategy' – the use of reason to undermine reason.[75] Berkeley owned the 1704, 1706 and 1730 editions of the *Opticks* and both the first and second editions of the *Principia* and read and understood Newton's works better than most of those thinkers who claimed Newton as their mentor.[76] He was excellently placed to expose the logical inconsistencies in Newton's reasoning, which he summed up in a most perspicuous manner: in short, Berkeley revealed that Newton, while postulating a hypothetical aethereal medium as a universal causal principle (queries 17–24), in the same work denied that there could be progress in natural philosophy through the employment of such principles.

This latter view had first been printed in the Latin edition of the *Opticks* in 1706. Here, Newton remarked that

> Nature will be very conformable to her self and very simple, performing all the great Motions of the heavenly Bodies by the Attraction of Gravity which intercedes those bodies, and almost all the small ones of their Particles by some other attractive and repelling Powers which intercede the Particles.[77]

Newton went on to explain that 'active principles' caused these forces and declared, 'These Principles I consider, not as occult Qualities . . .

[74] A. J. Kuhn, 'Nature Spiritualised, Aspects of Anti-Newtonianism,' *Journal of English Literary History* 41 (1974). See Cantor and Hodge, *Conceptions of Ether*: David C. Lindberg and Geoffrey Cantor, *The Discourse of Light from the Middle Ages to the Enlightenment* (Los Angeles, 1985), chapter. 2; Wilde, 'Hutchinsonian Natural Philosophy'.

[75] Cantor, 'The Analyst Revisited', pp. 675–80.

[76] *A Catalogue of the Library of George Berkeley Sold by Auction by Leigh and Sotheby on 6 June 1976 and on Five Following Days*. Copies in the British Library and the Keynes Collection, King's College, Cambridge.

[77] Newton, *Opticks*, Query 31, p. 397.

but as general Laws of Nature', adding in 1717 'their Truth appearing to us by Phenomena, though their Causes be not yet discover'd.[78] In 1717 Newton was concerned to counter Leibniz's charge that the cause of gravity was occult, therefore he stated emphatically that 'occult Qualities put a stop to the Improvement of natural Philosophy'.[79] While in query 31 Newton spurned the notion that the cause of gravity was occult, in query 28 he rejected mechanical causes. All matter, even the most subtle, resists motion, because the resistance arising from the *vis inertia*

> is proportional to the Density of the Matter, and cannot be diminish'd by dividing the Matter into smaller Parts, nor by any other means than by decreasing the Density of the Medium.[80]

Therefore, 'to make way for the regular and lasting Motions of the Planets and Comets, it's necessary to empty the Heavens of all Matter'.[81] Thus gravity cannot have a mechanical cause. Now in 1717, Newton claimed that both gravity and the refraction of light were caused by the density gradient of an 'Aethereal Medium', and that the vibrations of this medium were responsible for the 'alternate Fits of easy Transmission and Reflexion' of light in addition to the whole gamut of physiological phenomena – from nervous sensation to muscular motion. In order that the 1717 queries be consistent with his earlier statements, Newton made important changes to queries 28 and 31. In 1706, it was sufficient to qualify the emptiness of the heavens of all matter 'except perhaps some very thin Vapours, Streams of Effluvia, arising from the Atmospheres of the Earth, Planets and Comets', but in 1717 it became necessary to add to this list 'and . . . such an exceedingly rare Aethereal Medium as we described above'.[82] Having altered query 28 in order to accommodate his non-inertial, quasi-spiritual and fundamentally hypothetical aether, Newton, taking his cue from the Ancients, in the same query decried all natural philosophers who 'feigning Hypotheses for explaining all things mechanically', referred 'other causes to Metaphysics'. He insisted that,

> the main Business of natural Philosophy is to argue from Phenomena without feigning Hypotheses, and to deduce Causes from Effects, till we come to the very first Cause, which is certainly not mechanical.[83]

Berkeley was intent on exposing Newton's deceit. He began his critique with the following: 'it is the opinion of Sir Isaac Newton that

[78] *Ibid.*, Query 31, p. 401. For 1717 alterations see H. G. Alexander (ed.), *The Leibniz–Clarke Correspondence* (Manchester, 1956). [79] Newton *Opticks*, Query 31, p. 401.
[80] *Ibid.*, Query 28, pp. 365–6. [81] *Ibid.*, Query 28, p. 368.
[82] *The Leibniz–Clarke Correspondence*, p. 172.
[83] *Ibid.*, Query 28, p. 173.

somewhat unknown remains *in vacuo*, when the air is exhausted. This unknown medium he calls aether' (223), and continued by providing a characterisation of this aether, derived from queries 17–24, listing the functions Newton had attributed to it in 1717. Berkeley painted a mechanical picture of the 1717 aether, as his eighteenth-century opponents, notably Robinson, had done before him. Referring to query 21, Berkeley remarked that 'it is supposed to grow denser and denser continually, and thereby cause those great bodies to gravitate towards one another' (223) and that

> The extreme minuteness of the parts of this medium, and the velocity of their motion, together with its gravity, density and elastic force, are thought to qualify it for being the cause of all the natural motions in the universe. (224)

Berkeley pointed out that on the one hand it was impossible for such an aether to cause gravity because it would itself gravitate (225), and on the other that 'such a medium . . . seemeth not to be made out of any proof, nor to be of any use in explaining phenomena' (238). Put more palatably, the 1717 aether was both mechanical and hypothetical. It was totally unqualified to be a universal cause and should not be equated with active principles, for Newton had after all demanded that 'Hypotheses are not to be regarded in experimental Philosophy.'[84]

In 1717 Newton had ascribed to his aether the gravity and cohesion of bodies, the refraction of light, the fits of easy transmission and reflection, fermentation, animal motion and sensation. Referring to query 31, Berkeley reflected that 'All the phenomena that were before attributed to attraction, upon later thoughts seem ascribed to this aether, together with the various attractions themselves' (224). In justification of this claim, Berkeley drew on query 28 to point out that in 1706 the fits of easy transmission and reflection were as well explained by the vibrations excited in bodies by light rays, and the refraction of light was explained by the attraction of bodies. Taking his contrast between the two editions of the *Opticks* further, he concluded 'to explain the vibrations of light by those of a more subtle medium seems an uncouth explanation' (225). We should not be seduced into thinking that the Newton of 1706 fared better with his critic than the Newton of 1717, for although Berkeley was not opposed to invoking laws of attraction and repulsion, so long as they were regarded 'only as rules or methods observed in the production of natural effects' (231), he would not tolerate them as explanations: 'Attraction cannot produce, and in that sense account for the phenomena, being itself one

[84] Newton, *Opticks*, Query 31, p. 404.

of the phenomena produced and to be accounted for' (243). Berkeley's criticisms amounted to the accusation that, in 1706, Newton's universal causal principle was occult and, in 1717, it was mechanical. By treating the 1717 aether as mechanical Berkeley was able to impute to Newton the same failure Newton had faced in 1706 – that of being unsuccessful in his attempt to avoid the pitfall of infinite regress regarding the problem of causation. Berkeley delivered his final blow when he dismissed the very need to account for force, claiming that force 'whether attracting or repulsing, is to be regarded only as a mathematical hypothesis, and not as anything really existing in nature' (234). For 'sympathies' and 'oppositions' depend 'merely and altogether on the good pleasure of the Creator' (239).

Berkeley thus undermined the quest for the cause of forces, the research programme at the root of eighteenth-century Newtonianism. He showed that no mechanical aether could serve as such a cause, that the very existence of forces was itself hypothetical, and that the most that natural philosophers could do was make empirical generalisations concerning natural phenomena.[85] Berkeley brought the central Matthew strategy in his argument to a close when he playfully echoed Newton, declaring, 'it is one thing to arrive at general laws of nature from a contemplation of the phenomena, and another to frame an hypothesis and from thence deduce the phenomena' (228). And it is the latter enterprise that Berkeley was accusing eighteenth-century Newtonians of undertaking.

Although Berkeley matched his opponents' flair for manipulating natural-philosophical weaponry, he was none the less disadvantaged on the theological battleground, for High Church Anglicans faced the problem that natural reason could never prove the existence of the Trinity, that God is both three and one. Men of Latitude exploited this problem in their support of a rational theology which found its natural-philosophical justification in their advocacy of the 1717 aether as a universal causal principle, for this aether, once equated with active principles, could function as God's vice-regent in the natural world. For Berkeley, that a universal, material (and in some cases mechanical) aether was regarded as God's instrument was no less than blasphemy. A material aether implied that progress in natural philosophy was achieved independently of revelation and tradition, and that there was nothing in nature beyond reason, nothing mysterious, in other words, that God's activity was constrained by the natural order. Berkeley's own voluntarist belief was that the natural order was itself the result of

[85] Berkeley had expressed this view in 1710, *Principles*, section 66.

God's benevolence, and its maintenance a result of his direct and sustained intervention. Berkeley was committed to the belief that although nothing in religion is irrational, some things are above reason. His adherence to the view that natural philosophy cannot find causal explanations of natural phenomena was a result of his contention that man cannot rationally understand how God acts in the world. For Berkeley, Newtonian natural philosophy was the ultimate expression of Low Church Unitarianism: a material aether functioning as God's instrument in the natural world amounted to an identification of the aether with Christ as subordinate and created. There was no salvation for those eighteenth-century thinkers for whom the *Opticks* had become the Bible, no redemption for those physicians and natural philosophers, who, claiming to be priests, proceeded to treat of theology.

Berkeley replaced the 1717 aether with his own 'fine subtle spirit' (150) or some 'subtle active substance; whether it be called fire, aether, light, or the vital spirit of the world' (147). This aether was a universal cause:

> Being always restless and in motion it actuates and enlivens the whole visible mass, is equally fitted to produce and destroy, distinguishes the various stages of nature and keeps up the perpetual round of generations and corruptions, pregnant with forms which it constantly sends forth and resorbs (152).

Berkeley's aether did the work Newton had attempted to do with his own fluid. It accounted for 'The phenomena of light, animal spirit, muscular motion, fermentation, generation and other natural operations' (229). This aether was nothing less than 'an instrument or medium by which the real Agent doth operate on grosser bodies' (221).

Such a characterisation of the aether has led Peter Heimann to claim that 'Berkeley has thus assimilated Newton's concept of the aether to the universal active "aether" or fire developed by Boerhaave.'[86] Although in *Siris* Berkeley frequently expressed admiration for Boerhaave, his 'pure aethereal spirit' is not to be equated with Boerhaave's fire. For the chemist, fire was a material substance, and although Berkeley referred to the aether as an 'active substance', the word 'substance' did not imply material. We have seen that a material aether cannot serve as God's instrument in the natural world, indeed in *Alciphron* Berkeley had already attacked Boerhaave's materialism. It is therefore necessary to consider the ontological status which Berkeley attributed to his aether. It must be established whether Berkeley was

[86] Heimann, 'Nature is a Perpetual Worker', p. 14. For Boerhaave's materialism see R. E. Schofield, *Mechanism and Materialism* (Princeton, 1969).

thinking with the learned and speaking with the vulgar or whether he had introduced a novel category into his ontology.[87] We need to understand in what way Berkeley's aether can be said to exist.

Ian Tipton maintains that Berkeley's rejection of Boerhaave in *Alciphron* amounts to 'a refusal to resolve the soul into fire rather than a rejection of the fire theory as a whole'.[88] So in order to argue that Boerhaave's fire theory is compatible with Berkeley's idealism and explain how Berkeley came to accept 'that fire may be regarded as the animal spirit of this world',[89] he claims that Berkeley's unperceived aether is ideal, in the sense that it is in principle perceivable, unlike Locke's corpuscles, which for Berkeley were theoretical in the strongest sense – that is, in principle unobservable. Tipton presupposes that in *Siris* as in the *Principles*, the word 'thing' designates only spirits or ideas, and in order to read Berkeley as consistent, he forces the aether into the second category as a potential idea.

Tipton's argument amounts to the claim that in 1744, as in 1710, Berkeley was thinking with the learned and speaking with the vulgar. But as a mature text, representing a deepened and extended philosophy, *Siris* offers a new ontology compatible with true religion. The aether is not ideal in the way that matter is ideal, rather, it is ideal in the Platonic sense of the word. In *Siris* Berkeley frequently relied on Plato's authority, he stated that,

> Plato . . . held original ideas in the mind, that is, notions which never were or can be in the sense, such as being, beauty, goodness, likeness, parity. Some, perhaps, may think the truth to be this, that there are properly no ideas or passive objects in the mind but what were derived from sense; but that there are also besides these her own acts or operations; such are notions (308).

Berkeley reminded his readers that the Pythagoreans and Platonists had maintained that 'the soul is the place of forms', and revealed that his aether was 'determined by the soul, from which it immediately receives impression, and in which the moving force truly and properly resides' (171). By adopting the Platonic doctrine of ideal forms, Berkeley was able to maintain that his invisible, immaterial aether could truly be said to exist. Of fundamental importance in such an argument, is Berkeley's distinction between perceptions by ideas and perceptions by notions, since it is only to the former that the doctrine of 'esse est

[87] Berkeley, *Principles*, section 51. Berkeley quotes from Bacon's *De Augmentis Scientiarum* asserting that natural philosophers should 'think with the learned and speak with the vulgar,' p. 92.

[88] Ian Tipton, 'The Philosopher by Fire in Berkeley's *Alciphron*' in *Berkeley, Critical and Interpretive Essays*, ed. Colin. M. Turbayne (Manchester, 1982), p. 163.

[89] Berkeley, 'First Letter to Prior', p. 176.

percipi' applies.[90] We cannot have ideas of spirit – ideas being perceived and passive and spirit being unperceived and active – rather we have notions of spirit.[91] Thus the aether as an invisible spirit exists in reality because we can have notions of it; it is a substance in the sense that it is a thing. In the *Principles* Berkeley allowed for the existence of spirits – God and wills – and ideas, serving as 'marks or signs' for God's creatures. Now in *Siris* Berkeley introduced the aether as God's instrument, not to serve for the benefit of mankind as a signifier, but to aid God in his maintenance of the natural order. We might say that Berkeley's mature philosophy exhibits a theocentric rather than anthropocentric ontology.[92]

While Newton's aether was hypothetical and structurally nearer to gross matter than to spirit, the aether Berkeley extolled in *Siris* was not only immaterial or spiritual in nature, significantly it was phenomenal. It had a phenomenal manifestation in tar-water: 'Tar-water serving as a vehicle to this spirit' (218). Moreover Berkeley affirmed, in his 'First Letter to Prior' that the aether was responsible for tar-water's medicinal virtues.[93] Tar-water was literally a vital fluid, capable of purging away ill-manners and irreligion. On the theme of Berkeley and living waters, David Berman draws attention to the religious symbolism in Berkeley's repeated use of the fountain analogy. In his *Proposal*, Berkeley had referred to St Paul's College in Bermuda as a 'Fountain or Reservoir of learning', and in John Simbert's painting, 'The Bermuda Group' of 1729/30, a fountain is depicted in the background. Berman claims that the portrait 'graphically expresses the "Proposal's" extended metaphor'.[94] The fountain motif appears again as the frontispiece to *Alciphron* and in two later paintings of Berkeley (see plate 3). Yet again in his 'Second Letter to Prior', Berkeley employed the fountain analogy, when he wrote: 'The virtue of tar-water, flowing like the Nile from a secret and occult source, brancheth into innumerable channels conveying health and relief wherever it is applied.'[95] Berman points out that the Nile was called 'Siris' by ancient Egyptians. In short, his thesis is that 'Tar-water is the closest natural thing to drinkable

[90] Berkeley, *Principles*, sections 1–6. See also Harry M. Bracken, *The Early Reception of Berkeley's Immaterialism* (The Hague, 1965), esp. pp. 64–70.

[91] Berkeley, *Principles*, sections 29–30. See also Daniel E. Flage, *Berkeley's Doctrine of Notions; a Reconstruction Based on his Theory of Meaning* (London, 1987).

[92] G. Dawes Hicks, *Berkeley* (London, 1932), pp. 213–33.

[93] Berkeley, 'First Letter to Prior', section 16, pp. 176–7.

[94] David Berman, 'Bishop Berkeley and the Fountains of Living Waters', *Hermathena* 128 (1980), pp. 21–31, see p. 22.

[95] Berkeley, 'Second Letter to Prior', published in Prior's *Authentic Narrative*, *Works*, vol. 5, section. 15, p. 185.

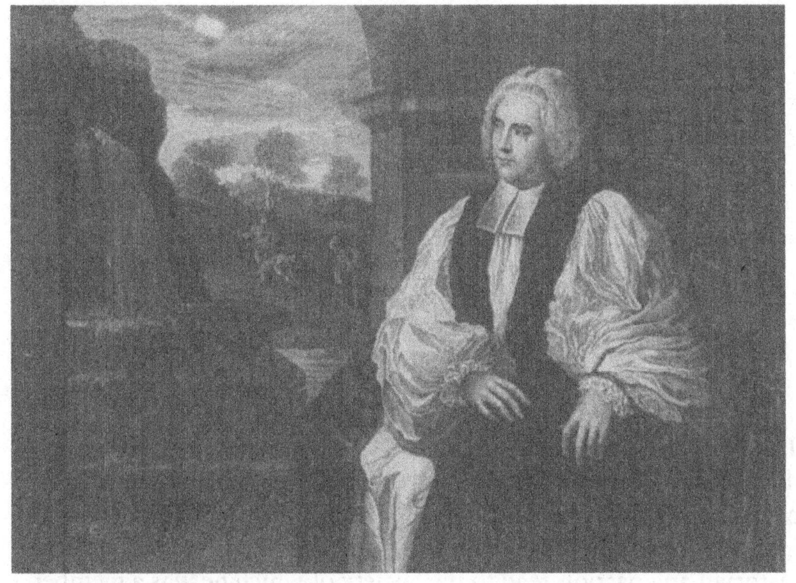

3 The Rt. Revd George Berkeley, Bishop of Cloyne

God.'[96] Rather than representing God, it is certainly arguable that tar-water represents Christ in its role as a healing and vivifying cordial: after all for Anglicans, the notion of imbibing Christ was routinely manifested in the performing of communion. We have seen that the Bishop was not prepared to tolerate the Unitarian notion that Christ was subordinate and created, and that he believed that the Newtonians' material aether gave ultimate expression to Low Church doctrines. Berkeley's spiritual aether, in its role as God's vice-regent, confronts the opinion that Christ was created and therefore subordinate to God. This aether symbolises Berkeley's attempt to demonstrate the existence of the Trinity, appropriating from his opponents the authority of natural philosophy. It represents his desperate bid to provide a rational basis for a belief which had previously been dependent on revelation alone. As such, *Siris* must be seen, in the true spirit of improvement, as the pinnacle of Berkeley's campaign to purify the polluted waters of eighteenth-century religion and morality.

[96] Berman, 'Bishop Berkeley', p. 26.

8

North America, a western outpost of European medicine

HELEN BROCK

The Medical Society of South Carolina, formed in 1789, had 'resolved that the new century should be introduced by recapitulating what had been done by and for the profession in the old'. Accordingly, on the first day of the nineteenth century, Dr David Ramsay, physician, historian and patriot, read to the Society of which he was a member a *Review of the Improvements, Progress and State of Medicine in the Eighteenth Century*, which afterwards was published.

Having won the War of Independence, Americans at this time were fiercely nationalist and anxious to demonstrate not only their political but also their cultural independence, particularly of Britain. If they could they would have severed their connections with European medicine. In 1806 *The Medical Repository and Review of American Publications on Medicine* announced that:

> We are content with the honour of being associates and fellow labourers with a band of distinguished physicians in the United States who have endeavoured to secure truth from perversion and to demolish errors to which time, prejudice and the authority of some respectable names on the other side of the Atlantic had lent a pernicious ascendency.

American physicians were preparing to produce a purified American medicine.

Therefore it might have been expected that Dr Ramsay would have dwelt principally on developments that had taken place in medicine in North America over the last century. There was in fact material from which he could have made an interesting talk, showing the evolution of medicine in the colonies from an unorganised profession staffed by poorly trained practitioners to a profession that in certain aspects compared very favourably with that in Britain. But sincere patriot as he was, he was broadminded enough to see the evolution of medicine in a much wider context. Educated at the college of New Jersey (now

Princeton) and at the Medical School of the College of Philadelphia, widely read in medical literature, he was admirably suited to review for his audience the advances that had taken place in anatomy, physic, surgery, midwifery and those parts of chemistry and botany that related to medicine and which had resulted from European research. His audience was reminded of the dominant position of European medicine in the medicine they practised in North America.

When Ramsay at the end of his lecture, turned briefly to medicine and doctors in North America there was little he could put forward as an American contribution to medical advancement. He instanced a number of American medical publications, but these were either by immigrant medical doctors or by native-born Americans who had been educated medically in Europe. In fact he did not do justice to the extent of American medical publications for he omitted contributions in the *Philosophical Transactions* of the Royal Society, in *Medical Observations and Inquiries of a Society of Physicians in London*, and in Edinburgh medical journals, publications with a wide circulation and likely to be more influential than books and pamphlets published in America. Though these publications often contained interesting observations they cannot be said to have provided any real contribution to medical advancement.

He praised the founding of the Philadelphia Hospital, the first real hospital in British North America and the medical schools founded at Philadelphia in 1765 and at King's College, New York in 1768. Both of these medical schools were founded on the pattern of the Edinburgh University medical school and were institutions aimed at bringing medical education in America into line with that in Scotland and on the continent of Europe. After the Revolution two other medical schools were founded, at Harvard in 1783 and at Dartmouth, New Hampshire in 1798.

The one area in which Ramsay thought that eighteenth-century America had made a real contribution to medical advancement was in demonstrating the use of inoculation in reducing the effect of epidemics of smallpox. Alas Genevieve Miller[1] has shown that inoculation in Britain developed concurrently with its use in America. Ramsay acknowledged that as yet America had made little if any contribution to medical progress but looked forward to the first day of the twentieth century when some member would entertain the Society with great improvements and brilliant discoveries made by Americans in the century ahead.

[1] Genevieve Miller, *The Adoption of Inoculation for Smallpox in England and France* (Philadelphia, 1957).

It is hardly surprising that medicine in North America amongst the white settlers was dominated by traditional European medicine. In many instances medical men were encouraged or officially appointed to accompany the first settlers, and immigrant doctors from Britain continued to arrive in America up to the War of Independence. After the early 1640s, as the English Civil War began to engage the energies of the English Puritans, immigration to New England declined and of the nearly 1,600 doctors who practised in Massachusetts between the founding of the colony in 1620 and 1800, fewer than 100 were immigrants.[2] In the eighteenth century only 3.9 per cent of doctors were immigrants. Immigration to the middle and southern colonies throughout the seventeenth and eighteenth centuries was much heavier, and with the immigrants came many doctors. Though no numerical estimation is possible, in Maryland immigrant doctors dominated the profession till the middle years of the eighteenth century. They came to the colonies for a variety of reasons: a few to escape political or religious persecution, but the majority came hoping to 'improve themselves'. And it was not only medical men from Britain who came. Wars, persecutions and poor economic conditions drove men, including some doctors, from various European countries to look for a better life in North America.

Through the seventeenth century there was little to attract to America well educated and dedicated physicians or men who were prospering at home. Those who came were, for the most part, the less skilled and less successful practitioners. Most were surgeons, a few were apothecaries, and hardly any could claim to be physicians.

In the eighteenth century, at least in London, the medical profession was divided into physicians licensed by the Royal College of Physicians to practice in the city and as medical graduates entitled to call themselves doctors; surgeons who were members of the Barber-surgeons' Company; and apothecaries (members of the Society of Apothecaries) who officially were allowed to practice. But many practised without a licence or membership. In the provinces though licensing or membership of guilds was still called for, the division of the profession had largely broken down and patients were attended by apothecary-surgeons (or general practitioners) who provided all branches of medical care. In the colonies, from the start, such a division of the professions was impossible, and medical men, whatever their qualifications, were general practitioners and early assumed the title 'doctor'.

[2] Eric H. Christianson, 'Medicine in New England' in *Medicine in the New World*, ed. Ronald Numbers (Knoxville, Tennessee, 1987).

Men born in the colonies who wished to become doctors to begin with had little opportunity to obtain, in North America, a good medical education. The apprenticeship system, though it existed, was unorganised and unregulated, for there were no craft or trade guilds or companies in any of the colonies to impose regulations. Of the 140 or so men practising in Massachusetts in the seventeenth century only about 20 per cent had been apprenticeship trained. By the eighteenth century 36.6 per cent had undergone a medical apprenticeship but it had rarely lasted more than a year. In the same period in England at least 80 per cent of practitioners had undergone a three-year apprenticeship. Massachusetts at least was concerned about medical education and as early as 1647 John Eliot had hoped to get support from England for setting up a medical school in the colony. The General Court affirmed the old principle of English Common Law that a judge might sentence the body of a murderer to dissection and on petition of President Henry Dunster of Harvard College agreed 'that such as studies physick or chirurgery may have liberty . . . to anatomize once in four years some malefactor in case there be such as the Courte shall alow of'.[3] But little came of these efforts. Though Harvard College, founded in 1636, never had a medical school till 1783, even in the seventeenth century a number of native-born doctors had attended college, and in the eighteenth century of the 1,370 practitioners, 399 had attended either Harvard College or Yale (founded in 1701) and 360 held BA degrees.[4] Most of these men intended to become ministers of religion but, either through private study or with a mentor, had acquired sufficient medical knowledge to enable them to care for both the souls and bodies of their parishioners. No other colony, till the middle of the eighteenth century, had been so concerned with the provision of medical education nor had so generally well educated doctors as Massachusetts. The vast majority of native-born doctors began practice, even if they had received an apprenticeship training, without the opportunity of learning anatomy except from picture books or having any proper training in surgery except what their masters could give them, the masters themselves being rarely skilful. Many offered medical advice and services having received no training at all.

By the eighteenth century the social evolution of the colonies made them more attractive to men of education. After the Act of Union

[3] John B. Blake, *Public Health in the Town of Boston* (Cambridge, MA, 1959).
[4] Christianson, 'Medicine in New England'.

between England and Scotland in 1707, which permitted Scotsmen to trade with the colonies and accept official employment there, considerable numbers of enterprising young Scotsmen emigrated to the colonies and with them came some Scottish doctors who saw in the colonies opportunities not available to them in their poor homeland. One of the earliest Scottish immigrant doctors, William Douglass, MD of Utrecht, settled in Boston in 1716 and became an important figure in Boston medicine. After the opening of the medical school at Edinburgh University in 1726 and medical teaching at Glasgow University from the 1740s, a number of the immigrant doctors were medical graduates and were to have a profound influence on American medicine. These men in the different colonies became leaders of the profession and in general achieved a social position above that enjoyed by members of the profession in earlier years.

Except in New England, where there were few immigrant doctors, there was little to attract native men of good families into the profession. For very few, even at the end of the colonial period, could make a reasonable living by the practice of medicine alone. The level of sickness in North America was such that doctors might have expected large and lucrative practices. But relatively few colonists could afford to employ a doctor. Medical fees tended therefore to be high as doctors attempted to obtain from their few patients as much as they hoped they could be persuaded to pay. Legislation attempted to control medical fees and patients went to court, often successfully, to have their medical bills reduced. As a result, even the wealthy generally relied on home remedies in the treatment of common complaints and endemic infection, for which they soon developed favourite medicines and only called in the doctor as a last resort or in an emergency.

William Douglass MD in Boston in 1718 claimed that he 'could live handsomely by the incomes of his Practice and save some small matter'.[5] Alexander Stenhouse in Baltimore in 1775 claimed to make *£707.16s.6d.* by his practice, and another £270 by his drug store and inoculating[6] when the salary of the Governor was only £1,000. It was only a very few town-based men who were in such a fortunate position. The rest, if they wished to prosper, had to become also merchants, farmers, planters, accept public office, keep an inn, speculate in land or some other activity. Provincial English doctors also sometimes

[5] Blake, *Public Health*.

[6] Bernard C. Steiner, 'New Light on Some Maryland Loyalists', *Maryland Historical Magazine* 2 (1907), pp. 133–7.

supplemented their earnings by various activities.[7] Affluent London doctors, like William Hunter, were not averse to financial speculation.[8]

Some doctors through their various activities became wealthy, but to this wealth medicine had not contributed greatly. Dr Charles Carroll, an Irishman who arrived in Maryland in 1715, became one of the wealthiest men in the colony, but this was through his extensive trading activities and his involvement in iron production in the colony. For most of the colonial period, except in New England where, up to 1700, 22 per cent of all doctors came from medical families of two or more generations,[9] relatively few sons, even the sons of doctors who had prospered, followed their fathers into the profession, for they saw prosperity lay in other activities. Nor were the sons of prosperous merchants, planters or lawyers attracted to the profession, for they too saw prosperity was possible without the added time and expense of acquiring a medical education, which was not obtainable in the colonies, at least at a level that would satisfy them.

Even the Scottish doctors generally had to resort to trading and other activities, which some did with great success, becoming rich. Their education, professional and social standing and wealth made them acceptable amongst the wealthy elite colonial families who by the eighteenth century controlled the commerce and politics of North America. Sons of these wealthy colonial families by the middle of the eighteenth century now saw medicine as an acceptable profession provided their parents could afford a medical education that would make them professionally equal to the Scottish immigrants.

It was in Maryland, South Carolina and Virginia that these Scottish immigrants had the greatest influence. These colonies had close links with Scotland; Maryland and Virginia through the tobacco trade and South Carolina through actively promoted Scottish immigration to the colony. Since therefore these colonies contained considerable Scottish communities, they attracted Scottish doctors.

Through the eighteenth century, Maryland had eighteen, South Carolina twenty and Virginia at least twenty-nine Scottish doctors, amongst whom were the leaders of the profession. Though twelve Scottish doctors settled in Massachusetts only William Douglass

[7] Margaret Pelling, 'Occupational Diversity, Barbersurgeons and the Trades of Norwich' *Bulletin of the History of Medicine* 56 (1982), pp. 484–551.

[8] C. H. Brock, 'The Happiness of Riches' in *William Hunter and the Eighteenth Century Medical World*, ed. W. F. Bynum and Roy Porter (Cambridge, 1985).

[9] Christianson, 'Medicine in New England'.

achieved prominence. New York had nine with Cadwallader Colden and Peter Middleton outstanding. Philadelphia had only seven.[10] Yet even without a number of influential Scottish doctors in these colonies, a number of young men, stimulated perhaps by an awareness of the improving status of the medical profession not only in the colonies but also in England, and a knowledge of exciting developments that were taking place in medicine, and growing colonial wealth that made European education increasingly possible, wished to enter the profession.

A very few colonists from the early years of the eighteenth century, had gone abroad to obtain a good medical education. After 1740 increasing numbers crossed the Atlantic to attend British and continental medical schools. Between 1740 and 1800, over 300 attended the Edinburgh medical school, but all did not graduate. Some chose to graduate at Glasgow where the expense was less and no Latin thesis was required. Others obtained a recommendation to an Aberdeen degree. Men from New England generally chose to study in London, for this was where these colonies had trade connections. At least fifty from Massachusetts studied abroad, thirty-eight in London, yet twelve went to Edinburgh, attracted there by the reputation of the medical school. Thirty-eight men from Pennsylvania went to Edinburgh and many of them also attended anatomy and midwifery lectures in London and walked the London hospitals. These widely educated Pennsylvanians not only became the leaders of the profession in the colony, but came to dominate American medicine.

By 1765 a medical school was opened in Philadelphia. Its establishment was mainly the work of two Pennsylvanians, William Shippen and John Morgan, both medical graduates of Edinburgh who had also studied in London. John Morgan had also visited physicians and medical institutions on the continent. It was founded on the pattern of the Edinburgh medical school and except for the professor of clinical medicine, Thomas Bond, who had attended lectures at the Hôtel Dieu in Paris, all the professors till the end of the century were Edinburgh graduates. In 1768 another medical school opened at King's College, New York, again founded on the Edinburgh model and staffed by Edinburgh graduates. The medical school of Philadelphia survived the Revolution and eventually amalgamated with the University of Penn-

[10] C. H. Brock, 'Scotland and American Medicine' in W. R. Brock, *Scotus Americanus* (Edinburgh, 1985).

sylvania in 1791. The medical school of King's College was disrupted by the Revolution but was re-established in 1792 by the trustees of Columbia University which replaced King's College.

Philadelphia had established a hospital in 1752, the first real hospital in British North America, and this was used for clinical teaching. By 1771 New York started raising money for a hospital but in 1775 when the building was nearing completion it was virtually destroyed by fire, and before the hospital could be rebuilt, the Revolution had broken out.

Now Americans need no longer go abroad for a university education. Though the Revolution hindered the further development of medical schools, Harvard medical school opened in 1783 at the end of hostilities, and in 1798 another medical school opened at Dartmouth, New Hampshire.

By the 1770s native-born graduates, and well-educated native doctors were joining graduate immigrant doctors in the leadership of the profession in the different colonies. This was to be of importance to American medicine for when the Revolution broke out, and many leading immigrant doctors either joined the British forces or left America, the profession was by no means left leaderless, and the improvements that had taken place in the proficiency of the profession were maintained.

American doctors were well able to keep in touch with medical developments in Europe. While popular medical works, like William Buchan's *Domestic Medicine*, were reprinted many times in the colonies and were easily available, for the profession more specialised books were imported, sometimes reaching the colonies within a year of publication and often forming part of the stock in trade of the numerous drug stores that were established in almost all towns in the eighteenth century, The *Philosophical Transactions* of the Royal Society circulated widely, copies of *Medical Observations and Inquiries* and the Edinburgh *Medical Essays* were advertised for sale. Local newspapers carried items of medical news and the *Gentleman's Magazine*, which often carried medical articles, was also widely available. It was also to these journals that Americans were contributing papers on their medical observations. Between 1730 and 1760 there were at least forty-three papers from Americans in the *Philosophical Transactions* though these were not all on medical subjects, while four Americans had papers in *Medical Observations and Inquiries*.

Immigrant doctors and Americans trained in Europe were educated in the European materia medica and this is what they continued to use in America. Some of the necessary plants had become transplanted to America and some experiments were made with indigenous plants, but by and large doctors depended upon imported drugs and medicines. Even in Massachusetts, it was traditional European medicines that were used.[11] Where something is known of the stock of medicines held by private families for home treatment of their ills,[12] it was imported medicines and drugs that filled the medicine cupboard. To meet this demand, by the eighteenth century, drugs stores, which also stocked imported surgical instruments, medical books and later electrical apparatus, had become established in most towns, often by the medical profession, though it was also looked on as a profitable commercial activity by men outside the profession. Local newspapers carried advertisements of the arrival of fresh cargoes of drugs and of sources of patent medicines. This reliance on imported medicines was to cause great problems at the beginning of the Revolution, when imports from Britain were cut off.[13] It was not till the French had come to the aid of the Patriots and drugs were arriving from Europe that the situation was relieved.

Now that the number of medical graduates, both immigrant and native-born was increasing, they found it was frustrating that they, who were fully qualified to call themselves doctor, could not distinguish themselves from 'all those who by the courtesy of *America* are stil'd Doctors because it is well known that Surgeons, Apothecaries, Chemists and Druggists or even mere smatterers in any of them are all promiscously call'd by that Title as well as real Physicians'.[14]

By the end of the eighteenth century, while the leaders of the medical profession approached in competence the qualified practitioners in Britain, below these the number of men who had been trained by apprenticeship, and that a much shorter apprenticeship than in Britain,

[11] J. Worth Estes, 'Therapeutic Practice in Colonial New England' in *Medicine in Colonial Massachusetts 1620–1820*, ed. P. Cash, E. H. Christianson and J. Worth Estes (Boston, 1980).

[12] Landon Carter, *The Diary of Landon Carter of Sabine Hill, 1752–1778* ed. Jack P. Green, 2 vols. (Charlottesville, 1965).

[13] George B. Griffenhagen, 'Drug Supplies in the American Revolution', *Contributions from the Museum of History and Technology* 225 (1961), pp. 110–33.

[14] Adam Thomson, *A Discourse on the Preparation of the Body for the Smallpox and the Manner of Receiving the Infection* (Philadelphia, 1750).

was very much smaller, and many became doctors without any formal training. Williams Smith's well-known complaint in 1757[15] was that

Quacks abound like locusts in Egypt, and too many have been recommended to a full practice and profitable subsistence; this is less to be wondered at, as the profession is under no kind of regulation. Loud as the call is, to our shame be it remembered, we have no laws to protect the lives of the King's subjects from the malpractice of pretenders. Any man at his pleasure, sets up for physician, apothecary, and surgeon. No candidates are either examined, licenced or sworn to fair practice.

Local papers provided the quacks with facilities for advertising their accomplishments and their panaceas for all ills and undoubtedly many fell victim to their claims.

The authorities were not unaware of the problem. Even in the seventeenth century both Massachusetts and New York had attempted to prohibit the activities of the ignorant. In 1760 New York and in 1772 New Jersey, in attempting to grapple with the problem, introduced legislation requiring all those who practised in these colonies to be examined and licensed. New Jersey went further, prohibiting doctors from setting up stalls and selling 'cure alls'.[16] But they had no effective means of enforcing their legislation, which depended mainly on the public reporting offenders. If a patient obtained relief from a quack he was unlikely to report an offender.

Americans returning from a British medical education, convinced of the advantages of a licensing system, and undoubtedly anxious to eliminate competition from uneducated practitioners, pressed for more rigid control of the profession. Virginian students requested the House of Burgesses to introduce legislation to prevent 'any one for the future from professedly practicing medicine who had not received a public testimony of his abilities, by being properly licenced and honoured with a doctor's degree'.[17] John Morgan in Philadelphia attempted in 1768 to found a Medical Society, which he hoped would function like the Royal College of Physicians in London. It was to provide a centre for the exchange of medical knowledge, encourage medical research and establish and enforce standards of professional conduct. Though established in Philadelphia its scope was to be intercolonial, and licensing of practitioners, which it proposed to undertake, was to carry authority in all British North American colonies. Morgan asked the Proprietor, Thomas Penn, for a charter to

[15] William Smith, *History of the Province of New York*, vol. 1 'From the First Discovery to the Year MDCCXXXII', ed. Michael Kamman (Cambridge, MA, 1972).

[16] F. R. Packard, *History of Medicine in the United States*, 2 vols. (New York, 1934).

[17] Wyndham B. Blanton, *Medicine in Virginia in the Eighteenth Century* (Richmond, 1931).

convert the Society into a College of Physicians. Penn asked for advice from Dr John Fothergill in London who had taken a great interest in Philadelphian medicine and the establishment of the medical school, and Fothergill suggested that the time was not yet right for such an institution,[18] and no College of Physicians was established in Philadelphia till 1787 (which attempted no international licensing). As a result of the experience in England in the sixteenth and seventeenth centuries of monopolies granted by the sovereign in return for favours either received or requested, which invariably forced up the price and restricted the availability of goods and services, the colonists were opposed to any measures that might create a monopoly. It was this hostility to legislation that could be viewed as creating a medical monopoly, that prevented the establishment of an effective control of the medical profession till well into the nineteenth century.

Eighteenth-century Americans, unless they had moved into sparsely inhabited frontier regions, generally had access to a doctor, for the ratio of doctors to the population was high. In New England it rose from 1 to 1,000 in 1700 to 1 to 417 in 1800,[19] though the significance of this ratio is uncertain. For in the first place many of the people were too poor to employ a doctor, and those who could just afford medical advice probably obtained it from quacks or untrained men who were not included in the count of doctors, though they were an important component of medical provision.

By the end of the eighteenth century there were only two general hospitals in what was now the United States, at Philadelphia and New York. This was far behind hospital provision in Britain where by the end of the century most towns, some no bigger than American towns, had established hospitals. It was not that America had no need of such institutions, but that initially when the population had been small, it was possible to organise otherwise the care of the sick poor. There seems to have been little tradition of doctors providing treatment of the poor free of charge.[20] Those who fell sick and could not look after themselves were cared for in private homes at public expense, a levy being made for their support on those who paid taxes. Even those who could pay for their own treatment, but who had no one to look after

[18] Whitfield J. Bell Jr, *John Morgan, Continental Doctor* (Philadelphia, 1965).

[19] Christianson, 'Medicine in New England'.

[20] Whitfield J. Bell Jr, 'A Portrait of the Colonial Physician' in *The Colonial Physician and other Essays* (New York, 1975).

them, would contract with a doctor to take him into his home and look after him. By the eighteenth century many towns or communities appointed salaried doctors to look after the poor in their own homes. But it became increasingly difficult to find private homes that would take them and many communities established alms or work houses where the indigent could be taken in and those who were sick looked after, but they did not provide the specialist services possible in a proper hospital. The insane were generally housed in prison or in alms houses where they were available, but in 1767 Virginia founded the first asylum for 'Idiots, Lunatics and other persons of unsound mind'.[21] New York in 1799 opened the first lying-in hospitals for indigent expectant mothers.[22] Philadelphia in 1786, New York in 1790 and Boston in 1791[23] followed the London example[24] of establishing public dispensaries which provided out-patient treatment for the sick poor.

It was not only the poor who sometimes required care or treatment beyond what was conveniently provided in the home, and by the end of the century some private hospitals had been established, two in Virginia[25] and there may well have been similar establishments in other colonies.

The French and Indian Wars of 1753–63 and the Revolution gave Americans some experience in the organisation of military hospitals and the care of the military sick and wounded, but it was a hardly won experience and in the early years of the Revolution the hospital services were totally chaotic. Like the English wars of the seventeenth and eighteenth centuries,[26] the Revolution provided military surgeons with a greatly increased experience in dealing with a wide variety of medical problems and emergencies which helped a general improvement in the profession. They were also able to learn from the generally more skilful French surgeons who worked alongside them and even from British surgeons, for sometimes American and British wounded were looked after in the same hospitals.[27] But the Revolution was also important in showing up the shortcomings in the profession and promoting improvements.

There was at the beginning of the Revolution no body to which the military command could appeal for authoritative advice on the organisation of medical support for the troops, or the control of camp

[21] Blanton, *Medicine in Virginia.*

[22] John Duffy, *History of Public Health in New York* (New York, 1968).

[23] Blake, *Public Health.* [24] See the chapter by Robert Kilpatrick (below).

[25] Blanton, *Medicine in Virginia.*

[26] Geoffrey Holmes, *Augustan England: Professions, State and Society, 1680–1730* (London, 1982). [27] Blanton, *Medicine in Virginia.*

diseases, nor was there any register recording the availability of doctors from which men could be called up for military duty. Such a register had been attempted in 1756 in Maryland,[28] but the necessary legislation was blocked. The army had to rely on volunteers and pay and conditions were such that there was little enthusiasm for volunteering.

Between 1783 and the end of the century, a determined effort was made to improve the profession. Though it was still impossible effectively to control who provided medical advice and services, and there was no legislation governing apprenticeships, facilities for medical education improved through increased university provision and through private lectures on various medical subjects. Though there had been previously a few medical societies, mainly in Massachusetts, in New Jersey and New York, and a student medical society in Philadelphia, formed from Dr Thomas Bond's clinical students,[29] in the post-Revolutionary period a number of societies came into existence aiming at an improvement in the profession.

Not till the slaves had introduced tropical diseases from Africa did the colonial doctors have to deal with complaints that were unfamiliar to European practice and for which there were no accepted therapies, for the infections from which the colonists suffered had all been brought with them from Europe. The indigenous Indians suffered from no infectious diseases they could pass on to the colonists.[30] Dysentery and typhoid, well known in England, to begin with caused the greatest havoc for they were easily brought in by human carriers not necessarily showing signs of illness. The lack of hygiene in the early settlements led to their early establishment as endemic complaints in their new home. Each summer in swampy ground and stagnant pools there bred millions of *Anopheles* mosquitoes capable of taking over from their European cousins the transmission of *Plasmodium vivax*, the cause of malaria.[31] Dysentery, typhoid and malaria are diseases in which one

[28] The Archives of Maryland (Baltimore 1883 –),vol. 52, p. 468.

[29] Whitfield J. Bell Jr, 'An Eighteenth Century Medical Manuscript' in *The Colonial Physician and Other Essays* (New York, 1975).

[30] Lucile E. Hoyme, 'On the Origins of New World Paleopathology' *American Journal of Physical Anthropology*, new series, 31 (1969), 295–302 and Saul Jarcho, 'Some Observations on Disease in Prehistoric North America' *Bulletin of the History of Medicine* 38 (1964), pp. 1–19.

[31] Darrett B. Rutman and Anita H. Rutman, 'Of Agues and Fevers: Malaria in the Early Chesapeake' *William and Mary Quarterly*, third series, 33 (1976), pp. 31–60.

attack induces little immunity to subsequent attacks, so that the colonists over and over again fell victims to these diseases.

It was not long before the full range of European infectious diseases were imported into America and were superimposed on top of the endemic complaints. Smallpox, measles, diphtheria, whooping cough, scarlet fever, mumps, influenza, tuberculosis, typhus, rabies and almost certainly anthrax and tetanus came to afflict the colonists. Whether or not venereal disease was introduced into Europe from America, it certainly came back again with the colonists. Even when doctors were confronted with the African diseases, yaws and yellow fever, medical theory of the day was able to determine the appropriate treatment. Yaws had early been recognised as related to syphilis and therefore the appropriate treatment was with mercury.[32] Yellow fever, believed to result from some corruption in the body, was treated by purgings and bleedings.

The level and character of the disease situation in the different colonies depended on climate, geography, pattern of immigration, mode of settlement and economic activity. In New England where the climate was temperate and where immigration had been mainly in family groups that settled in small townships and villages, and employed themselves in agriculture, endemic diseases were not as devastating as they were in the middle and southern colonies where the summers were hotter and the settlement pattern different. In Virginia and Maryland, given over to the cultivation of tobacco, many immigrants were indentured servants. The tobacco plantations were established mainly along the rivers that served not only as a source of water for domestic purposes but as a sewage and garbage disposal system as well and were a constant source of infection.

Diseased passengers, landing at ports, sometimes children suffering from the English endemic childhood diseases of smallpox, measles and similar infections, which were not yet endemic in the colonies, were often the starting point for epidemics in North America. These spread easily where there were urban developments and where non-immune populations had developed between epidemics. Boston and the other ports and towns of New England had suffered from smallpox, measles and diphtheria epidemics in the seventeenth century. Maryland, with no urban development till the eighteenth century, where the population had settled on isolated plantations and which had many immigrant

[32] Royal Society, Journal Book, IX, 188.

servants and young adults who had survived childhood infections and were therefore immune to further attacks, was long spared epidemics. It was not till ports and towns were developed to deal with developing and changing economic developments, and a large native-born, non-immune component of the population had come into being by the 1730s that Maryland started to suffer from smallpox epidemics.

Medical advances through the seventeenth and eighteenth centuries had done little to improve therapy. While the approved treatment of the endemic diseases by purging and bleeding, if the cases were mild was not greatly harmful but did little to relieve, in severe cases it was highly likely to be lethal. Relief of dysentery was acknowledged as being very difficult,[33] and some managed to make comfortable fortunes from colonial legislatures by claiming a reward for publishing their cures. Richard Bryan got £250 out of the Virginian legislature. Supposed cures for yaws were also rewarded. Joseph Howard received £3,000 out of the South Carolina Assembly in his cure of 'yaws or almost any corrupt blood etc'.[34]

Dysentery, typhoid and malaria continued to plague Americans right through the eighteenth century. In the middle and southern colonies malaria was seen as the most common complaint; in New England malaria by the eighteenth century had largely died out. By the beginning of the eighteenth century cinchona was available in America for the treatment of malaria. It was sometimes of poor quality or adulterated and some doctors lost faith in it. Since they believed that malaria was a liver complaint they preferred to treat it by purging and bleeding. Its use by the poor was prohibited by the cost and its potential for relieving malaria was never fully realised. In the large ports of Philadelphia, New York and Boston tuberculosis was becoming endemic and a main cause of death amongst the poor.[35]

Knowledge of inoculation against smallpox had reached Massachusetts about 1720 in copies of the *Philosophical Transactions* containing the paper of Emanuel Timonius[36] about its use in Constantinople. A copy had been lent to the Reverend Cotton Mather who had also learnt about its use from his Negro servant. Massachusetts from 1620, the year of its foundation, had suffered smallpox epidemics, Cotton Mather tried to persuade the medical profession of the value of

[33] William Cockburn, 'A Discourse on the Difficulty of Curing Fluxes', *Philosophical Transactions* 38 (1732), pp. 385–93.

[34] Francisco Guerra, *American Medical Bibliography 1639–1783* (New York, 1962).

[35] Guerra, *American Medical Bibliography*.

[36] Emanuel Timonius, 'Letter from Emanuel Timonius from Constantinople', *Philosophical Transactions* 29 (1713), pp. 72–6.

inoculation but almost to a man they rejected the treatment on moral as well as medical grounds. Only one doctor, Zabdiel Boylston, was interested and when Boston was engulfed in an epidemic in 1721 inoculated his own and Mather's children and others brave enough to try the new protection. In a Boston population of 10,700, there were 5,750 cases of natural smallpox with 842 deaths (146 deaths per 1,000 cases); of the 287 people who were inoculated there were only six deaths (21 deaths per 1,000 inoculated).[37] Thereafter, though inoculation was often opposed by legislatures, mainly because of the danger of inoculated patients starting epidemics, it was widely practised and undoubtedly saved many lives. Some colonies followed the London example and established inoculating hospitals where the patients could be held to prevent them spreading the disease.

Other diseases also caused epidemics, particularly measles, diphtheria and what was probably influenza,[38] often affecting New England in the seventeenth century where there was the largest concentration of population. By the eighteenth century, with population growth and urbanisation, these infections appeared more frequently in the middle and southern colonies. Since none of these diseases became endemic many escaped infection till they were adult, reacting to them more severely than did children, and this was one of the causes of high mortality in these epidemics.

Massachusetts particularly, and New York, had tried actively to control disease. There were believed to be two types of epidemic disease, those that like smallpox and measles were contagious, and those like malaria that were caused by miasmas or bad air. The colonies followed the European practice of attempting to control the introduction of contagious disease by quarantining ships or traffic from places of infection. In 1665 both Boston and New York quarantined ships from London to prevent the introduction of the plague; thereafter quarantine was frequently imposed on incoming ships not only in these two ports but in most colonial ports. But once infection was introduced then isolation of the infected had to be imposed, restricting the sick to their homes, impressing nurses to look after them and placing guards on the door to prevent contact with the outside. In 1717 Boston established a pest house on Spectacle Island to which infected cases could be removed. New York did not establish a pest house till 1760.

Attempts to control by legislation the miasmas that resulted, par-

[37] Blake, *Public Health*.

[38] John Duffy, *Epidemics in Colonial America*, reissue (Port Washington, New York, 1972).

ticularly in hot weather, from rotting garbage and stagnant water, and which were believed to cause the summer rise in agues, were ineffective, for there were no means of enforcing laws relating to street cleaning, siting of privies and slaughter houses etc. Yellow fever is caused by a virus transmitted by the mosquito *Aedes aegypti* and had caused small epidemics in various ports from 1698 to 1768; thereafter North America was free from the infection till 1793 when there was a devastating epidemic in Philadelphia, followed in 1794 by epidemics in Baltimore and New Haven and in Boston in 1795, and few ports were free of it for the next few years. A controversy broke out as to whether it was contagious or a virulent form of malaria caused by miasmas. Quarantine was imposed on vessels coming from the West Indies which was in fact the main source of the disease, but most believed that it was caused by miasmas and citizens and officials were driven to enormous efforts to eliminate all causes of miasmas. In Philadelphia, Baltimore, New York and Boston, health committees or health officers were appointed to oversee the cleaning of the streets and disposal of garbage. This was the beginning of an active concern with public health, pre-dating the introduction of a Public Health Bill and the appointment of Officers of Health in England by fifty years.[39]

Through the seventeenth century middle and southern colonial doctors were confronted by a level of disease giving higher infant mortality and shorter life expectancy than in provincial England. In New England where health generally was better and the climate and way of life less exacting, life expectancy was greater than in England.[40] By the eighteenth century colonial health had improved, but not through any active attempt at improvement beyond laws introduced, in towns like Boston[41] and New York,[42] to control miasmas and bad smells. Improved general health resulted mainly from better housing and an improved and more varied diet which increasingly contained vegetables and fruit and the availability of beer or cider as a drink instead of polluted water. But the usual method of cooking, particularly amongst the poor, was to boil meat and vegetables together, destroying any sources of vitamin C. Mild scurvy was a common complaint. Cadwallader Colden believed it affected most families[43] and this is also suggested by the advertisements in local papers for

[39] Arthur Swinton, *The History of Public Health* (Exeter, 1965).

[40] Lorena Walsh and Russell R. Minard, 'Two Life Tables for Men in Early Colonial Maryland', *Maryland Historical Magazine* 69 (1974), pp. 211–27.

[41] Blake, *Public Health*.

[42] Duffy, *Public Health in New York*.

[43] Saul Jarcho, 'Cadwallader Colden as a Student of Infectious Diseases', *Bulletin of the History of Medicine* 29 (1955), pp. 9–115.

antiscorbutic toothpastes. The health of the colonists at no time was as bad as that in the slums of the large European cities.

While a study of doctors and disease is of itself of interest, the effect of disease on social, economic and political development is of much greater interest. While few records exist that provide firm demographic and statistical measurements, because populations generally were smaller and social organisation was simpler, it is possible to make reasonable suggestions as to the effect of disease on colonial development.

Except in New England, the level of disease was such that through the seventeenth century population growth was possible only through continual immigration. Constant sickness amongst the work-force, even in the eighteenth century, must have affected economic development. When towards the end of the seventeenth century the supply of indentured servants to the southern colonies began to give out through improved economic conditions in England and the demand created for soldiers for the English wars, their place was taken by African slaves. More expensive than servants, they were only an economic proposition if they survived considerably longer than the five years for which servants were indentured. Few first generation slaves survived more than two or three years. It was not till a population of second generation slaves had built up with longer life expectancy that they became financially acceptable.

In the seventeenth century no money was available in the colonies for capital investment for few men lived long enough to become rich. There was little social division in the colonies based on wealth and North America was looked on as a land of opportunity. The eighteenth century brought increased life expectancy and more men had time to become rich. But still little of this increasing wealth went into industrial development which was discouraged by Britain, or public works, and most of it was used for personal financial improvement. The rich in the different colonies established themselves as an elite and exclusive body of men who increasingly controlled colonial commerce. They cemented their position by intermarriage, and with the reduction in child mortality increasingly had a son to inherit their wealth and position.

The majority of immigrants in the seventeenth century were men of little education and no experience of administration and politics, yet the control of the colonies was largely in the hands of such men, who died off before they learnt how to govern. So colonial politics were often chaotic. In the eighteenth century with an increasing population of native-born colonists knowledgeable about their colony and with more years to learn the skills of government, politics became more professional and organised. But increasingly the wealthy elite gained control of politics and administration and men outside this exclusive group found themselves excluded from influence in colonial affairs.[44]

But disease had more than an economic and political effect. In small and rather homogeneous communities, the people were well aware of the effect of endemic and epidemic sickness. In New England, where sickness was looked on as God's punishment for evil-doing, religion, death and prospects of everlasting damnation lay heavily upon the people. Prayer and religious exercises were essential adjuncts to medical treatment. Maryland had no established church till 1702. Here with ever present disease and none to remind them of the Day of Judgement, the colonists lived only from day to day. Scattered plantations relieved the inhabitants from some of the restraints on behaviour imposed by public opinion in Britain. Conditions of life and restrictions placed on marriage of indentured servants hardly promoted high moral standards. Drunkenness was widespread, fornication common, 10 per cent of children born in the colony were illegitimate, infanticide often practised, sometimes by the most revolting methods, and cruelty to servants and slaves sometimes beyond belief. For many outside the sophisticated life in the capital, Annapolis, life was nasty, brutish and short, even in the eighteenth century, and in Virginia conditions were little better.

Medicine in North America is seen generally as an extension of British medicine, but the British were not the only Europeans established in North America – California had long been part of the Spanish American Empire as had Florida. At the end of the Seven Years War, Florida became a British possession, but in 1783 the British were driven out and it once more belonged to Spain. The Dutch had settled along the Hudson river in what they called New Holland but it had been conquered by the English in 1664. The French had long been established in Canada and round the mouth of the Mississippi river in Louisiana. Canada was acquired by the British at the end of the French and Indian Wars in 1763, while Louisiana had gone to Spain. Medicine in these possessions also was dominated by the traditional medicine of

[44] David W. Jordan, 'Political Stability and the Emergence of a Native Elite in Maryland' in Thad. W. Tate and David L. Ammerman, *The Chesapeake in the Seventeenth Century* (Chapel Hill, 1979).

the mother countries, but British, French and Spanish medicine were essentially European medicine. Spain and France however maintained a much greater control over the practice of medicine in their colonies than did the British. Medicine in Spanish New World colonies[45] and French colonies[46] has been recently very fully discussed and will not be considered here.

There were other medical traditions operating in North America besides European medicine. The Indians had their own highly developed medicine, largely employing local herbs and described as particularly successful in treating wounds, undoubtedly of great use amongst a very warlike people. If there had been any infectious diseases which the Indians could have transmitted to the colonists, and to which the colonists had no immunity but for which the Indians had cures, the course of colonial history and medicine might have been changed. The Indians might have transmitted the disease but withheld the cure so that colonisation might have been reduced if not prevented. If on the other hand the Indians had handed over the cure, then Indian medicine might have had a greater impact on colonial medicine. The situation was, however, reversed. The colonists transmitted to the Indians, sometimes it is believed intentionally, European diseases to which the Indians had no immunity, and certainly did not provide them with inoculation when it became available, and probably not with cinchona or any other European medicines, so that by the eighteenth century the Indians of the Eastern seaboard were virtually wiped out. As Cotton Mather put it in 1702 'the woods were almost cleared of those pernicious creatures to make room for a better growth'.

The Spaniards had early introduced into Europe some American plants with medicinal properties learnt from the Indians. Sassafras, believed to be effective against a variety of complaints including rheumatism and venereal disease, became an important export from America: the first export in 1603 from the New England region was a cargo of sassafras (*Laurus sassafras*). In 1770 England imported some seventy-seven tons and it became part of the English Pharmacopoeia as did snake root (*Polygala senega*) and ginseng (*Panax trifolium*). There was little fraternisation between the Indians and the colonists and the Indians were reluctant to divulge their medical secrets, but the Indian uses of some local plants became known. Nicholas Monardes had

[45] G. Risse, 'Medicine in New Spain' in *Medicine in the New World*, ed. Ronald Numbers (Knoxville, Tennessee, 1987).

[46] Tony Gelfand, 'Medicine in New France' in *Medicine in the New World*, ed. Ronald Numbers (Knoxville, Tennessee, 1987).

published a book on American medicinal plants, some of which grew in North America, and this in 1577 had been translated as *Ioyfvll Nevvs Ovt of the Newe Founde Worlde*. In the seventeenth and eighteenth centuries various works like John Josselyn's *New England Rarities* (1675) and John Bartram's *Descriptions Virtues and Uses of Sundry Plants of These Northern Parts of America* (1751) gave useful information about Indian cures. The Royal Society in London had an ongoing interest in Indian medicine. The Reverend John Clayton in Virginia wrote to the Secretary of the Royal Society, Nehemiah Grew, in 1687, describing a number of Indian practices and claimed his life was saved by an Indian herbal cure.[47] They were provided with information from Dr Richard Brooke of Maryland who in 1752 was using some Indian cures in his practice. John Fothergill wrote to John Bartram in Pennsylvania to ask what use was made of Indian cures by doctors and ordinary people. He replied that the Indians had discovered the use of many plants but the inexpert use of them by the colonists made people discard them as useless.[48] Benjamin Rush, the prestigious Philadelphian doctor, in 1774 declared 'We have no discoveries in the materia medica to hope for from the Indians of North America.'[49] The European materia medica was too firmly entrenched in North American medicine to welcome in Indian medicines of doubtful use. Even during the Revolution, when European medicines became hard to get, little use was made of Indian herbal cures.

There was even a third medical tradition in operation. The slaves brought their own medical beliefs with them and a few amongst them were known as doctors. A form of inoculation had long been practised in Africa and it was not only Timonius's paper in the *Philosophical Transactions* but also what he learnt about its use from his African servant that persuaded Cotton Mather in 1721 to advocate its use.

The health of the slaves was the responsibility of their masters and when they fell ill they were subjected to European medicine. While they were more resistant to malaria and smallpox than European immigrants, they suffered greatly from chest infections in the unfamiliar cold winters. For minor complaints they probably treated themselves according to their own traditional cures and some of these for common illnesses were made public in local newspapers and yearly almanacs.

[47] Edmund Berkeley and Dorothy Berkeley, *The Reverend John Clayton, a Parson with a Scientific Mind* (Charlottesville, 1965).

[48] William Darlington, *Memorials of John Bartram and Humphrey Marshall* (Philadelphia, 1894).

[49] Benjamin Rush, *An Inquiry into the Natural History of Medicine Amongst the Indians of North America and a Comparative View of Their Diseases and Remedies With Those of Civilised Nations* (Philadelphia, 1774).

Yaws, a complaint with which the slaves must have been well acquainted, was generally treated with mercury, but James Pawpaw, a Virginian slave, was granted his freedom and an annual pension for his cure of yaws which became widely used in America.[50] Though yellow fever was certainly an African disease, there is no record of slaves providing any cure for it.

It is even possible to suggest the development of a fourth medical tradition. While care was organised for the poor who were really sick, there were many less serious conditions that they had to deal with themselves. Some popular books like William Buchan's *Domestic Medicine* had been frequently reprinted in America and gave helpful advice, but they were European books relying on medicines available in Europe. Josselyn's or Bartram's books would have informed them of local alternatives but they were unlikely to have access to such books. Local almanacs also gave what may have been helpful advice on the treatment of common ills, but the use made of this advice is unknown. Some English folk medicine practices can be traced in America.[51] But if the necessary English herbs could not be obtained in America then the colonists had to rely on old beliefs; for instance that plants that look alike have the same medical properties. Thus American pennyroyal was endowed with the capacity to cure snake bites and even kill snakes that belonged to Cretan ditany. Alternatively, the medical properties of plants were believed to be indicated by their form and colour, yellow flowers being useful for jaundice and walnuts appropriate for complaints of the brain. But such folk medicine as developed amongst the white settlers would have been transmitted by word of mouth and left no written record and now lies beyond the reach of history.

By the eighteenth century Europeans and European medicine dominated not only eastern North America but parts of the South and West as well and was penetrating into the interior. In spite of occasional professional interest in Indian medicine little had been accepted into American practice. At the beginning of the century the organisation and control of medicine within the British colonies, and its personnel and practice, particularly in surgery, was of a low standard. By the end of the century great improvements had been made. The standard of competence at the top of the profession approached that in the larger British provincial towns, though, with no effective control over who

[50] Thomas C. Paramore, 'Non-venereal Treponematosis in Colonial North America,' *Bulletin of the History of Medicine* 44 (1970), pp. 571–81.

[51] Edward Eggleston, *The Transit of Civilisation from England to America in the Seventeenth Century* (New York, 1901).

entered the profession, there were still many ignorant and dangerous men who managed to make a living in medicine. With four university medical schools the situation compared favourably with Britain's two Scottish medical schools and some medical teaching at Oxford and Cambridge, but opportunities for hospital training particularly of surgeons was well behind that in Britain. Without any regulation of apprenticeship training, many Americans still entered practice poorly prepared. Nor was there as yet much interest in North America in medical research.

The Indians were everywhere in retreat, devastated by European diseases to which they had no immunity and by alcohol fed to them by the Europeans. Indian medicine never before up against epidemic diseases of this kind had no ready cures nor was time provided for finding suitable treatments. Europeans offered them no help, only too pleased to see them so easily removed as a hindrance to their take-over of the land. Slaves officially were subjected to European medicine but undoubtedly held on to some of their traditional practices. Poor whites developed their own medicine compounded from many traditions. These traditions, of great importance to those that relied on them, are neglected by historians of American medicine.

9

John Haygarth, smallpox and religious Dissent in eighteenth-century England

FRANCIS M. LOBO

To the few modern historians who have studied him, Dr John Haygarth (1740–1827) seems to be many things. Modern scholars have hailed this late-eighteenth- and early-nineteenth-century physician as an 'apostle of sanitation', a 'pioneer of demography', or simply a "medical pioneer'.[1] Such a variety of praise stems from Haygarth's many and apparently unrelated activities as a physician. Through an analysis of these medical projects, however, and by keeping in mind both Haygarth's cooperators and their place in late-eighteenth-century England, one can uncover what Haygarth truly was: a physician working with the conviction of the 'philanthropic' responsibility of the 'wealthy and opulent' in society for the 'poor and ignorant'. The notions of philanthropy, reform and improvement were central to all of Haygarth's projects to relieve the misery of the poor. Although it has been said that Haygarth was 'ahead of his time', his attitude towards the poor and the work arising from it are tied to a definite time and place, clearly reflecting the religious, political and socio-economic conditions of England at the time of the American and French Revolutions.

This chapter won the Osler Medal of the American Association for the History of Medicine, 1988.
Acknowledgements: I would like to thank Dr Adrian Wilson and Dr Andrew Cunningham of the Wellcome Unit for the History of Medicine at the University of Cambridge, for, respectively, the inspiration and the guidance I received in originally preparing this paper as my M.Phil. dissertation. I am also grateful to Dr Thomas R. Forbes, Dr Arthur J. Viseltear and Dr John H. Warner of the Yale University School of Medicine for their helpful critiques. Finally, I must thank the Thouron-University of Pennsylvania British–American Exchange Program, whose munificence enabled me to undertake this project.

[1] John Elliot, 'A Medical Pioneer: John Haygarth of Chester,' *The British Medical Journal* (1 Feb 1913), pp. 235–42, and George H. Weaver, 'John Haygarth – Clinician, Investigator, Apostle of Sanitation. 1740–1827,' *Bulletin of the Society of Medical History of Chicago* 4 (1928–35), pp. 156–200. These, along with the paper in note 2, are the only secondary materials that deal exclusively with Haygarth's life and work.

In this chapter, I will demonstrate that Haygarth's most ambitious and personally most important project, his plan to eradicate smallpox, originated, as did many of his various activities, in the agenda for reform advanced primarily by religious Dissenters. This integration of Haygarth's plan with the ideals of those who were so publicly critical of the established religious and political institutions determined in large part the plan's ultimate fate. Indeed, because of their exclusion from political power, Haygarth's Dissenting friends found it necessary to advance their philanthropic programmes among a definable set of predominantly Dissenting organisations and individuals, here termed the 'Dissenting intellectual network'. The names and deeds of Haygarth's friends – William Cullen, John Fothergill, Thomas Percival, John Coakley Lettsom, John Aikin, James Currie, to name a few – have attracted much more modern attention than Haygarth, with the result that much information about Haygarth can only be obtained through the biographies of these men. Unlike them, Haygarth neither left behind an adoring crowd of students to write his biography, nor did he, as a member of the Church of England, have a crowd of fellow Dissenters ready to exalt his memory. This chapter, then, will show that Haygarth both shared their philanthropic ideas and was at least their equal in working to implement those ideas.

I intend here to lift Haygarth from the footnotes of other histories by describing the plan that he proposed to conquer smallpox. The background to this discussion will consist of a search through his early life and education for those seminal events that caused him to undertake such a mammoth task. It will also contain a picture of the political and religious divisions in Haygarth's England, as well as an account of the practice of inoculation against smallpox up to Haygarth's time. This will give a good contemporary perspective on the arguments, accomplishments and proposals detailed in Haygarth's two works on smallpox, *An Inquiry How to Prevent the Small-pox and Proceedings of a Society for Promoting General Inoculation at Stated Periods, and Preventing the Natural Small-pox in Chester* (1784) and the *Sketch of a Plan to Exterminate the Casual Small-pox from Great Britain and to Introduce General Inoculation* (1793). The *Inquiry* described Haygarth's notion of the nature of the 'variolous (smallpox) distemper' and the successful prevention of its spread in Chester which, according to Haygarth, proved his notion correct. The *Sketch*, written as a sequel to the *Inquiry*, expanded the measures of the Chester Smallpox Society to a nationwide scale, involving compulsory inspection of homes and general inoculation. The conclusion of Haygarth's work regarding smallpox will then be found in Edward Jenner's discovery of the preventive powers of the 'vaccine inoculation', of which Haygarth and many of his medical friends soon became zealous advocates. The contrast between what Haygarth and Jenner offered was sharp: Haygarth proposing an expensive nationwide system of surveillance and inoculation with the 'natural smallpox', with its attendant dangers, at a time of a draining war with Revolutionary France and fears of a similar upheaval at home, as opposed to the miraculous, apparently danger-free vaccine from Jenner, a man lacking the religiously and politically suspicious associates that surrounded Haygarth. In 1802, Parliament voted Jenner an unprecedented £10,000 reward, triggering the international glorification of Jenner with which modern readers are very familiar. The demise of Haygarth's plan, however, did not result from the advent of Jenner's vaccination. In fact, Haygarth's proposal died for want of attention several years before the disclosure of Jenner's discovery. In the reactionary political climate of England in the 1790s, Haygarth could get no hearing from England's rulers for a plan that had attracted the support of many of the kingdom's most infamous religious Dissenters.

John Haygarth was born in Garsdale, a small village in the West Riding of Yorkshire, in 1740. His father owned a small manor house and was probably of the yeoman class of lesser landed gentry. It can be gathered from his correspondence that Haygarth had several sisters and a brother, presumably older and the inheritor of the family property, whose family remained in Garsdale.[2] As was the case with the younger sons of gentry families, Haygarth was intended for a respectable profession, which, for young John, was to be medicine. Haygarth attended the nearby Sedbergh School, a renowned grammar school possessing formal links with St John's College, Cambridge.[3] Haygarth's immediate family members were not Dissenters, and so it was probably at Sedbergh that he mingled with Dissenters for the first time. The extent to which Dissenters were admitted to Sedbergh is not known, but the physician John Fothergill, the son of Quakers and an immensely important figure in Haygarth's life, attended Sedbergh twenty years before Haygarth.[4] Anthony Fothergill (no relation to, but a good friend of the above), a Quaker who later helped to found the Humane Society, was at Sedbergh about five years before Haygarth.[5] After his last year at Sedbergh, Haygarth was tutored in mathematics by the self-taught mathematician and surgeon, John Dawson.

[2] George H. Weaver, 'John Haygarth – Portrait, Letter, and Descendants,' *Bulletin of the Society of Medical History of Chicago* 4 (1933), pp. 264–7.
[3] B. Wilson (ed.), *The Sedbergh School Register 1546 to 1909* (Leeds, 1909), pp. 4 and 179.
[4] *Ibid.*, p. 163. [5] *Ibid.*, p. 178.

Although a distant kinsman of Haygarth, Dawson came from a very poor, Dissenting family. His fame as a mathematician became so great during his lifetime that he was sought out by students bound for Cambridge, coaching at least eight future senior wranglers at the university. Haygarth remained his lifelong friend and admirer, using Dawson's calculations in his arguments on behalf of inoculation and of the benefits of eradicating smallpox. Haygarth matriculated at St John's College, Cambridge in 1759, and graduated MB in 1766. He later wrote that he spent some of those years before obtaining the MB training in London and Edinburgh.[6] Where and when he studied in London remains unknown. His time at the University of Edinburgh, however, was probably between the years 1763 and 1765, and was spent under the tutelage of the great Professor William Cullen.

William Cullen was certainly one of the most influential men in Haygarth's life, as indeed he was to a whole generation of Edinburgh medical students. Many of those who would later cooperate with Haygarth were his classmates at Edinburgh: Drs Percival, Matthew Dobson, William Falconer and William Irvine. Drs. Aikin, Lettsom, Currie and Benjamin Waterhouse followed afterwards by several years. At the time of Haygarth's studies there, Cullen held the sole professorship in chemistry, a position which he used to promote chemistry as a branch of natural philosophy in its own right.[7] Cullen found chemistry's greatest virtues in its firm grounding in the observation of natural phenomena and in the medical, industrial and other utilities in each of its discovered truths.[8] Cullen's object was to make chemistry appeal as a study to all gentlemen of a philosophical disposition, to demystify it by cutting through and rendering comprehensible the complex jargon which had previously intimidated so many learned men. Industry and the development of commerce was of great importance to Scottish intellectuals of the time, including Cullen and, most notably, his intimate friend Adam Smith, who was the Professor of Moral Philosophy at Glasgow when Cullen held the chair in chemistry at that university. 'Chemical philosophy', according to Cullen, was the philosophy of industry, which made it of pre-eminent importance to philosophical gentlemen.[9]

[6] John Haygarth, *A Letter to Dr. Percival, on the Prevention of Infectious Fevers; And an Address to the College of Physicians at Philadelphia on the Prevention of the American Pestilence* (Bath, 1801), p. 125.

[7] John Thomson, *An Account of the Life, Lectures, and Writings of William Cullen, M.D.* (Edinburgh, 1859), vol. 1, p. 97.

[8] A. L. Donovan, *Philosophical Chemistry in the Scottish Enlightenment* (Edinburgh, 1975), pp. 102–10.

[9] Cullen MSS, Glasgow University Library, quoted in *ibid.*, p. 60.

Chemistry was the way of understanding nature for the purpose of practical application, making it, in Cullen's opinion, a necessary study for a philosophical Scottish gentleman at this time of burgeoning Scottish industry. Cullen consequently opened his chemistry lectures, which he gave in English instead of Latin, to the whole student body, both at Glasgow and at Edinburgh. The students responded with great enthusiasm. By Cullen's reasoning, chemistry's great utility was its qualification to be an object of philosophical enquiry. Cullen held that the 'laws' of 'chemical philosophy' must be arrived at by generalisation from empirically observed facts and then tested through experimentation. But, as his friend David Hume proposed, the real philosophical measure of these truths was their utility.[10] To philosophers of a different time or place, such a measure might seem the very antithesis of philosophical reasoning, yet to the thinkers of the 'Scottish Enlightenment', who ridiculed the search for 'final causes' or some intrinsic order in nature, the utility of truths derived from the various philosophies in controlling future events provided those studies with their only meaning. As Haygarth was to later argue by quoting Francis Bacon, 'For the fruits and effects are the sureties and vouchers, as it were, for the truth of philosophy.'[11]

Cullen impressed more upon his students than simply a new respect for chemistry. He also taught them to respect the broad responsibilities of the medical profession. Cullen presented his students with a comprehensive account of disease based on the acting of 'proximate' and 'remote' causes upon the human body.[12] Thus the relationship between man and environment, the source of remote causes, became an object of medical study, and such conditions as uncleanliness, overcrowding and the natural formation of the environment became objects of medical concern in the attempt to prevent contagion.[13] These conditions should be sought out in places like hospitals, prisons and, in the case of the remote cause of 'marsh miasma', in the natural formations of a particular location.[14]

The type of physician to follow Cullen's search for remote and

[10] *Ibid.*, pp. 60–1.

[11] John Haygarth, *An Inquiry How to Prevent the Small-pox, and Proceedings of a Society for Promoting General Inoculation at Stated Periods, and Preventing the Natural Small-pox, at Chester* (Chester, 1784), p. 216. Haygarth quotes Bacon in Latin.

[12] Thomson, *William Cullen, M.D.*, pp. 333–6.

[13] Christopher Lawrence, 'Ornate Physicians and Learned Artisans: Edinburgh Medical Men, 1726–1776,' in W. F. Bynum and Roy Porter (eds.), *William Hunter and the Eighteenth-Century Medical World* (Cambridge, 1985), p. 172.

[14] William Cullen, *First Lines of the Practise of Physic*, ed. James C. Gregory (Edinburgh, 1829), pp. 55–6.

proximate causes was one of a much broader general education and interests. As his former student and chief biographer John Thomson remembered, Cullen believed that the prospective physician should acquire a superior philosophical, literary and general scientific education, a point which Cullen pressed in addition to his crusade for higher standards in the granting of Scottish medical degrees.[15] Pursuant to this interest, Cullen was active in the Philosophical Society of Edinburgh and, with his legendary paternal attention to his students,[16] presumably encouraged them to do likewise. As will be described below, societies such as the Philosophical Society of Edinburgh provided intellectual fora for a variety of people – from the leading unorthodox philosophers of Cullen's generation, to physicians inspired by Cullen, to prominent Quaker merchants – with the common characteristics of standing outside conventional religious, social and political circles, and with the common interest of exchanging useful knowledge.

In late 1766, the year of his graduation with the degree MB from Cambridge, Haygarth was elected physician to the Chester Infirmary by the governors of that charity. The Chester Infirmary had been founded in 1755, providing, along with the several other provincial infirmaries founded at that time, a respectable opportunity for prominent members of the community to group themselves, usually along the religious and political lines that governed all social interactions, in a structured and highly visible charitable project. As has been demonstrated regarding the similar charitable infirmary in the City of Manchester,[17] the Chester Infirmary also showed some political partiality among its subscribers, particularly in Haygarth's later years there, suggesting the use of the charity by political partisans to display their collective merit to the community. At the time of Haygarth's election, Chester politics were dominated by the Grosvenor family, who controlled Chester's two seats in Parliament nominally in the Tory interest, but who were noted for an 'independent and unpredictable' stance in the House of Commons.[18] From what is known about the political views of the approximately 1,000 voting freemen in Chester (from a population of about 15,000), the politics of the Grosvenors accorded

[15] Thomson, *William Cullen, M.D.*, pp. 505–6. [16] *Ibid.*, pp. 135–7.

[17] J. V. Pickstone and S. V. F. Butler, 'The Politics of Medicine in Manchester, 1788–1792: Hospital Reform and Public Health Services in the Early Industrial City,' *Medical History* 28 (1984), pp. 227–49.

[18] B. E. Harris (ed.), *The Victoria History of the Counties of England; A History of the County of Chester*, vol. 2 (Oxford, 1979), p. 135.

well with local popular opinion.[19] Although at the beginning of a period of decline, Chester was a prosperous port town in which the generally Whig industrialists never appeared on any significant scale, as they did in nearby Manchester and Liverpool. Chester's position in national politics was consequently supportive of Tory values – older money, the church, and the King.

It may seem surprising then that Haygarth, with the contacts and friendships which he had already formed with many Dissenters who held what can only be called extreme political opinions, should settle in Chester. Yet there were actually several good reasons for Haygarth to choose Chester. First, there was his friendship with William Falconer, who was studying for his medical degree at Edinburgh during Haygarth's time there, and who graduated MD also in 1766. Falconer's father, William Falconer, Esq., was the Recorder of Chester, and as such was part of the Grosvenor oligarchy in the town. He was also one of the founders of the Infirmary charity, holding the important office of Treasurer in 1755, its first year of existence.[20] Sir Richard Grosvenor, later first Earl Grosvenor, was Chairman of the charity in that year.[21] Dr Falconer's older brother, Thomas Falconer, Esq., became a governor of the charity in 1765, and was rotating in the chairmanship of the weekly board meetings at the Infirmary in the years around Haygarth's election. As William Falconer was elected physician to the Infirmary in the same year as Haygarth,[22] it is likely that Haygarth took advantage of the influence of his friend's family to secure a position as a colleague. Although William Falconer resigned from the Infirmary in 1769, moving his practice to Bath, Haygarth remained on intimate terms with the brothers, both of whom were to be valuable co-workers in his later projects. The influence of Cullen's doctrines of disease and contagion would also have made philosophically disposed physicians like Haygarth and Falconer seek out infirmary positions as an opportunity for further study. One must also remember that an appointment to one of the nation's few charitable infirmaries provided an excellent means of gaining a reputation and a clientele among the elite of the community. Haygarth did indeed do well in Chester,

[19] *Ibid.*, p. 135, and Joseph Hemingway, *A History of the City of Chester* (Chester, 1831), pp. 37–41.

[20] Chester Royal Infirmary, Minutes of Board Meetings and General Meetings, vol. 1 (1755–8), Chester City Records Office, p. 20.

[21] *Ibid.*, p. 20.

[22] Joseph Hemingway, *History of the City of Chester* (Chester, 1831), p. 199. It is unfortunate that the minutes of the Infirmary board meetings of late 1766 to early 1768 are missing.

becoming a significant local property owner.[23] Equally, Haygarth must have looked like an attractive candidate to the laymen governors of the Infirmary, for, in addition to his personal contacts with Infirmary luminaries, he was also a medical graduate of Cambridge and a member of the Church of England. These personal characteristics certainly qualified him for acceptance in all of Chester's conventional circles, and would help explain why Haygarth in Chester was able to implement many of the projects of the mostly Dissenting network of physicians with greater ease and speed than his Dissenting colleagues in other provincial towns and cities.[24]

To see how Haygarth maintained his contacts with like-minded colleagues, one must note the astonishing network of mostly Dissenting intellectuals that existed throughout the latter half of the eighteenth century. The personalities contained in this 'Dissenting intellectual network' included the most famous, and, to some, infamous, people outside of government in eighteenth-century England. That they were not in government is significant in any explanation of the network's existence, for the Dissenting congregations of England were still being officially excluded from full political power, both on the local and on the national level, by the Corporation Act of 1661 and the Test Act of 1673, neither of which was repealed during Haygarth's lifetime. The intellectual network provided the leading Dissenting figures with an arena for presenting their own plans and ideas for improving English society. If one were to work out an agenda from their various proposals, it would certainly reflect their interests as prominent industrialists, prosperous merchants and professionals, and evangelical divines, all sharing a new, religiously inspired perspective on society.

The basic unit of the intellectual network was a 'society' which, although located in a particular city, often had overlapping membership with societies of different cities, creating an extensive circuit through which the Dissenters' ideas could be passed. For the generation preceding Haygarth, Percival and Falconer, there was the Lunar Society of Birmingham, founded by, among others, the Unitarians Josiah Wedgwood and Joseph Priestley, of whom the former was the

23 Haygarth owned a large piece of land near the centre of Chester, on which he planted an extensive garden. His residential property was highly valued by his parish, and he also owned property in other parts of the town. Documents CR69/3/125–59, Chester City Records Office.

24 Pickstone and Butler, 'Politics of Medicine in Manchester.' Pickstone and Butler tell of the difficulties faced by Dissenting physicians in implementing reforms in the Manchester Infirmary.

founder of the pottery dynasty and the latter Percival's dear mentor at the Dissenting Warrington Academy.[25] The Lunar Society, so named because it met on nights of the full moon, hosted on occasion Priestley's friend Benjamin Franklin, who, when visiting Great Britain in 1759, travelled to Edinburgh to see his friend and correspondent Cullen.[26] Both Cullen and Franklin had tight bonds of friendship with the Quaker John Fothergill, with whom Franklin worked in late 1774 and early 1775, in league with the Quaker merchant David Barclay, Lord Hyde and the colonial secretary Lord Dartmouth, to avert hostilities between England and the American colonies.[27] Fothergill was both a member of Cullen's Philosophical Society and a financier of Priestley's natural enquiries.[28] Percival, undoubtedly inspired by his idols Priestley and Cullen, founded the Manchester Literary and Philosophical Society in 1781, conducting meetings in a Unitarian chapel in Manchester.[29] Haygarth read at least two papers before this society. One of these, read in 1781 in conjunction with Thomas Henry, the Unitarian chemist, surgeon and later correspondent with Haygarth on the smallpox project, was entitled 'On the preservation of Sea Water from putrefaction by means of quicklime; with an account of a newly invented machine for impregnating water or other fluids with fixed Air, &c.',[30] and was very much in the spirit of Cullen's chemical investigations. The Unitarian physicians John Aikin and James Currie, both of whom became proponents of their friend Haygarth's plan to exterminate smallpox, contributed papers to the Manchester society. Haygarth's former tutor and mathematical correspondent on smallpox, John Dawson, was made an honorary member both of the Manchester society and of Cullen's Philosophical Society in Edinburgh. Other contemporary societies with predominantly Dissenting interests and influence were the Medical Society of London, founded by Haygarth's Quaker physician friend John Coakley Lettsom, the Bath Literary and Philosophical Society, before which Haygarth read his 'On the Prevention of the American Pestilence',[31] and the Society for Bettering the Conditions of the Poor of Liverpool, to which

[25] See, Robert Schofield, *The Lunar Society of Birmingham* (Oxford, 1963).
[26] Thomson, *William Cullen, M.D.*, p. 139.
[27] R. Hingston Fox, *Dr. John Fothergill and his Friends* (London, 1919), pp. 323–37.
[28] *Ibid.*, p. 215.
[29] See, H. J. Fleure, 'The Manchester Literary and Philosophical Society,' *Endeavour* 6 (1947), pp. 147–51.
[30] *Manchester Philosophical Society Memoirs* 1 (1789), pp. 41–53. Also, John Haygarth, 'Description of a Glory,' *Manchester Philosophical Society Memoirs* 3 (1790), pp. 463–6.
[31] See, Haygarth, *Letter to Dr. Percival.*

Haygarth contributed papers later in life.[32] And all of the physicians mentioned above were Fellows of the most distinguished of the philosophical societies, the Royal Society of London, continuing the Dissenting tradition started at that institution by Lord Willoughby de Parham and propagated by those under his patronage, notably Priestley and Percival.[33] On his election to the Royal Society in 1781,[34] Haygarth joined the likes of the Dissenting minister and political writer Dr Richard Price and the Quaker 'philanthropist' John Howard. The former of these was influential in Haygarth's three studies on mortality and population in Chester, one of which was printed in the Royal Society's *Philosophical Transactions* in 1778.[35] Through Howard's writings, Haygarth's innovations in infirmary fever wards received wide renown.[36]

But just as important as the formal structure of the philosophical societies were the friendly meetings and personal correspondence between Haygarth and others of similar interests. The friendship which he struck up with John Fothergill became an important source of inspiration from his early years at Chester until Fothergill's death in 1780. Fothergill had purchased a country house, Lea Hall, about twenty miles distant from Chester, to use every autumn as a retreat from his busy London practice.[37] As his later writings tell, Haygarth periodically visited Lea Hall, where he met on occasion Fothergill's young second cousin, Benjamin Waterhouse.[38] Waterhouse, a native of America, was under Fothergill's supervision during his three years in Britain, 1775 to 1778, years which he spent studying medicine in

[32] John Haygarth, Letter to Sir Robert Peel and Sir J. Newport, 1818, in the Peel Papers, General Correspondence, vol. 95, British Library manuscripts collection. Haygarth is writing as 'a stranger' to advise them on a parliamentary bill dealing with typhous fever in Ireland. He refers them to his publication in the *Reports of the Society for Bettering the Condition of the Poor*, no. 9, p. 147. Haygarth also contributed articles to this journal on the subject of education for the poor.

[33] See, P. J. W. Higson, 'The Lancashire Barons Willoughby de Parham and their Connections with Protestant Dissent, 1640–1785', unpublished Ph.D. thesis (Liverpool University, *c.*, 1965) in Royal Society of Arts, London.

[34] Haygarth was elected FRS on Feb. 8, 1781. His election certificate lists those who nominated him as: Dr William Heberden (the elder), Dr John Fothergill, Dr William Watson, Dr Patrick Russell, Mr Owen Salusbury-Brereton, Sir George Shuckburgh and Mr William Seward. Of these seven men, only Heberden and Fothergill can with certainty be called intimates of Haygarth's.

[35] John Haygarth, 'Observations on the Population and Diseases of Chester, in the Year 1774', *Philosophical Transactions* 68 (1778), pp. 131–54.

[36] John Howard, *An Account of the Principal Lazarettos in Europe; with Various Papers Relative to the Plague; Together with Further Observations on some Foreign Prisons and Hospitals* (Warrington, 1789), p. 208.

[37] Fox, *Dr. John Fothergill*, p. 23.

[38] John Haygarth, *A Sketch of a Plan to Exterminate the Casual Small-pox from Great Britain; and to Introduce General Inoculation* (London, 1793), pp. 320–1.

London and at the University of Edinburgh. Waterhouse returned to America in 1782, having received his medical degree at Leyden, and in the next year became the first Professor of Medicine at the newly founded school of medicine at Cambridge (later Harvard) University in New England.[39] Haygarth and Waterhouse became permanent friends and prolific correspondents on the smallpox question. Haygarth additionally wrote of his 'frequent and delightful interviews at Frodsham' with John Aikin, during which the two discussed medical affairs.[40] Haygarth also continued his intercourse with his Edinburgh classmates. A letter from Percival, in Manchester, to Cullen, dated 11 November, 1770, tells of a special arrangement among the old professor's former students:

> Drs. Dobson, Bostock, Haygarth, and myself have agreed to meet, for our mutual improvement, every three months at Warrington, which lies in the centre between Liverpool, Chester, and Manchester. Glad shall I be to receive any medical intelligence from you, that I may communicate it to our Society. Our next interview will be on the 2nd of December.[41]

Haygarth kept Professor Cullen informed and sought his advice on his works regarding the 'variolous contagion.'[42] In 1772, Thomas Falconer visited Cullen, carrying a letter of introduction from his friend Haygarth:

> Dear Sir, *Chester, June 1772*
>
> As I have always observed that men of superior abilities entertain a particular regard and esteem for each other, I think myself extremely fortunate in having the opportunity of introducing to you Mr. Falconer, brother to the Doctor, your late pupil. You will soon find that Mr. Falconer has acquired an uncommon degree of knowledge in every branch of both ancient and modern learning and in natural history. He is very desirous of becoming personally acquainted with men of genius in our sister kingdom, who have become so justly celebrated for their excellent publications in every part of polite literature; and, on this account I think myself most fortunate in introducing him to one who is so intimately known, and so highly respected by them all.[43]

In addition to revealing the respectful nature of Haygarth's friendship for Thomas Falconer, this letter indicates that Falconer, who laboured faithfully with Haygarth in the operation of the Chester smallpox society, shared some of the philosophical inspiration which Haygarth felt, even if he lacked Haygarth's vast knowledge of the smallpox disease. Whether Haygarth first introduced Falconer to the great network of Dissenting reformers is uncertain. He did, however, become known to wider Dissenting circles. Anna Seward, the poet of Lichfield and an intimate of the Lunar Society, dubbed Falconer, an

[39] Fox, *Dr. John Fothergill*, p. 375. [40] Haygarth, *A Sketch*, p. 214.
[41] Thomson, *William Cullen, M.D.*, p. 635. [42] *Ibid.*, pp. 639–40. [43] *Ibid.*, p. 638.

accomplished classicist and a patron of literature, the 'Maecenas of Chester.'[44]

The projects which this group of Dissenting reformers discussed and tried to implement embodied the eighteenth-century notion of 'philanthropy.' John Howard, through his efforts to improve the conditions in England's prisons and to investigate the use of lazarettos in preventing the plague, became perhaps the most widely known 'philanthropist' of his time. John Fothergill, who worked throughout his lifetime on various projects to relieve human misery, was also popularly known as a 'philanthropist.' Haygarth himself received the compliment late in life of 'philanthropic physician' from Dr Lettsom, who was also considered a great 'philanthropist.'[45] They earned this title by their common support of or participation in a set of projects designed to improve society in line with their religious convictions. The Protestant Dissenters, encompassing Unitarians, Quakers, Baptists, Methodists and others, as well as some of the evangelical Anglicans, regarded themselves as a revived source of Christian love, charity and morality in an age of corrupting excess and spiritual decay. The way in which they would help their fellows was not by lofty utopian planning, but rather by simple, direct, workable acts of 'philanthropy.' The life of simplicity and industry which they led made them efficient businessmen, and brought many of them great fortunes. But this too was good in their eyes, for their factories would provide character-building useful employment for the poor, and they would demonstrate responsibility and compassion in their position of economic power.[46] Of course, some of them forgot this ethic when they had made their fortunes, but in the cases of the great 'philanthropists', this belief permeated their work. Although the movements for reform drew support from several types of Dissenter, most of those regarded as 'philanthropists' in the eighteenth century were Quakers. Perhaps their relative reticence in political matters made them more appealing to the public than the high-profile Unitarian Dissenters, like Price, Priestley, Aikin and Currie, who, although advocating the same philanthropic projects, explicitly and vocally backed such extreme causes as American independence, the French Revolution and parliamentary reform.

[44] See, 'Thomas Falconer, Esq.', '*Dictionary of National Biography* (Oxford), vol. 6, p. 1,026.

[45] John Coakley Lettsom, *Hints Designed to Promote Beneficence, Temperance, and Medical Society* (London, 1801), vol. 1, p. 277.

[46] Isabel Grubb, *Quakerism and Industry before 1880* (London, 1930), preface. Also see: R. V. Holt, *The Unitarian Contribution to Social Progress in England* (London, 1938); H. McLachlan, *English Education under the Test Acts* (Manchester, 1931); and R. H. Tawney, *The Radical Tradition* (London, 1964).

Perhaps the most successful philanthropic endeavour was the campaign for prison reform, championed by John Howard, which achieved much more livable conditions for prisoners. Howard expanded his institutional survey to include infirmaries, and found his ideal in the clean and well-arranged Chester Infirmary under the 'ingenious Dr. Haygarth.'[47] The movement to abolish the slave trade, uniting the efforts of, among others, the Anglican evangelical William Wilberforce, MP, Quakers Fothergill and Lettsom, and Unitarians Priestley, Wedgwood and Currie, was warmly applauded by Haygarth in the *Sketch of a Plan to Exterminate the Casual Small-pox* as an outstanding example of the English 'spirit of humanity.'[48] On a much smaller scale, a group of mainly Quaker and Unitarian physicians formed in 1774 a society for the recovery and resuscitation of drowned persons in London, which has since survived as the Royal Humane Society.[49]

Haygarth, through his influence at the Chester Infirmary, and certainly with inspiration from Fothergill and Lettsom in London, instituted a similar society as a subdivision of the Chester Infirmary Charity in 1776, citing for the governors of the charity the examples of such organizations in London, Edinburgh and Liverpool.[50] Bathing, a practice limited to the upper classes of society, was advocated by Fothergill and his friends as an important hygienic measure for the poor. The Chester Infirmary, undoubtedly at Haygarth's instigation, built both warm and cold baths over the years from 1771 to 1773, which were available to needy members of the public for a modest fee.[51] Haygarth's further advocacy of basic education for the poor, fully outlined in his *Letter to Bishop Porteus* of 1812, was in the same spirit as the morally educating children's tales published for popular consumption by the Unitarian Percival.[52]

The conviction of holding a purer and truer view of the Christian ministry was the primary motivation behind the Dissenters' philan-

[47] Howard, *Account of Principal Lazarettos*, p. 208. [48] Haygarth, *A Sketch*, pp. 21–2.

[49] Fox, *Dr. John Fothergill*, pp. 225–7.

[50] Chester Royal Infirmary Minutes, vol. 4 (1773–8), pp. 196, 198 and 209 (meetings of 18 Oct. and 22 and 17 Dec. 1776). At the 17 Dec. meeting, orders were given for three iron hooks for pulling bodies from the water to be made 'on the same plan as the one sent from Liverpool.' The plan may have come from Haygarth's friends in that city, Drs Dobson and Currie.

[51] *Ibid.*, vol. 3 (1768–73), pp. 157 and 242, and vol. 4 (1773–8), p. 29, (meetings of 5 Feb., 1771, 25 Aug. 1772, and 28 Sept., 1773). At the 5 Feb., 1772 meeting, Haygarth was requested to 'apply to some Friend in London for a plan or plans for a hot Bath.'

[52] See, John Haygarth, *A Private Letter Addressed to the Right Reverend Dr. Porteus, the Late Lord Bishop of London; to Propose a Plan, Which Might Give a Good Education to All the Poor Children in England, at a Moderate Expense – Printed at his Lordship's Desire* (London, 1812).

thropic deeds. This conviction made them regard the poor multitudes of eighteenth-century England as the proper objects of compassion, material charity and evangelisation. But, as mentioned above, in order to fully understand the actions of Dissenters in the eighteenth century, one must consider their continued exclusion from full participation in government by the Test and Corporation Acts. In light of the Dissenters' continual campaign for repeal of these acts, their philanthropy may be seen to serve the additional purpose of advancing them in the estimation of the ruling Church of England establishment. What few allies they did have within the establishment were Whigs, and extreme Whigs at that, which might place the politically active Dissenters as Whig extremists. They certainly opposed the 'Church and King' Tories, celebrating instead the 'constitutional' aspect of British government, which, they argued, should ensure full political entitlement for them. For this reason many Dissenting leaders applauded the Revolutions in America and France, in which they saw the births of constitutional governments without state religion. Haygarth, while not expressing his political views as publicly as his Unitarian friends Currie and Aikin, made no attempt to conceal his admiration for American society, his intimate contacts in America, and his correspondence with leading physicians inside Revolutionary France. In placing Haygarth in this political and religious menagerie, it should be remembered that he was a lifelong member of the Church of England, which itself encompassed a wide range of beliefs.[53] It thus seems that Haygarth, through his friendships with a number of the most inspired Dissenters of his day, from the days as John Dawson's student, through his time at Edinburgh, to the years of Fothergill's nearby presence, adopted the political views and the philanthropic vision of the Dissenting community, while remaining in the Church of England.

One great endeavour of the philanthropists with a direct bearing on Haygarth's smallpox activities was the establishment of registrations of births, marriages, deaths and causes of death throughout the kingdom to supersede the spotty and inaccurate records kept in local parishes. Fothergill, Price, Percival, Cullen and Haygarth all displayed intense active interest in this movement. For Price in particular, such a register would verify his theory, first advanced in his *Observations on Reversionary Payments* of 1771, that the turpitude of eighteenth-century England, reflected in the kingdom's unprecedentedly large national debt, irresponsibly indulgent rulers and unsound governmen-

[53] Haygarth had his children baptised in the Church of England; see L. F. Farrall, *Parish Register of the Holy and Undivided Trinity in the City of Chester, 1532–1837* (Chester, 1914), pp. 221, 223, 226, 230 and 235. His son John went on to become Rector of a church at Upham.

tal policies, had resulted in a great decline in the nation's population during the century.[54] Price could also use the register in his calculations on the values of reversionary payments and life insurance. All of these men would find such information valuable as a means of investigating the relationship between health and a person's environment and personal status. Haygarth, certainly with the personal encouragement of Fothergill and Percival, conducted surveys of the Chester Bills of Mortality from the city's parishes for the years 1772, 1773 and 1774. In the 1772 study, Haygarth explained the value of the work:

A faithful and minute register of mortality, and of the various diseases most fatal to mankind, at different ages, must evidently be of the most important consequence, to the politician, the philosopher and the physician, in their several endeavours to relieve the miseries, and promote the happiness of human nature.[55]

Furthermore, wrote Haygarth, this register could 'confirm or confute' the opinion of 'a writer, of distinguished abilities in political arithmetic, [Price, who] has offered many arguments, which give too much cause to apprehend that England, in about 70 years, has lost near a quarter of her people.' Haygarth also agreed with Price on the value of the register in determining 'the doctrine of annuities to widows . . . the value of reversionary payments, and of assurances on lives, and other important questions in civil society.' In the survey for 1773, Haygarth acknowledged Price's involvement in his work, writing, 'At the request of Dr. Price, author of the very ingenious essays on annuities, &c. an improvement is made', whereby Haygarth detailed deaths over the age of eighty, to make calculations on annuities for people of that age of 'tolerable exactness.'[56]

The register for 1772 also shows the influence of Cullen on Haygarth's preparation of the study. Haygarth wrote:

In the Table of diseases . . . the technical are added to the vulgar names, and the arrangement of a justly celebrated professor is adopted, in order to convey more distinct ideas to the faculty, and to place disorders of a similar nature nearest each other, for their mutual illustration.[57]

[54] See Richard Price, *Observations on Reversionary Payments; on Schemes for Providing Annuities for Widows, and for Pensions in old Age; on the Method of Calculating the Values of Assurances on Lives; and on the National Debt*, second edition (London, 1772); and Peter Brown, *The Chathamites* (London, 1967), pp. 111–86, for a short study of Price and of his political and economic theories.

[55] John Haygarth, 'Observations on the Bills of Mortality in Chester, for the Year 1772,' in James H. Cassedy (ed.), *Mortality in Pre-Industrial Times – the Contemporary Verdict*, Pioneers of Demography Series (Westmead, 1973), p. 67.

[56] John Haygarth, 'Bill of Mortality for Chester for the Year 1773' in Cassedy (ed.) *Mortality in Pre-Industrial Times*, p. 86.

[57] Haygarth, 'Observations on the Bills of Mortality . . . 1772,' p. 75.

He was referring to his old mentor's nosological classification of diseases, a system created by Cullen both as a didactic aid and as a means of showing the generic divisibility of diseases. The four 'classes' of the *Morborum Genera* were 'I. Febrile Diseases, II. Nervous Diseases, III. Diseases of Habit and IV. Local Diseases', of which the first, 'Febrile Diseases', included smallpox under the 'order' of *exanthemata* ('eruptions').[58] All of the 'Febrile Diseases', such as 'jail fever', 'consumption', 'measles' and the deadly but simply named 'fever', were those that were accompanied by fever and, as Haygarth later argued, could be grouped together as 'infectious distempers.'[59] Cullen had a personal interest in Haygarth's population study, as shown in the letter that Thomas Falconer carried to Cullen in 1772:

> Mr. Falconer will give you a plan for a register of births, &c. in Chester. You will observe that no distinctions are attempted but such as a parish-clerk might understand. Any improvement you would be so kind as to communicate, I shall be glad to adopt.[60]

Two other former students of Cullen's, Dr Percival in Manchester and Dr Dobson in Liverpool, were conducting the same investigations in their respective cities.[61] Both were in close contact with Haygarth, and both had felt the same motivations that compelled their colleague in Chester to observe population there. All of these men had made the mental correlation between a healthy and large population and a healthy and large growth in industry, an enterprise in which the Dissenters were very prominent and which they regarded as vitally important for the nation's welfare. Haygarth, lamenting over the small number of children per marriage in Chester, later wrote, 'One cause of this small proportion is probably the want of manufacturers (in Chester).'[62] Percival recorded the converse situation in Manchester,

[58] *Ibid.*, p. 89. Also, see letter from Haygarth to Cullen in Thomson, *William Cullen, M.D.*, p. 642. In the letter, dated 'Chester, October 16, 1780,' Haygarth thanks Cullen for a complimentary copy of his *Synopsis Pharmacopiae*, adding, 'I always highly admired your method of arranging disease. But the last edition of your Synopsis greatly exceeded my expectation. It is a book that will ever be in my hands, for I keep in concise Latin the cases of all of my patients, and afterwards arrange them into genera according to your system.' Also see Cullen, *First Lines*, p. 27.

[59] *Ibid.*, p. 89. Also, Haygarth, *An Inquiry*, p. 134. Haygarth claims that the 'facts' from any other 'infectious disemper,' such as 'jail fever,' could be used to support his smallpox doctrine.

[60] Thomson, *William Cullen, M.D.*, p. 639.

[61] Thomas Percival, 'Observations on the State of Population in Manchester,' reprinted in *Population and Disease in Early Industrial England*, ed. Bernard Benjamin (London, 1973), p. 19.

[62] Haygarth, 'Observations on the Population ... 1774', p. 145. *The Oxford English Dictionary* shows that the word 'manufacturer' was taking on the meaning of 'factory' in the late seventeenth and early eighteenth centuries.

writing, 'yet the flourishing state of our manufactures cannot fail to promote the population, by affording plentiful means of subsistence to the poor.'[63] To these men, population and 'manufacturers' were naturally linked, and just as Cullen had always looked to help the nation by applying the 'chemical philosophy' to the needs of industry, so did his former students try to promote the welfare of the nation by using observations on mortality to learn the state of the population and, hence, the state of industry. Percival wrote:

The number of inhabitants and progress of population in the kingdom; the increase or decrease of certain diseases; the comparative healthiness of different situations, climates, and seasons; and the influence of particular trades and manufactures on the duration of life, are subjects of the highest importance to the community; and equally interesting to the statesman, the philosopher, and the physician.[64]

Dr Lettsom later argued for the lower classes' worthiness of compassion and of material help resulting from their usefulness, in numbers, to industry:

This class, who labour with industry, *become from their poverty the very pillars of the state*; for, a labour is necessary to the existence of all governments, and as it is from the poor only that labour can be expected or such as have no surplus in store, so far from being an evil, under the proper regulations, it is a blessing to have a number of poor inhabitants.[65]

The philosophical physicians, Haygarth and Percival especially, thought that their philanthropic enterprises on behalf of population would naturally have a beneficial effect on industry, and, because industry would provide useful employment for the poor, consequently promote the material and spiritual welfare of England.

A smallpox epidemic in Manchester in 1773 probably made Percival the first to recognise the impact of this disease on the kingdom's rate of mortality. Percival recorded in detail both the mortality of smallpox and the ages of those who succumbed to the disease. In a work completed in February of 1775, he also claimed to have helped direct Haygarth's attention to smallpox.

My friend Dr. Haygarth, to whom I communicated the preceding *Tables of the comparative mortality of the small-pox, &c.* had adopted the plan, and pursued the same inquiry at Chester. His statements will show how exactly our observations agree.[66]

The information which Haygarth subsequently gathered was published in the Royal Society's *Philosophical Transactions* as a part of his

[63] Percival, 'Observations on the State of Population', pp. 61–2. [64] *Ibid.*, p. 17.

[65] Lettsom, *Hints Designed to Promote Beneficence*, p. 184.

[66] Thomas Percival, 'On the Small-pox and Measles,' reprinted in Benjamin, *Population and Disease*, p. 77.

'Observations on the Population and Disease of Chester in the Year 1774'. Above all, it showed a dramatic increase in smallpox mortality in Chester during an epidemic in 1774. In 1772, the disease had killed sixteen persons and in 1773 only one, but in 1774, it infected 1,202 persons, of whom 202 died.[67] He calculated that the proportion of deaths by the 'natural small-pox' to all deaths in 1774 was in a ratio of one to two and seven tenths. Smallpox had suddenly become responsible for more than one quarter of all deaths in Chester. Furthermore, Percival and Haygarth both found that smallpox had an extraordinarily high mortality among young children, such that one quarter of all smallpox fatalities were children under one year of age.[68] Percival concluded from this information that inoculation is best performed on infants at two to three months of age. If performed any earlier, Percival noticed that the infant system would not respond, and, if delayed any longer, the young child could catch the natural smallpox with fatal consequences. This conclusion reveals the common intention of Haygarth and Percival in constructing the study of smallpox mortality. Haygarth wrote that he conducted these inquiries into the 'proportional fatality of the natural small-pox, in order to demonstrate the advantages of inoculation, and to discover at what age this operation should be performed that it may become the most extensively beneficial to society.'[69] Haygarth and Percival thus together turned their attention to inoculation as the best means of lowering the mortality of smallpox.

In the reports by Percival and Haygarth, one can see their segment of the Dissenting intellectual network in action. As smallpox had been epidemical in Manchester in 1773,[70] resulting in a heavy loss of life, Percival saw this disease as a major cause of any possible population decrease. Percival gathered information about smallpox mortality from surrounding communities, contacting Mr John Aikin, father of Dr John Aikin and tutor at the Dissenting Warrington Academy, to obtain the mortality figures for the town of Warrington, where smallpox was also epidemical in 1773.[71] The smallpox epidemics of Manchester and Warrington were then undoubtedly discussed at the quarterly meetings, in Warrington, of Haygarth, Percival, Bostock and Dobson. It was probably here that Percival 'communicated' the table of comparative smallpox mortality to Haygarth, with the result that

[67] Haygarth, 'Observations on the Population . . . 1774', p. 142. [68] *Ibid.*, p. 143.
[69] *Ibid.*, p. 142
[70] Percival, 'On the Small-pox and Measles', p. 69. Percival records that in 1773, 139 died of smallpox in the parish of the Collegiate Church, Manchester, against 66 in 1772 and 87 in 1774. [71] *Ibid.*, p. 71.

Haygarth was ready to observe the mortality of the disease when it became epidemical in Chester the next year. Haygarth and Percival, faced with ravaging epidemics in their respective cities and in close conference together, first expressed at this time their common conviction that smallpox had to be dealt with on a large scale by what was then the only available preventive measure, inoculation.

At the time of the Chester epidemic, inoculation had been established as a practice in England for over half a century. But since the time of its introduction in the 1720s through the royal patronage of Caroline, Princess of Wales, inoculation was regularly performed only upon the wealthy. In the early years of inoculation, the complicated process, including deep incisions, long preparatory and recovery periods, special regimens, and consequently high costs, made the procedure particularly unrealistic for a poor labourer. Additionally, an infection or a case of virulent or 'natural' smallpox often followed these early inoculations, so that many of the wealthy who could afford the operation were, understandably, frightened of the attendant risks, only feeling compelled to undergo inoculation when faced with the greater danger of a smallpox epidemic.[72] Inoculators also faced hostility from some communities which rightly feared that those sick from the inoculated smallpox could spread the natural form of the disease to others. Inoculation even endured considerable, but quickly diminishing, opposition from religious authorities, who regarded inoculation as sinful because it was 'distrusting Providence' and a deliberately incurred risk of death.[73]

In spite of these countervailing forces, however, inoculation grew in popularity and availability over the next few decades. As the practice of inoculation passed into the hands of a larger number of operators, including 'amateurs' and 'itinerants,'[74] the price of the operation fell within the reach of some of the lower classes. But their inoculations were without the care, both before and after the operation, given to the wealthy by the surgeons, who performed the actual inoculations, and by the physicians, who supervised the whole process. There were examples of *gratis* inoculations for the poor, occurring, for the most part, when parish authorities found the cost of an amateur inoculator to be less than the costs of nursing and burial for those who caught the natural smallpox.[75] Sometimes a successful inoculator would offer differential rates for the operation, so that parish authorities could pay for mass inoculation of their poor. Among the famous eighteenth-

[72] Peter Razzell, *The Conquest of Smallpox* (Firle, 1977), p. 41. [73] *Ibid.*, p. 42.
[74] *Ibid.*, p. 49. [75] *Ibid.*, pp. 45–50.

century inoculators to do so were the Quaker surgeon Thomas Dimsdale, later created a Baron of the Russian Empire for his inoculation of the Empress Catherine II[76] and the surgeons of the Sutton family, whose new and far less dangerous method of inoculation, which Dimsdale also employed, did much to increase the demand for inoculation throughout the 1760s.[77]

The only institution dedicated solely to combating smallpox before Haygarth's activities was the London Smallpox Hospital, founded in 1746, which both inoculated recommended poor persons in the hospital and admitted as patients people suffering with smallpox, who were as a rule excluded from other infirmaries. The London Smallpox Hospital did, however, restrict admission to persons over seven years of age,[78] by which time, Haygarth and Percival realised, most persons would have already had the disease. The required three- to four-week stay in the hospital for inoculation certainly would have strongly dissuaded those labouring poor adults who were yet vulnerable to smallpox from coming in for the operation.[79] The Smallpox Hospital was consequently regarded by some contemporaries as a charity simply for the inoculation of the subscribers' servants, who were largely immigrants from the countryside and thus somewhat less likely to have been previously infected with smallpox.[80] By the mid 1770s when smallpox began to preoccupy John Haygarth, the practice of inoculation had received wide approval. In provincial parts, some of the poor were given the benefits of inoculation at the discretion of various parish authorities. But in urban areas, from the teeming capital, through smaller cities like Manchester, Liverpool and Chester, the London Smallpox Hospital, with its unique regulations, represented the only notable and sustained attempt to provide inoculation for the poor. Thus throughout the whole of England generally, and particularly in the cities, inoculation was still a preserve of the rich. Haygarth later wrote of the destructive effect of this 'partial inoculation':

> It removes from society all opposers of the progress of the small-pox. Before inoculation was known, a gentleman's family, liable to the distemper, was held in continual terrour of its visitation; watched its approach into the neighbourhood with careful solicitude; took early, and often successful measures to prevent its introduction into the town or village which was situated in or near the place of their residence. These exertions . . . would frequently prevent its communication into larger towns, and thus

[76] Fox, *Dr. John Fothergill*, pp. 81–91.
[77] Derrick Baxby, *Jenner's Smallpox Vaccine* (London, 1981), pp. 26–7.
[78] M. C. Buer, *Health, Wealth and Population in the Early Days of the Industrial Revolution* (London, 1926), p. 184. [79] *Ibid.*, p. 184. [80] *Ibid.*, p. 184.

diminish its fatality among the inhabitants. But, this time, and in this neighbourhood, all who dread the distemper are inoculated; whence the community are wholly deprived of the benefit of these salutary precautions.[81]

Haygarth concluded that the 'intelligent and opulent, whose families enjoy the inestimable blessings of inoculation, ought certainly, in generosity, and even in justice, to promote measures to preserve the weak, and defenceless multitude from the calamities to which *they* alone are exposed.'[82]

Haygarth, Percival and Dobson were all now watching the mortality of smallpox, convinced both of its extraordinary destructive effects on population and that in inoculation they had the medical means to combat it. But Haygarth had a professional position in Chester that was certainly superior to the Dissenter Percival's in Manchester and probably better than what Dobson had in Liverpool before poor health forced his retirement to Bath in 1780, helping Haygarth to accomplish all of the things that he recorded in his books of the next two decades. As the successful execution of the projects to provide bathing facilities (1771–3) and to recover drowned persons (1776) show, Haygarth had become sufficiently influential among the charity's subscribers to make them share some of his priorities and concerns. Even the Corporation which governed the city of Chester saw some value in Haygarth's work, paying him '£10.10' for his 1774 mortality survey.[83] His good friend Thomas Falconer was a prominent figure among the subscribers, regularly serving as chairman of the weekly board meetings.[84] From this secure position, Haygarth pondered the great problem of smallpox on which the epidemics of 1772 to 1774 had helped to focus both his attention and the thoughts of Percival and Dobson. Haygarth noticed in 1774 that the 'natural smallpox' was 'dreadfully fatal' to the poor of Chester, a situation which 'made a deep impression on my mind, especially when I considered that it was possible to prevent such destruction.'[85] 'Ever since that time,' he wrote, 'it has been an object of my most anxious wishes to preserve their lives by inoculation.'[86] Haygarth spent the next few years thinking about the prevention of smallpox in Chester both through mass inoculations and through an understanding of the nature of the 'natural small-pox.' In addition to the conferences with Percival and Dobson, he discussed his ideas on these matters with Fothergill, Aikin, his old teacher Cullen

[81] Haygarth, *A Sketch*, pp. 37–8. [82] *Ibid.*, p. 38.
[83] Assembly Book 1740–1786, Chester City Records Office.
[84] Chester Royal Infirmary Minutes, vol. 3 (1768–73), vol. 4 (1773–78), and vol. 5 (1778–82), Chester City Records Office. [85] Haygarth, *An Inquiry*, p. 8. [86] *Ibid.*, p. 8.

and his other 'medical and philosophical acquaintances,'[87] gathering their remarks and, undoubtedly, their encouragement.

By 1777, when smallpox was again epidemical in Chester, Haygarth had formulated his smallpox doctrine and upon this had built a plan to eliminate the disease through inoculations and through a series of regulations on the habits and movements of infected persons. Haygarth gave a detailed account of the plan in his 1784 book *An Inquiry How to Prevent the Small-pox and Proceedings of a Society for Promoting General Inoculation at Stated Periods, and Preventing the Natural Small-pox, in Chester*. As the title indicates, Haygarth and his cooperators, most notably Thomas Falconer, founded a charitable society, supported by private subscriptions, for the sake of financing and implementing his programme. The Chester Society was to oversee a two-pronged attack on the disease. First, the Society would pay for general inoculations of the poor and then distribute rewards to those families nursing inoculated children. This was thought necessary because, in addition to the expense of caring for a sick child, the 'poor and ignorant' had to overcome their fear of inoculation itself, which, Haygarth wrote, had a mortality rate of one in one hundred, compared with the one in five mortality of the 'natural small-pox.'[88] Secondly, the Society would use monetary rewards and paid informants to compel members of an infected household to obey a set of rules, the so-called 'Rules of Prevention,' which Haygarth believed would prevent the spread of the disease.

Haygarth's 'Rules of Prevention' were in fact the practical applications of his theory on the nature of the smallpox contagion. They formed the vital second leg of his plan, and so deserve quotation in full:

Rules of Prevention

I Suffer no person, who has not had the small-pox, to come into the infectious house. No visitor who has had any communication with persons liable to the distemper, should touch or sit down on anything infectious.

II No patient, after the pocks have appeared, must be suffered to go into the street, or other frequented place.

III The utmost attention to *cleanliness* is absolutely necessary: *during* and *after* the distemper, no person, clothes, food, furniture, dog, cat, money, medicines, or any other thing that is known or suspected to be daubed with matter, spittle, or other infectious discharges of the patient, should go out of the house till they be washed; and till they have been sufficiently exposed to fresh air. No foul linen, or any thing else that can retain the poison, should be folded up and put into drawers, boxes, or be otherwise

[87] *Ibid.*, p. 10.
[88] Haygarth, 'Observations on the Population ... 1774', p. 142 and Haygarth, *An Inquiry*, p. 154.

shut up from the air, but immediately thrown into water and kept there till washed. No attendants should touch what is to go into another family, till their hands are washed. When a patient dies of the small-pox, particular care should be taken that nothing infectious be taken out of the house so as to do mischief.

IV The patient must not be allowed to approach any person liable to the distemper, till every scab is dropt off, till all the clothes, furniture, food, and all other things touched by the patient during the distemper, till the floor of the sick chamber, and till his hair, face, and hands, have been carefully washed. After every thing has been made perfectly clean, the doors, windows, drawers, boxes, and all other places that can retain infectious air should be kept open till it be cleared out of the house.[89]

The 'Rules' were ultimately based on Haygarth's theory that smallpox was an 'infectious distemper' which was spread by identifiable contacts with the 'variolous poison.' Using the type of chemical reasoning that Cullen propounded, Haygarth postulated that 'variolous poison' was simply that portion of 'variolous matter,' that is, the pus or scab of a smallpox pustule, that had 'dissolved' in the air, yielding a transparent but odoriferous 'solution.' Haygarth regarded 'transparency' as 'a *test* of solution . . . founded upon a very exhaustive and uniform induction of facts.'[90] Haygarth observed that 'opaque bodies,' such as metals, could yield transparent solutions when dissolved in their 'proper menstrua,' while, on the other hand, two transparent substances, such as 'water and oil,' could result in an opaque mixture.[91] The transparency of solutions, Haygarth argued, rested upon so many 'uniform facts' that it was a 'chemical principle or *law* of nature.'[92] (Haygarth was using the method exactly prescribed by Cullen for establishing a chemical law, that is, generalisation from a multitude of observed phenomena, or 'facts'.)[93] This 'law' could be applied to the 'universally allowed' fact that the natural smallpox is 'always communicated thro' the air.'[94] Haygarth maintained that the 'pestilential effluvia, or *miasms*' existed in the air only in close proximity to the 'variolous matter' in the eruptions on the skin of a smallpox patient.[95] Proof of this was to be found in the '*peculiar* and offensive stench' surrounding a smallpox patient, for just as taste revealed solutions in liquid, so could smell reveal the solution of variolous poison in air.[96] But the full proof of the original proposition was evident in the observation that air which is 'strongly impregnated with various miasms, is perfectly transparent.'[97] If, however, the 'solvend,' that is, the variolous poison, should be placed in a quantity of 'menstruum' too small to dissolve the whole, 'supersaturation' would

[89] Haygarth, *An Inquiry*, pp. 118–20. [90] *Ibid.*, p. 17. [91] *Ibid.*, p. 18. [92] *Ibid.*, p. 18.
[93] Donovan, *Philosophical Chemistry*, p. 109. [94] Haygarth, *An Inquiry*, p. 19.
[95] *Ibid.*, p. 19. [96] *Ibid.*, p. 20. [97] *Ibid.*, p. 20.

result, with a portion of the poison remaining undissolved. Haygarth believed this to be the case inside the small corked vials in which inoculators kept the variolous pus. In the small containers, the pus might even remain in a half-fluid state for several months, as the quantity of air was not 'sufficient to dissolve the moisture.'[98] Haygarth found his solubility theory confirmed by 'extensive and uniform analogy,' for just as the perspiration of men and plants, and all kinds of 'invisible odours,' dissolved transparently in the air, so did the variolous poison form a transparent and 'odiferous' solution in air.[99]

Haygarth later disclosed that in the preparation of the *Inquiry*, he formulated the chemical solution theory with the help of 'the judicious discrimination of Dr. Cullen,' who had pointed out the differences between a 'chemical mixture' and a 'solution,' the former altering the properties of the bodies and the latter preserving them.[100] Cullen held that among the fumes floating in the air were 'bodies with which the air may be impregnated [that is], all these that may be taken up with water in the way of solution.'[101]

A previously uninfected and hence susceptible person could then contract the disease by inhaling concentrated variolous poison as would be found in the air close either to the pustules on a smallpox patient or to any variolous matter that the victim might have deposited on objects surrounding him, such as furniture or the family dog. Alternatively, and preferably, the susceptible person could have a small amount of variolous matter, that is, the 'undissolved' pus or scab from an inoculator's vial, poked into the skin and become immune through the milder inoculated form of the disease. It was because of this infectiousness of the 'variolous poison' arising from 'variolous matter' that Haygarth stressed both the isolation of the patient and the careful washing of all things touched by the patient. Haygarth saw a great problem in inducing the poor to practise such cleanliness, writing that many of the articles enumerated in the 'Rules' coming from an infectious house 'find their way unsuspected in to all families of a certain rank. The poison is quickly and universally dispersed among the lowest class of people, whose poverty renders them dirty.'[102] For this reason, the Chester Small-pox Society would issue a 'Promissory Note' for at least one half crown to an infectious family to be paid when the Society's 'inspectors' were satisfied that the 'Rules' had been obeyed and the infection not spread during the course of the disease.

Although William Cullen's influence over this work was clearly

[98] *Ibid.*, pp. 22–3. [99] *Ibid.*, pp. 23–4. [100] Haygarth, *A Sketch*, pp. 317–18.
[101] Donovan, *Philosophical Chemistry*, p. 148. [102] *Ibid.*, p. 61.

great, it is striking that his name is not mentioned at all in the *Inquiry*. The answer to this apparent mystery comes in a letter from Haygarth to Cullen, dated 'Chester, 11 Sept., 1779,' in which Haygarth was thanking Cullen for the latter's comments on Haygarth's variolous theories:

> Most respected Professor
> With sentiments of warmest gratitude, I return my sincerest thanks for the favour of your friendly and philosophical remarks upon my paper concerning Variolous Contagion. A reluctance to engage unnecessarily any of your time, which is so honourably and usefully employed, was my motive for delaying so long these most cordial acknowledgements, and a request for your farther criticisms on some alterations and additions to the Inquiry . . .
> Whether you approve or disapprove of the doctrine I advance, you may be assured that no uncandid nor improper use shall be made of your remarks, they shall be regarded as a *private* and sacred token of friendship . . .
> I shall expect with much anxiety your remarks on the enclosed papers, and particularly I request, as a private favour, your explicit answer to the queries at the conclusion. Your opinion shall be regarded, as it ought, with the utmost deference.[103]

Perhaps Cullen did not want to have a public reputation for officiousness in regard to the activities of his former students, in spite of his obviously great interest. At any rate, the silence in the *Inquiry* about Cullen's comments was not Haygarth's choice but rather the old professor's.

In March 1778, shortly after the end of the 1777 smallpox epidemic in Chester, Haygarth's 'Small-pox Society' started offering rewards for adherence to the 'Rules of Prevention' by infectious people. A general inoculation was first held in early 1780 and was further offered in the spring seasons of 1781 and 1784. Up to 1784, the year of the *Inquiry*'s publication, the Society enjoyed what Haygarth regarded as vindicating success. The Society had virtually eliminated smallpox from the city, with only sporadic, localised cases of the disease and no city-wide epidemics during the six years of the Society's operation. Furthermore, the general inoculations in Chester had inspired similar programmes in Liverpool, presumably the work of Drs Dobson and Currie, and in Leeds.[104] In 1784, however, the Society's fortunes turned sour. Haygarth later wrote:

> The proceedings of the small-pox society at Chester, were suspended, soon after my former publication on that subject (i.e., the *Inquiry*) was sent to press. The suspension was occasioned, neither by any medical deficiency nor by a deficiency in the voluntary subscriptions, but solely by the ignorance and delusion of the populus.[105]

[103] Thomson, *William Cullen, M.D.*, pp. 639–40. [104] *Ibid.*, p. 208.
[105] Haygarth, *A Sketch*, p. 481.

Indeed, only one child was inoculated in the 1784 general inoculation compared with 213 in the previous inoculations. Perhaps there was more to the Society's collapse than a lack of cooperation from the populus, perhaps some political strife among the subscribers on which Haygarth was silent. Or it is conceivable that Chester's pool of willing participants had been exhausted by the first two general inoculations. It can not be known with certainty. But Haygarth was not daunted by the failure of his voluntary society plan to combat smallpox. He had larger plans, plans that would eliminate the fractional participation inherent in voluntary programmes.

As disappointing to Haygarth as the 1784 inoculation must have been the fact that only general inoculation was instituted in Leeds and Liverpool. This certainly dismayed Haygarth, for he had formulated an equally important weapon against smallpox in his 'Rules of Prevention,' which any city following Chester's example should surely institute along with general inoculations. The only other application of the 'Rules' was by Percival in Manchester, where they were adapted to fight an outbreak of typhus fever in 1789.[106] But the omission by the former cities of anything like the 'Rules of Prevention' from their smallpox programmes, in addition to the rejection of general inoculation by the poor of Chester, probably brought Haygarth to see 'civil regulation' as the only means of ensuring widespread observance both of the 'Rules' and of the practice of inoculation. The details of these 'civil regulations' subsequently formed the core of his second book on smallpox, *A Sketch of a Plan to Exterminate the Casual Small-pox from Great Britain; and to Introduce General Inoculation*, published in 1793. The emphasis on prevention extended even to the title, in which, instead of the 'natural small-pox,' the 'casual small-pox' appeared, for contracting smallpox was, Haygarth believed, a preventable 'casualty . . . as (is) a fractured limb.'[107]

In the *Sketch*, Haygarth appealed to the 'philosophy and philanthropy' of all 'patriotic' Englishmen in his quest for the creation of a 'Publick Establishment' to oversee general inoculations and to enforce the 'Rules of Prevention.' His invocation of patriotism and philanthropy, and the book's dedication to King George III, who 'graciously condescended to patronize the following proposal,'[108] show that Haygarth was trying to make what was primarily the programme of

[106] Pickstone and Butler, 'The Politics of Medicine', pp. 236–7.

[107] Haygarth, *A Sketch*, p. 1.

[108] *Ibid.*, p. iii. Haygarth may have obtained this patronage through his friend William Heberden (the elder), himself a friendly acquaintance of the King, as it seems unlikely that Haygarth would have any direct connection with the monarch.

his Dissenting friends into the concern of every patriotic Englishman, for Haygarth and all of his Dissenting associates believed that their activities were most conducive to the spiritual and material well-being of the kingdom. Haygarth accordingly wrote that it would require a 'truly patriotick prince' to effect the legislation necessary for the 'Publick Establishment' to combat smallpox.

Haygarth proposed a three-tiered hierarchy of officials for the 'Publick Establishment.' At the bottom, 500 surgeon or apothecary 'inspectors' would, as in the Chester Society, conduct house-to-house inspections throughout the nation. The kingdom was to be divided into 500 districts, one for each Inspector, based on population density. Haygarth suggested using the number of militia men usually raised from given areas as indicators of their populations, and assigning the Inspectors accordingly. On the next level, fifty physicians, one for every ten Inspectors, would act as 'Directors,' making certain that the Inspectors were properly performing their duties. Haygarth thought that the King or the Royal College of Physicians should have the prerogative of appointing men at this level. To oversee the entire operation, Haygarth envisaged a 'Commission' of five physicians in London and three physicians in Edinburgh, again appointed by the King or the Royal College of Physicians. Professor Cullen would surely have approved of such great responsibility being vested in medical men. The 'Publick Establishment' would be empowered to issue rewards for information about outbreaks of smallpox and for proper observance of the 'Rules of Prevention' by needy families. For those above want who had observed the 'Rules,' public thanks would be given in local newspapers. Transgression of the 'Rules' would be punished by a stiff fine, or, if the transgressor should be too poor to pay a fine, by public display as a 'wicked villain' in the nearest market town.

Haygarth thought that the salaries of the Directors and Inspectors (the Commissioners would receive no salary) should be supplied from the county rates, while rewards given to the poor for either information or observance of the 'Rules' should come from parish funds. Haygarth was, however, surely convinced by Price's writings of the evils of national excess and national debt. He consequently pointed out that the 'Publick Establishment' would actually save money for the nation. Haygarth first emphasised that the cost was 'trifling' to begin with, amounting 'but to a small fraction of the *interest* of the *extra* expences of a single year's war.'[109] Yet, as the 'Publick Establishment'

[109] *Ibid.*, p. 149.

saved an increasing number of poor children's lives, every year it would be concomitantly saving society 'the charge of bearing, nursing, and burying the 30,000 (poor children) who die before they become useful to society, being all of it lost to the publick.'[110] The savings would increase yearly, as fewer people incurred the distemper, more than paying the expenses of the 'Publick Establishment.' Besides, when the day came that smallpox was finally eradicated from Great Britain, the 'Publick Establishment' and its expenses would naturally be suspended.

In arguing for a national programme, Haygarth also made explicit his concern for the kingdom's population. He asked his friend John Dawson to compute the increase in the population of Great Britain that would result from the eradication of smallpox based on the smallpox mortality figures from Chester, Liverpool and Manchester, generalised over an entire population of about eight million. Dawson, using what he considered very conservative figures, calculated that the population of Great Britain would increase by about one million persons in fifty years.[111] Haygarth rejoiced at such a prospect:

> Political writers indulge various hypothetical notions concerning the cause of different degrees of population in different nations. But, in spite of all fanciful speculations to the contrary, I cannot but think that a measure which would so remarkably increase the number of children to be added to society, must forward population in a great degree, and probably not less than Mr. Dawson's calculation. Britain is in a rapid state of improvement. Such an increase of youth of both sexes could not be a hindrance but a help to her prosperity.[112]

And he had further praise for the state of affairs in America:

> I have long thought that the astonishing increase of population in America was owing, in a great measure, to the effectual care there taken to preserve the people from the ravages of the small-pox.[113]

Haygarth even compared the effect of smallpox on population with the legendary mortality of 'the Plague,' claiming that smallpox, because it was a constant presence, had killed many more.[114] He estimated that 'during the last thousand years, the small-pox alone has destroyed a full tenth, and probably a larger proportion of the whole human race!'[115] Haygarth had apologised in the preface to the *Sketch* for transgressing his rule of not stating 'political' views by inserting comments on so political an issue as population. Haygarth's friend Price, in fact, had done much to make population a political issue. That Haygarth did not remove his thoughts on population from the *Sketch*

[110] *Ibid.*, p. 151. [111] *Ibid.*, pp. 144–5. [112] *Ibid.*, pp. 146–7. [113] *Ibid.*, pp. 148–9.
[114] *Ibid.*, pp. 160–3. [115] *Ibid.*, p. 8.

simply shows how central they were to all of his efforts against smallpox.

The greatest portion of the *Sketch* was taken up by Haygarth's correspondence with his medical friends (see plate 4), mostly Dissenters, in which they gave their solicited comments on the efficacy of Haygarth's 'Rules of Prevention.' Haygarth had sent a 'circular letter' to these men – Dawson, Aikin, Professor William Irvine of Glasgow, Percival, Professor Martin Wall of Oxford, Waterhouse in America, Thomas in Manchester, Dr James Clark in New Castle, Dr Odier in Geneva and Currie in Liverpool – asking them to point out any deficiency in the 'Rules of Prevention.' While several of them, particularly Waterhouse, disagreed with Haygarth's theory of 'solution' as the specific chemical means by which the variolous poison became aerial, none of them took issue with the 'Rules' which Haygarth had built upon his theory of smallpox contagion. They all fundamentally agreed that smallpox was an infectious distemper, which was enough of a theoretical concordance for all of them to enthusiastically endorse the 'Rules of Prevention' and, consequently, Haygarth's entire plan. Haygarth sent the circular letter to Cullen in 1787,[116] but the aging professor, if he did at all reply, may have entreated Haygarth once again to silence about his comments. Haygarth also received a letter in 1791 from the Magistrates of the Republic of Geneva requesting his advice on their efforts to control smallpox in their city. Haygarth admitted being greatly encouraged by their trust in him and in the principles originally published in the *Inquiry*, just as he had been encouraged to further his plans to combat smallpox upon learning that the *Inquiry* had been deemed worthy of translation into German, by Dr Cappel of Berlin, and into French, by Dr La Rocher of Paris.[117] Among all of this encouragement, however, there was one foreboding note, coming significantly in James Currie's reply of 1792:

> Whether your proposals will meet with the general attention they deserve I will not presume to say. I have my doubts whether knowledge and philanthropy are as popular at present as they ought to be. In the mean time, however, your book will receive the approbation of those who are judges of its merit, and its principles will doubtless be called into action, if the happy period so confidently foretold should ever arrive, 'when the powerful shall be subjected to the wise'.[118]

Haygarth wrote that he foresaw the greatest danger to his plan in the prospect of it being labelled 'a "visionary scheme"; "an extravagant and dangerous innovation"; "an invasion of personal liberty"; "an

[116] Thomson, *William Cullen, M.D.*, pp. 640–1. [117] Haygarth, *A Sketch*, pp. 464–70.
[118] *Ibid.*, pp. 453–4.

A

SKETCH

OF A PLAN TO EXTERMINATE THE

CASUAL SMALL-POX

FROM GREAT BRITAIN;

AND TO

INTRODUCE GENERAL INOCULATION

TO WHICH IS ADDED, A

CORRESPONDENCE

ON THE NATURE OF VARIOLOUS CONTAGION,

WITH

Mr. DAWSON,	Profeſſor WATERHOUSE,
Dr. AIKIN,	Mr. HENRY,
Profeſſor IRVINE,	Dr. CLARK,
Dr. PERCIVAL,	Dr. ODIER,
Profeſſor WALL,	Dr. JAMES CURRIE:

AND ON THE BEST MEANS OF

PREVENTING THE SMALL-POX, AND PROMOTING INOCULATION, AT GENEVA;

WITH THE

MAGISTRATES OF THE REPUBLICK.

BY JOHN HAYGARTH, M.B.

F.R.S. Lond. F.R.S. and R.M.S. Edinb. and of the American Academy of Arts and Sciences.

LONDON,

Printed for J. JOHNSON, N° 72, St. Paul's Church-Yard

MDCCXCIII.

4 Title-page of John Haygarth, *A Sketch of a Plan to Exterminate the Casual Small-pox from Great Britain* (London, 1793)

expensive project"; &c.'[119] But Currie's apprehensions were, considering the mood of England's rulers in the 1790s, perhaps a bit more sober, for Haygarth's plan did not receive any notable attention from governmental officials. With such famed contributors to the *Sketch*, and with the book's dedication to the King, the silent demise of the plan deserves some explanation. To understand the failure of Haygarth's plan to attract support or even attention from those in power, one must recognise the central political fact of Europe in the 1790s, namely, the mighty ambitions of Revolutionary France. While the politically active Dissenters, particularly Price, were watching the events in France of 1789 and 1790 with unabashed enthusiasm, most of England's governors were reflecting with great unease on the possibility of such a thing happening in England. The Dissenters saw in France the potential that they thought England had possessed at the time of its Revolution of 1688, the potential to become a nation without distinctions in entitlement based on the dominance of a State church. Price expressed these opinions in his published sermon of November 1789, 'On the Love of Our Country,' through which he became one of England's most widely recognised exponents of the virtues of the French Revolution. Price's sermon subsequently became an object of Edmund Burke's abuse in his *Reflections on the French Revolution* of 1791. A wide spectrum of English political leaders, including Prime Minister William Pitt the Younger and Burke, regarded the French Revolution as an unnatural and improper usurpation of power which should not happen in Great Britain. Projects for reform, particularly for parliamentary reform, became suspicious enterprises to most Members of Parliament. In 1790, proposals for both parliamentary reform and relief for Unitarians were soundly defeated. William Wilberforce could not even get a hearing on a slave trade reform proposal in 1792, and the situation was rapidly deteriorating. By 1793, when Haygarth's *Sketch* was published, France had declared war on England, hoping to take the Revolution across the Channel. In the next year, Parliament suspended the Habeas Corpus Act, and a wave of trials of suspected subversives followed. In this climate of extreme political sensitivity, in which the interests of all of those outside of the ruling establishment had suddenly become subversive, Haygarth put forth a grand proposal for a medical reform which depended on the works and testimony of a number of well-known Dissenters, including the 'celebrated and ingenious Dr. Price.'[120] Among the other correspondents in the *Sketch*, Dr Aikin had been forced to move from Great Yarmouth in 1792 because

119 *Ibid.*, p. viii. 120 *Ibid.*, p. 33.

his Unitarian religion and sympathy with the French Revolution enraged the 'Church and King' local citizenry. Dr Currie, who had warned Haygarth in his correspondence about national opinion, was known to be the author, under the alias of 'Jaspar Wilson,' of an open letter to Pitt in 1793 that urged the Prime Minister to avoid declaring war on France. The people with whom Haygarth and his project were associated made the *Sketch*, even with its royal dedication, immediately dismissable, explaining why Haygarth's plan never came to be debated as a legislative possibility.

The final theme of Haygarth's smallpox activities can be found in the 'vaccine inoculation' discovered by Edward Jenner. In 1794, Haygarth was informed by The Revd. Dr Worthington, a close friend of Jenner's, about the early observations on 'the cow-pox.' Haygarth advised caution in his reply to Worthington, dated 'Chester, April 15th 1794':

> Your account of the cow-pox is indeed very marvelous; being so strange a history, and so contradictory to all past observations on the subject, very clear and full evidence will be required to render it credible.
>
> You say this whole rare phenomenon is soon to be published, but do not mention whether by yourself or some other medical friend. In either case, I trust that no reliance will be placed upon vulgar stories. The author should admit nothing but what he has proved by his own personal observations, both in the brute and human species. It would be useless to specify the doubts which must be satisfied upon this subject before rational belief can be obtained.
>
> If a physician should adopt such a doctrine, and much more, if he should publish it upon inadequate evidence, his character would materially suffer in the public opinion of his knowledge and discernment.[121]

It seems unlikely that Worthington did not show Haygarth's letter to Jenner. The date of Haygarth's reply suggests that Worthington wrote to him in early 1794. Perhaps Jenner and Worthington, having just read Haygarth's newly released *Sketch*, wanted to test the opinion of this obviously knowledgeable author about the cow-pox phenomenon.

In 1798, Haygarth, at the age of fifty-eight, left the Chester Infirmary with happy memories.[122] He settled in the curative resort town of Bath, as did many other physicians, where he could once again practice medicine in the company of his old friend William Falconer. In the same year, Jenner published *An Inquiry into the Causes and Effects of the Variolae Vaccinae*, detailing cases of cow-pox infection and inoculation from Jenner's experience. One of the persons to read Jenner's

[121] John Baron, *The Life of Edward Jenner* (London, 1827), pp. 134–5.
[122] Haygarth, *Letter to Dr. Percival*, pp. 127–8.

Inquiry in the months after its publication was Thomas Percival. Jenner had personally sent a copy to Percival. In his reply, dated 'Manchester, Nov. 20th, 1798,' Percival wrote:

The facts which you have adduced incontestably prove the existence of the cow-pox and its ready communication to the human species. But a larger induction is yet necessary to evince that the *variolae vaccinae* renders the person who has been affected with it secure during the whole life, from the infection of small-pox . . .

As soon as I had perused your work, several months since, I wrote to my excellent friend Dr. Haygarth (late of Chester, now of Bath) urging him to engage in a correspondence with you on his favourite and benevolent plan of exterminating the small-pox, of which your discovery points out a more probable means than any which has yet been proposed. Permit me to express a wish that you would confer with Dr. H., either personally or by letter, on this interesting subject.[123]

There is no direct evidence of either correspondence or a personal meeting between the two men, but it seems likely that they did communicate, for Haygarth soon became a zealous advocate of Jenner's vaccine inoculation. In the second edition of his *Inquiry*, published in 1801 (see plates 5 and 6) Haygarth wrote:

The discovery of Vaccine Inoculation by Dr. Jenner is the most fortunate and beneficial improvement that medical science ever accomplished. It does not, however, preclude the necessity of investigating the variolous poison, and of considering by what regulations its propagation may be prevented. In order to secure the unthinking multitude from this destructive Pestilence, measures to prevent the casual Small-pox should everywhere accompany Vaccine Inoculation . . .

I had the good fortune successfully to convey the first Vaccine Contagion to the inhabitants of America through Professor Waterhouse.[124]

Waterhouse also wrote of his vaccine connection with Haygarth. In a letter to Edward Jenner, dated 'April 24th, 1801,' he told of a bad portion of vaccine-infected thread from Haygarth:

The case at Geneva, under Dr. Odier, was ours exactly. One inch and a half of infected thread from Dr. Haygarth was the whole stock from whence perhaps 3,000 persons have been inoculated, but I fear the greatest part of them have been spurious.[125]

Haygarth was thus the supplier of vaccine to Waterhouse and Odier, both friends of his long before the discovery of vaccine. The enthusiasm which Haygarth showed suggests that he thought of the vaccine inoculation as an even better component of his plan than smallpox

[123] Baron, *Life of Edward Jenner*, pp. 157–8.

[124] John Haygarth, *An Inquiry How to Prevent the Small-pox and Proceedings of a Society for Promoting General Inoculation at Stated Periods, and Preventing the Casual Small-pox in Chester, a New Edition* (Bath, 1801), pp. 208–11. It should also be noted that the 'M.D.' which Haygarth placed after his name in this edition was an honorary degree given him by the new medical school at Cambridge (now Harvard) University in New England in 1794, presumably through the efforts of Waterhouse.

[125] Baron, *Life of Edward Jenner*, p. 440.

For the Cambridge Philosophical Society
JH

AN

INQUIRY

HOW TO PREVENT THE

SMALL-POX.

AND

PROCEEDINGS OF A SOCIETY

FOR

Promoting GENERAL INOCULATION at stated periods, and preventing the Casual SMALL-POX in CHESTER.

——— culpam compesce, priusquam
Dira per incautum serpant contagia vulgus.
VIRG. GEORG. iii. 468.

A NEW EDITION, WITH ADDITIONS.

BY

JOHN HAYGARTH, M.D.

F.R.S. LOND. F.R.S. AND R.M.S. EDINB. AND OF THE AMERICAN ACADEMY OF ARTS AND SCIENCES.

BATH, PRINTED BY R. CRUTTWELL,
FOR
CADELL AND DAVIES, STRAND, LONDON.

1801.

5 Title-page of the second edition of John Haygarth, *An Inquiry How to Prevent the Small-pox* (London, 1801)

i.			ii.	iii.	iv.	v.	vi.	vii.	viii.	ix.	x.	xi.
PATIENTS. Order.	Name.	No.	Street.	Occupation.	Small-Pox Fever began.	Date of Information.	Gratis Rules, or Promissory Notes.	Whence infected.	Date of Death, or Last Scab.	Washed and aired.	Infection communicated to	Rules observed or transgressed.
1.	E. Bryly	2	Sty-lane.	Fisherman.	1778, Jan.	Jan. 30.	P. N. Jan. 30.				none.	observed.
2.	M. Morris	2	Bridge-st.	Flour-dealer.	March 24.	April 3.	P. N. April 3.		April 25.	April 26.	Coleclough's 4th Family.	transgressed.
3.	A. Collier	2	Northg.-st.	Bricklayer.	April 7.	April 14.	P. N. Ap. 14.		L. S. Ap. 29.	April 30.	none.	observed.
4.	H. Coleclough	2	Bridge-st.	Labourer.	1st, Ap. 23. 2d, May 3.	April 26.	P. N. Ap. 26.	Morris's 2d F.			none.	observed.
5.	Mr. Smith	1	Bridge-st.	Watch-mak.	April 22.	April 24.	G. R. Ap. 24.		L. S. May 4.	May 5.	none.	observed.
6.	A. Singleton	2	Northg.-st.	Labourer.	May 6.	May 10.	P. N. May 10.	Liverpool.			Ashton's 7th F.	transgressed.
7.	E. Ashton	2	Northg.-st.	Labourer.	1st May 30. 2d June 14.	June 4.	P. N. June 4.	Singleton's 6th F.	June 23.	June 24.	none.	observed.
8.	H. Price	1	Gorse-St.	Shoemaker.	May 29.	June 8.	P. N. June 8.		July 6.	July 8.	none.	observed.
9.	E. Evans	2	Bars.	Cobler.	May 30.	June 13.	P. N. June 13.	Croughton.	June 27.	June 27.	10, 11, 12, 13, Families.	transgressed.
10.	A. Conolly	1	Bars.	Baker.	June 18.	June 23.	P. N. June 23.	Evans's 9th F.	July 10.	July 10.	none.	observed.
11.	C. Jones	1	Bars.	Weaver.	June 22.	June 25.	P. N. June 25.	Evans's 9th F.	July 14.	July 15.	none.	observed.
12.	H. Huxley	2	Bars.	Newsman.	June 20.	June 25.	P. N. June 25.	Evans's 9th F.	July 14.	July 15.	Smith's 17th F.	transgressed.
13.	Mr. Jenkin	1	Bars.	Tanner.	June 16.	June 26.	G. R. June 26.	Evans's 9th F.	July 14.	July 15.	Morris's 15th F.	transgressed.
14.	E. Alsop	1	Bars.	Soldier.	July 9.	July 11.	P. N. July 12.	10th, 11th, 12th, or 13th Families.	July 29.	July 29.	Downing 16 F.	transgressed.
15.	M. Morris	1	Forest-st.	Shoemaker.	July 20.	July 23.	P. N. July 23.	Jenkins's 13th F.	August 3.	Aug. 4.	none.	observed.
16.	A. Downing	1	Bars.	Sailor.	July 23.	July 27.	P. N. July 28.	Alsop 14th F.	August 2.	Aug. 4.	none.	observed.
17.	A. Smith	2	Bunce-la.	Glazier.	July 22.	Aug. 6.	P. N. Aug. 6.	Huxley 12th F.	August 21.	Aug. 21.	none.	observed.
18.	E. Tilston	1	Forest-st.	Shoemaker.	Sept. 10.	Sept. 26.	P. N. Sept. 26.		October 7.	Oct. 8.	none.	observed.
19.	E. Johnson	1	Gorse-St.	Labourer.	October 4.	Oct. 5.	P. N. Oct. 5.		October 14.	Oct. 15.	none.	observed.
20.	L. Bellis	3	Crooks-la.	Coachman.	1. Oct. 21. 2. Nov. 2. 3. —— 3.	Oct. 29.	P. N. Oct. 30.		Nov. 27.	Nov. 21.	none.	observed.

6 Table from the second edition of John Haygarth, *An Inquiry How to Prevent the Small-pox* (London, 1801)

inoculation, for smallpox inoculation was known by many contemporaries to occasionally be a source of infection with the virulent natural smallpox. One of vaccine's purported virtues was, of course, that it could not convey the smallpox contagion. It is significant, however, that Haygarth switched the emphasis in regard to preventive measures: whereas, in the *Sketch*, inoculation was meant to back up observance of the 'Rules of Prevention,' now the miraculous new vaccine held the dominant position. The new vaccine was 'a discovery which can effectively destroy the Small-pox, the most mortal enemy that ever afflicted mankind.'[126] Haygarth would never have claimed such a virtue either for inoculation alone, or solely for observance of the 'Rules of Prevention.' In this statement, Haygarth admitted that all he could do to combat smallpox would be done under the rubric of Edward Jenner's vaccine.

I have endeavoured to show that Haygarth's project to eradicate smallpox may, like his smallpox contagion itself, be explained in terms of Haygarth's identifiable circumstances and personal contacts. All of Haygarth's works originated from a network of interests which he had mostly adopted from his Protestant Dissenter friends: their religiously motivated 'philanthropic' interests in helping the poor; economically motivated interests in the welfare of population and industry; and possible political interest in portraying themselves as philanthropic persons, having a purely non-partisan concern for the welfare of humanity at heart. In addition, the way in which Haygarth demonstrated philanthropy – through medical projects directed by medical men with a medical understanding of disease and mortality – can be associated with the extraordinary education that he and many of his philanthropic friends received at Edinburgh under William Cullen. Haygarth's unique project to eradicate smallpox was simply one instance of a larger inspiration by a singular perspective on eighteenth-century England. The Protestant Dissenters saw England in dire need of improvement. Haygarth and his friends would improve their nation in a variety of ways: spiritually, by abolishing such offences against humanity as the slave trade and unbearable prison conditions; materially, by opening factories which would, in turn, confer grace upon the poor and ignorant multitudes in the form of productive work; and medically, by implementing programmes with the dual aims of augmenting the kingdom's population and of relieving the poor somewhat from their suffering.

[126] Haygarth, *An Inquiry*, *New Edition*, p. 210.

As for the project's demise, others who have treated Haygarth's plan have implied that Jenner's 'epoch-making discovery' rendered it useless.[127] But this is an historical elision, for Haygarth's plan met an end of its own making, saddled with the stigma of reform and Dissent in a decade politically hostile to anything outside of the conservative sphere of 'Church and King' orthodoxy. Through his adoption of the Protestant Dissenters' programme Haygarth's projects were integrally involved in the national politics of the late eighteenth century. In promoting these projects, Haygarth was identifying himself with nationally recognised extremist figures, most notably Price, Currie and Aikin. His project to eradicate smallpox, conceived in a Tory town, no less, during years of high hopes among the Dissenters, died as a result of a dramatic change in the nation's political mood in the years following the French Revolution.

[127] Elliot, 'A Medical Pioneer: John Haygarth', p. 238.

10

'Living in the light'
dispensaries, philanthropy and medical reform in late-eighteenth-century London

ROBERT KILPATRICK

The most striking feature of medical philanthropy in eighteenth-century London is that it found expression in two distinctive institutions – hospitals and dispensaries – and that their dates of founding fell into two widely separate periods over twenty years apart. The five general hospitals of eighteenth-century foundation were all established between 1720 and 1745, while thirteen dispensaries were opened in London between 1770 and 1800.[1] What accounts for this second explosion of philanthropic activity and why was it channelled through a new kind of institution?

Several reasons have been put forward to explain the appearance of

[1] This list has been compiled from Patrick Colquhoun's *Police of the Metropolis* (London, 1797), p. 380; Anthony Highmore's *Pietas Londinensis* (London, 1810), pp. 332 ff. J. J. Baddeley's *Account of St. Giles Cripplegate* (London, 1888), p. 213, and reports from various dispensaries.

1769 Dispensary for the Infant Poor, Red Lion Square (later Soho Square).
1770 General Dispensary, Aldersgate Street.
1774 Westminster General Dispensary.
1777 London Dispensary, Primrose Street.
1777 Surrey Dispensary, Union Street, Southwark.
1779 Metropolitan Dispensary, Fore Street, Cripplegate.
1780 Finsbury Dispensary, Union Street, Southwark.
1782 Eastern Dispensary, Alie Street, Whitechapel.
1783 Public Dispensary, Carey Street.
1785 St Marylebone Dispensary, Well Street, nr. Oxford Street.
1786 New Finsbury and General Dispensary, West Smithfield.
1789 City Dispensary, Bevis Marks.
1792 Universal Medical Institution, Old Gravel Lane, Ratcliffe Highway.
1793 London Electrical Dispensary, City Road.
1801 Bloomsbury Dispensary, 62, Great Russell Street.
1805 London Dispensary for Curing Diseases of the Eye and Ear.
1805 Middlesex Dispensary, Great Ailiff Street.
1805 Royal Universal Dispensary, Featherston Buildings, Holborn.
1805 St. James's Dispensary, Berwick Street. Soho.
1805 Ossulston Dispensary, Bow Street, Bloomsbury.
1805 Western Dispensary, Charles Street, Westminster.

the 'dispensary movement' in the last quarter of the eighteenth century. Irvine Loudon has argued that 'it was largely the manifest failure of the hospital to evolve, adapt and enlarge to meet the crisis in health at the end of the eighteenth century that led to the dispensary movement'.[2] But if there was indeed a 'crisis in health' at this time why was it not met by the foundation of new hospitals rather than dispensaries? We cannot blame the supporters of the voluntary-subscription hospitals in particular for not expanding; they were working with limited budgets and were constantly under threat of closure. The potential for expansion simply did not exist and even if it had been possible, would hospital governors have wanted to do so? We shall never know because the situation did not arise. What is certain however is that in the late eighteenth century a large number of people were committed to the founding and running of dispensaries. The question of whether such a crisis in health existed, and, if so, how it was perceived by the governors and physicians associated with the London dispensaries needs to be explored. These institutions should be looked at in their own right and not as improved versions of hospitals. If one considers eighteenth-century philanthropy in terms of medical care provision it is tempting to see the dispensaries as successes and the hospitals as failures, but in the long run it was the hospital that triumphed precisely because of its ability to be adapted to new social and political realities. Let us now turn our attention to the General Dispensary in Aldersgate Street founded in 1770 by the Quaker physician John Coakley Lettsom and look at its purpose and how it was organised and run.

The General Dispensary was the second institution of this kind to have been founded in eighteenth-century London but it was the model upon which all subsequent dispensaries were based. It was preceded in 1769 by the Dispensary for the Infant Sick Poor in Red Lion Square which had been founded by the physician George Armstrong.[3]

[2] I. Loudon, 'The Origins and Growth of the Dispensary Movement in England', *Bulletin of the History of Medicine* 55 (1981), p. 330. Very little is known about these medical charities, but for further background reading see: W. Hartston, 'Medical Dispensaries in Eighteenth Century London', *Proceedings of the Royal Society of Medicine* 56 (1963), pp. 753–8; Z. Cope, 'The Influence of the Free Dispensaries upon Medical Education in Britain', *Medical History* 13 (1969), pp. 29–36; H. E. Frank, 'The Background of the London Dispensary', *Journal of the History of Medicine* 20 (1965), pp. 199–221; A. Rosenberg, 'The London Dispensary for the Sick Poor', *Journal of the History of Medicine* 14 (1959), pp. 41–56.

[3] See Anon., *A General Account of the Dispensary for the Relief of the Infant Poor, Originally Instituted by Dr. George Armstrong in A.D. 1769* (n.p., n.d., *c.* 1772). For more recent accounts see W. L. Maloney, *George and John Armstrong of Castleton: Two Eighteenth Century Medical Pioneers* (London, 1954); F. N. L. Poynter, 'A Unique Copy of George Armstrong's Printed Proposal for Establishing the Dispensary for Sick Children, London 1769', *Medical History* 1 (1957), pp. 65–6.

Lettsom's dispensary was different from Armstrong's in one important respect: the General Dispensary was not restricted to children but accepted patients of all ages. While the various London dispensaries differed from each other in detail, they all shared many common features. The dispensaries usually started life in rented premises and as patient numbers and the volume of subscriptions grew they moved into larger houses which in some cases were purpose-built. Dispensaries were wholly financed by voluntary subscriptions and thus, in common with the voluntary hospitals, their financial state was often precarious and unstable. They were subject to the changing fashions of eighteenth-century philanthropy.

As at the voluntary hospitals, subscribers to the dispensaries were made governors on payment of a minimum contribution, and at the General Dispensary this was one guinea per year. Only patients sent to the dispensary with a letter of recommendation from a governor were seen by physicians, and subscribers were allowed to have one patient on the books in proportion to their donation (one patient per guinea subscribed). This points to an important difference between the voluntary-subscription dispensaries and hospitals. At the hospitals the number of beds restricted patient admissions, while the system of out-patient relief at the dispensaries meant that as many objects of charity could be seen as the governors were willing to send. In such circumstances it is not surprising that the dispensaries treated more patients than did the hospitals. For the governors of dispensaries, these institutions offered one inestimable advantage over the voluntary hospitals: they were able to give more charity per guinea and thus the dispensaries provided philanthropy on the cheap. The popularity of the General Dispensary in the first eight years of its existence, 1770–8, can be seen from Lettsom's own figures for the number of subscribers: 1770 (100); 1773 (300); 1775 (600) and 1778 (1,400).[4] Support from the public was overwhelming, probably in part attracted by the relatively low subscription charges which were about one-fifth of those at the voluntary-subscription hospitals.

But this cannot fully explain why dispensaries were founded and supported in the late eighteenth century because, although voluntary-

[4] J. C. Lettsom, *Medical Memoirs of the General Dispensary in London, for part of the years 1773–1774* (London, 1774), p. xvii. The subscription rates were relatively low; Lettsom's reasons for having cheap subscriptions were 'with a view to render the charity more extensive, and give the industrious poor an early opportunity of obtaining recommendations from their benevolent neighbours, on the earliest attack of sickness' (*Medical Memoirs*, p. xxi).

subscription hospitals and dispensaries were in competition with one another for funds, the hospitals did not collapse for want of governors; we will need to look beyond the lower subscription rates of the dispensaries to explain their popularity between 1770 and 1800. The key to unravelling this mystery lies in the fact that the dispensaries were fundamentally different from the voluntary-subscription hospitals in four important respects: (1) Dispensaries were founded and run by medical practitioners – largely Dissenting physicians – on behalf of the governors who did not play a direct and active role in the daily operation of these institutions; (2) All patients were seen on an out-patient basis (many in their own homes) and there were no beds; (3) Most cases of disease seen by the physicians were listed in the dispensary records as 'fever', a category excluded from the general London hospitals; (4) Few surgical patients were admitted to the dispensaries and no operations were carried out by surgeons on them – such patients comprised the bulk of admissions to the London hospitals.

Now that we are able to see that there were major differences in how hospitals and dispensaries were organised, run and the purposes they fulfilled, it is necessary to account for these and explain why *the dispensary model* became the predominate institutional form for the expression of medical philanthropy in late-eighteenth-century London. We need to explain why so many Dissenting physicians in London suddenly showed a new interest in the condition of the sick poor at this time and more particularly in the disease of 'fever'. I intend to explore the relationship between their knowledge and understanding of the causes of fever and how to study and treat it. Moreover I will show that it is possible to account for their medicine – and the institutions and societies they founded to advance it – in terms of their religious and political beliefs.

John Coakley Lettsom and his professional colleagues at the General Dispensary in the years 1770–5 had certain interests and experiences in common. The most important of these was that they were members of the Society of Friends, or Quakers, and they were part of a close-knit network of Dissenting physicians, philosophers and philanthropists which included John Fothergill, William Cullen, Thomas Percival, James Currie and others. Francis Lobo has shown (in this volume, pp. 217–53) how extensive this network was in his work on John Haygarth's scheme for smallpox eradication, and explained how these men supported each other in their various schemes and projects –

financial, philosophical and philanthropic. This network of Dissenters was bound together by a genuine concern to improve the health and living conditions of the labouring poor. Such philanthropy was a natural expression of their particular religious and political beliefs and for Lettsom it found an outlet in his activities as a physician. It is his role as a *Quaker philanthropist* that largely explains the kind of medicine that he practised and the institution he founded – the General Dispensary – to extend medical relief to the sick poor in London. Four aspects of Lettsom's life will need to be considered: (1) membership of the Society of Friends from birth; (2) training by apprenticeship to a surgeon-apothecary and later as a physician at the Universities of Edinburgh and Leyden; (3) his relationship with the Quaker physician John Fothergill (1712–1780); (4) his role as a leading philanthropist engaged in a variety of projects for social and political reform. The first of these experiences – as a Quaker – later influenced Lettsom's activities as a physician and philanthropist.

By turning to Lettsom's published writings and correspondence we are able to see that he wrote profusely on a wide variety of topics, but what united the apparent diversity was his concern to use philanthropy as a means of reforming society in accordance with Quaker beliefs. This is evident in everything he wrote, including books and papers on medical subjects.[5] Lettsom's Quaker ideals provide the consistent thread which runs through the bulk of his writing. His creation of the General Dispensary in 1770 and, later, the Medical Society of London in 1773, were part of a much larger programme of philanthropic reform which was consistent with and inspired by his concern to act for the public good. He proposed the creation of societies for the reform of prostitutes, for bettering the conditions of the poor, for promoting useful literature, and for the recovery of drowned persons. These were

[5] Lettsom was a prolific pamphleteer and wrote on the following subjects: *Hints Respecting the Distress of the Poor in the Years 1794, 1795*; *Hints Respecting a Samaritan Society*; *Hints Respecting Crimes and Punishments*; *Hints Respecting Wills and Testaments*; *Hints Respecting a Female Benefit Club, and Lying-in Charity*; *Hints Respecting a Village Society*; *Hints Respecting the Support and Education of the Deaf and Dumb Children of the Poor*, *Hints Respecting Employment of the Blind*; *Hints for Establishing a Society for Promoting Useful Literature*; *Hints to Masters and Mistresses Respecting Female Servants*; *Hints Respecting Religious Persecution*; *Hints Respecting Humane Societies, for the Recovery of Drowned Persons*; *Hints Respecting Female Character, and a Repository for Female Industry*; *Hints Respecting the Immediate Effects of Poverty*; *Hints Respecting the Society for Bettering the Condition, and Increasing the Comforts of the Poor; Hints Respecting the Society for the Discharge and Relief of Persons Imprisoned for Small Debts*; *Hints Respecting the Prevention and Cure of Infectious Fevers*; *Hints Addressed to Card Parties*; *Hints Respecting the Establishment of Schools for Extending Education to the Poor*, *Hints for the Establishment of a Medical Society in London*.

just a few of his many projects for reform and in *Hints Designed to Promote Beneficence, Temperance and Medical Science* we are able to see the breadth of his reforming zeal. To look at Lettsom's medical writings separate from the programme of social reform that inspired them is to misrepresent them. Lettsom was a Quaker first, a physician second and a philanthropist third. From what we know of his early life we are able to see just how important his membership in the Society of Friends was to his later activities as a philanthropist-physician.

Lettsom was born in 1744 in the West Indies to a middle-class Quaker family, and the formative years of his life were spent almost exclusively among the tight-knit community of the Society – a religious sect characterised by its in-marrying and close bonds of friendship. As a Quaker Lettsom acquired the values and social connections that were to determine the course of his professional career and guide him to seek a practical application of knowledge for the benefit of the public good. At the age of six he was sent to England and was placed in the care of the Society in Lancaster where he was befriended by the Quaker preacher Samuel Fothergill who soon became Lettsom's guardian. Fothergill arranged for Lettsom to attend a local Quaker school and in 1761 he was apprenticed for five years to Fothergill's distant relative Abraham Sutcliff, a Quaker surgeon-apothecary at Settle in Yorkshire. Because the Corporation (1661) and Test (1673) Acts were still in force at this time, Dissenters were excluded from most professions – the law, Parliament, commissions in the army and navy – so medicine became a well-trod pathway for social advancement.

Because Quakers were excluded from Oxford and Cambridge, many of them used their connections and acquaintanceships among the Society of Friends to secure apprenticeships and patronage at the commencement of their careers in medicine. Through the Society Lettsom was educated as a young man, apprenticed to Sutcliff and introduced by Samuel Fothergill to his gifted and highly successful brother, the Quaker physician John Fothergill. In 1766 at the age of twenty-two Lettsom came to London and became acquainted with the Quaker community there through John Fothergill. Lettsom enrolled as a physicians' pupil at St Thomas's Hospital where he followed the practice, probably at the suggestion of Fothergill who had spent two years there as a student between 1736 and 1738. The hospital was well known by the 1760s for the high calibre of the teaching of its medical and surgical staff, many of whom were Dissenters. But it was through his close friendship with Fothergill that Lettsom was directed towards philanthropy and the study of fevers.

Fothergill had been the first graduate of the University of Edinburgh to be admitted as a Licentiate of the College of Physicians of London in 1744.[6] He published books and papers on the subject of epidemics, the most important of which was *Account of the Sore Throat Attended with Ulcers* (1748) which presents the natural history of an epidemic of malignant sore throat or diphtheria which occurred in London in 1747. This was followed by *Observations on the Weather and Diseases of London* (1751–4) and in *Philosophical Transactions* he published a paper 'On the Epidemic Disease of 1775'. Fothergill served as a patron and role-model for the young Lettsom and it was through this association that Lettsom was first introduced to Quaker philanthropy.

> Fothergill's philanthropic efforts were partly connected with the public benevolence of the Society of Friends. He took an active part in the foundation of the school for Quaker children at Ackworth, to which he liberally contributed; he was interested in the funds raised for the relief of Spanish prisoners, and in numerous plans for improving the health, cleanliness, and prosperity of the working classes.[7]

Yet Fothergill also managed to cultivate one of the largest and most lucrative private practices in London, and when he left the city in 1770 he handed it over to Lettsom. Lettsom never forgot the debt that he owed to his patron and friend, and in 1773, soon after founding the Medical Society of London, he provided funds to pay for an annual award known as the Fothergillian Medal and three years after his mentor's death in 1780, Lettsom published *Memoirs of John Fothergill, M.D.* which included a biographical sketch and a complete collection of Fothergill's writings. A more detailed study of Fothergill's activities is beyond the scope of this chapter but he is an excellent example of how throughout the eighteenth-century many Quakers rose from humble backgrounds to positions of great wealth and influence.

Roy Porter says that the Quakers became 'closed and quietist and declined in numbers from about 38,000 in 1700 to about 20,000 in 1800. But this evaporation left them socially more select: the proportions of merchants and professional men rose and artisans declined.'[8] But their impact on the transformation of economic life in England in the late eighteenth-century was dramatic and Quaker families such as the Barclays, Lloyds, Darbys and Wilkinsons – to name but a few –

[6] Sir G. Clark, *A History of the Royal College of Physicians of London*, 2 vols., (London, 1964–6), vol. 2, p. 543; see also the biography by Lettsom in *The Works of John Fothergill*, 2 vols. (London, 1783).

[7] J. F. Payne, 'John Fothergill', entry in *Dictionary of National Biography* (Oxford), vol. 20, p. 67.

[8] Roy Porter, *English Society in the Eighteenth Century* (Harmondsworth, 1982), p. 199.

comprised 'a muster of undissipated industrial talent unmatched elsewhere in the eighteenth-century world.'[9] The changing experiences of Quakers in London was similarly striking and, as Raistrick shows, the proportion of merchants, dealers and skilled artisans in the capital had risen compared with the number of labourers and unskilled workers.[10] By 1780 many London Quakers were found in middle-class positions and were financially able to pursue philanthropic projects in accordance with their religious and political beliefs. To explain why the General Dispensary was founded in 1770 by Lettsom we need to look briefly at what it meant to be a Quaker at this time and how their view of man's relationship to God and to society influenced the way they implemented their programme of social reform.

The movement known as the Society of Friends was founded in the mid seventeenth century by George Fox (1624–91), son of a Leicestershire weaver.[11] He was apprenticed to a shoemaker and was brought up among artisans: it was to these people that his teaching was directed. He sought in his ministry to bring the relations of trade under the influence of Quaker standards of a spiritual life. About 1650–1 Fox travelled in the north of England, forming the first groups of 'seekers after truth' in Yorkshire and Westmoreland. The essence of the Quaker ethic was a belief that every person carried within them the Kingdom of God, known as the 'Inner Light', and in *A Brief Account of the Rise and Progress of the People, Call'd Quakers* (1694), William Penn wrote:

> That which People had been vainly seeking Without, with much Pain and Cost, they (the Quakers) by this Ministry found Within . . . For they were directed to the Light of Jesus Christ Within them, as the Seed and Leaven of the Kingdom of God. A faithful and True Witness and just Monitor in every Bosom.[12]

Because the Quakers believed that the 'Light of Christ' was in each person, they held that all people were equal in the sight of God. In accordance with this belief, Quakers eschewed the use of titles which

[9] *Ibid.*, p. 199.

[10] A. Raistrick, *Quakers in Science and Industry, Being an Account of the Quaker Contributions to Science and Industry During the Seventeenth and Eighteenth Centuries* (London, 1968), pp. 35–88.

[11] For further reading on Fox and Quakers see: J. S. Watson, *The Life of George Fox, the Founder of the Quakers* (London, 1860); A. C. Bickley, *George Fox and the Early Quakers* (London, 1884); Sir G. Newman, *George Fox, the Founder of Quakerism (Tercentenary of George Fox, 1624–1924)*, (London, 1924); V. Noble, *The Man in Leather Breeches (The Life and Times of George Fox)*, (London, 1953); H. E. Wildes, *Voice of the Lord. A biography of George Fox* (Philadelphia, 1965).

[12] W. Penn, *A Brief Account of the Rise and Progress of the People, Call'd Quakers* (Philadelphia, 1694), quoted in F. B. Tolles, *Meeting House and Country House: The Quaker Merchants of Colonial Philadelphia 1682–1763* (New York, 1963), p. 4.

acknowledged rank, refused to take oaths or pay tithes to the established church. The Quakers did not expect outsiders to help them – a view which came from their experiences as members of the closed and tight-knit 'Society', and their belief in the 'Inner Light'. Because of the existence of the 'Inner Light' within each person, man lived closest to God in a state of independence and liberty, free from any constraints on his ability to help himself and others. Quakers were actively opposed to the slave-trade and sought to abolish it throughout the British Empire. In 1767 Lettsom was left some property in the West Indies by his father, 'the most valuable portion of which consisted of fifty slaves, whom Lettsom, though possessed of no other resources, at once emancipated.'[13] Because of the presence of the 'Inner Light' within each individual regardless of their rank or colour, the Quakers believed that it was in a man's power to lead a truthful, responsible and moral life, and through cooperation to further the interests of other Friends. The Quaker ethic fostered an attitude that valued education, self-improvement, and the sharing of skills and knowledge. The practical application of knowledge for mutual benefit and the public good was sought by Quakers in their activities in industry, finance, trade, medicine and philanthropy.

Raistrick points to several characteristics of Quaker life that suited their experiences as skilled artisans and which contributed to their success and prosperity during the Industrial Revolution. He says that learning was highly valued as a means of success in every activity in life. Emphasis was placed on the importance of an enquiring mind, and value was placed on personal judgement and independent thought. Self-improvement was brought about through education, and the 'Society' established many schools in the eighteenth century. In such schools there was always a strong element of practical utility in the teaching and every subject was studied with an eye to its potential as a useful skill. Tolles says that

> Practical, methodical activity in the world was considered as evidence that one was indeed living 'in the Light'; the expenditure of physical energy and the handling of material objects was identified with industry, whereas abstract speculation and contemplations, when not directed towards purely religious questions, was equated with idleness.[14]

[13] *Dictionary of National Biography*. See: J. J. Abraham, *Lettsom: His Life, Times, Friends and Descendents* (London, 1933); T. J. Pettigrew (ed.), *Memoirs of the Life and Writings of John Coakley Lettsom*, 3 vols. (London, 1817). In 1772 Lord Mansfield ruled that the status of slavery was inadmissable on English soil.

[14] Tolles, *Meeting House and Country House*, p. 206.

And idleness was perhaps the worst charge that could be levelled at a Quaker. Such practical, methodical activity was directed towards the pursuit of knowledge with great success by many Quakers, and their achievements as businessmen, iron-masters, instrument-makers and physicians are startling by any standard. What characterised this group of Dissenters was that they were all self-made men: through their own industry and shrewd judgement they had built up successful family businesses, many of which still survive.[15]

The Quaker ethic and their political position as Dissenters in the eighteenth century led them to open up new areas of economic activity to their advantage. Success in business, commerce and trade contributed to their social advancement and by 1770 many Quakers were in positions of great economic power and influence. For Quakers 'living in the Light', such prosperity carried with it responsibilities for the welfare of others and a need to find practical expressions of their concern to improve the living conditions of the poor. Many Quaker industrialists, for example the Darbys of Coalbrookdale, pioneered schemes in their workshops and factories for the fair treatment of workers and provision for their spiritual and material welfare.[16] This coincided with the expansion of their industrial works and the transition from individual crafts to industrial organisation. As Dissenters they sought to reform society in ways which suited their economic interests and religious beliefs: the poor became an object of concern to these men not only because they were rich and in a position to do something about the living conditions of the poor, but also because they were Quakers.

Quaker philanthropy in the eighteenth century had several characteristic features. It was small-scale and sought to enable the labouring poor to help themselves to become self-supporting by providing just enough charity to carry them through periods of individual infirmity or economic decline. The freedom from constraint was always maintained because this was an essential ingredient of the Quaker ethic of 'living in the Light'. For this reason many Quakers were opposed to institutions such as prisons, madhouses and hospitals which confined or restrained their inmates and patients within their walls. As Andrew Scull has shown, the Tuke family and other Quakers in York founded an asylum in 1792 for Friends 'deprived of the use of their reason' and the moral therapy practiced at the York Retreat aimed

[15] Barclay's, Lloyd's, Wilkinson, Fry's, Cadbury's, Terry's and Rowntrees are a few examples.
[16] See A. Raistrick, *Dynasty of Iron Founders: the Darbys and Coalbrookdale* (London, 1953).

at minimizing external, physical coercion . . . Restraint might be necessary to prevent bodily injury, but it ought to be a last resort, and was never to be imposed solely for the convenience of the attendants. While Tuke did not think that restraint could be entirely done away with, he did insist on doing away with its most objectionable forms – gyves, chains, manacles – and his refusal to employ it as a routine measure was a marked departure from prevailing practice.[17]

Tuke sought to create conditions favourable to the return of reason in response to kindness and fair treatment. And the plan of the Retreat 'was designed to encourage the individual's own efforts to reassert his powers of self-control'[18] and in common with other Quaker attempts at reform, the treatment was conceived to respect the independence and dignity of the individual.

The universal system of 'giving thanks' found at the voluntary-subscription hospitals, which emphasised deference and marked the relations of power between the governors and patients, was never a part of Quaker-inspired charities. Quakers essentially trusted in the willingness and ability of the labouring poor to support themselves if suitable living conditions of cleanliness, orderliness and employment were made available to them. Although Quaker philanthropy was often palliative in its aims – seeking to remedy immediate problems of ill-health or unemployment – it also sought to alter the conditions in which the labouring poor were living. There was always a strong element of *prevention* in all Quaker philanthropy, and this was no less true of the General Dispensary.

For Fothergill, Lettsom, Howard and other Quaker philanthropists, the first step towards preventing unwholesome conditions in eighteenth-century England was to visit places where people were confined and deprived of their liberty: prisons, lazarettos, lunatic asylums and hospitals were obvious destinations for Quaker philanthropists, and the systematic visiting and recording of their observations occupied much of their time. Howard was concerned that such institutions corrupted the health and the morals of the people contained in them. The source of this influence, writes Howard in *The State of Prisons in England and Wales* (1777), is London. He says that it

is in this further reformation, that it will be absolutely necessary to begin with the capital; for as, in my former visits, when I have met with gaol fever in country prisons, I have been almost constantly told that it was derived from those in London; as the corruption of manners, also flowing from that great fountain, spreads far and wide its malignant streams.[19]

[17] A. Scull, *Museums of Madness: The Social Organization of Madness in Nineteenth Century England* (London, 1979), p. 68. [18] *Ibid.*, p. 68.

[19] J. Howard, *The State of Prisons in England and Wales* (London, 1777). For further biographical sources see: J. Aiken, *A View of the Character and Public Services of the Late John Howard*,

The ultimate aims of Howard's programme for the reform of prisons and other institutions of confinement were two-fold: (1) he sought to provide healthy living conditions in them to enable their inhabitants to become useful members of society; (2) to promote the salvation of individual souls. These aims are clear in *The State of Prisons* where Howard writes that he was 'not an advocate of extravagant and profuse allowance to prisoners. I plead only for necessities in such a moderate quantity as may support health and strength for labour.'[20] And many people died on the gallows and in prisons 'who might have been useful to the state'. Howard was convinced that many of these people

> might, by regular, steady discipline in a penitentiary-house have been rendered useful members of society; and above all, from the pleasing hope that such a plan might be the means of promoting salvation of some individuals – of which, every instance is, according to the unerring word of truth, a more important object than the gaining of the whole world.[21]

Driven by his Quaker sense of duty towards the poor, Howard often risked his own life to investigate the conditions in which the poor lived. He remarks that

> Trusting in Divine Providence, and believing in myself in the way of my duty, I visit the most infectious hospitals and noxious cells; and while thus employed, I fear no evil. In an offensive room, I avoid drawing my breath deeply; and on my return, sometimes wash my mouth and hands.[22]

Divine Providence must have failed him in 1790, for he succumbed to gaol fever and died.

Disease was seen as one factor among many that prevented the inmates in such places from becoming diligent and sober workers – an important concern of all Quaker philanthropy – and once inside these institutions men like Lettsom and Howard turned their attention to the disease that afflicted the poor. What they saw everywhere they looked was *fever*. Howard says that

> from my observations in 1773 and 1774 I was fully convinced that many more were destroyed by it, than were put to death by all the public executions in the Kingdom . . .

Esq., LL. D. (London, 1792); J. B. Brown, *Memoirs of the Public and Private Life of John Howard, the Philanthropist* (London, 1818); T. Taylor, *Memoirs of John Howard, Esq. F. R. S., The Christian Philanthropist* (London, 1836); J. Field, *The Life of John Howard* (London, 1850); J. Stoughton, *The Christian Philanthropist: A Memorial of John Howard* (London, 1853); H. Dixon, *John Howard, a Memoir* (London, 1854); E. C. S. Gibson, *John Howard* (London, 1901); M. Southwood, *John Howard, Prison Reformer: An Account of his Life and Travels* (London, 1958). [20] Howard, *State of Prisons*, p. 62. [21] *Ibid.* p. 27.
[22] *Ibid.* p. 18.

this frequent effect of confinement in prison seems generally understood, and shews how full of emphatical meaning is the course of a severe creditor who pronounces his debtor's doom to rot in Gaol.[23]

For many men and women who had avoided the scaffold, once entering a prison their executioner might very well be fever. Institutions of confinement might deprive prisoners of a degree of liberty as part of their punishment for criminal activity (often indebtedness), but with great frequency, claimed Howard, they lost their lives too. Howard, Lettsom and other Quaker philanthropists did not advocate the closure of all prisons but they sought a reform of their economy and management to ensure that the health and morals of prisoners were maintained to enable them to eventually return to employment. Such philanthropists did not enter hospitals and prisons looking for fever, but by seeking out the conditions within them they came to see that fever posed a threat to the lives of the poor. To understand how this group of Quaker reformers thought that fever should be treated and why the institution they founded for this purpose – the General Dispensary – took the form that it did we must turn our attention to Lettsom's experience as a medical student in Edinburgh where he came under the influence of Dr William Cullen (1710–90).

In 1768 Lettsom arrived in Edinburgh to study medicine at the university and enrolled in the popular course of lectures given by Cullen.[24] As a student under Cullen, Lettsom was taught that medicine was a proper object of philosophical enquiry, the aim of which was practical utility. The value of practical knowledge, the search for truth in the natural world and their usefulness in contributing to 'improvement' in all spheres of human activity, was part of the Quaker ethic that Lettsom was raised to accept. From Cullen, Lettsom learned to understand the causes and nature of 'contagion' and its effect – fevers – in a particular way which influenced his later work as a physician. Writing of contagion Cullen said that

it is now well known that the effluvia constantly arising from the living human body, if long retained in the same place, without having been diffused in the atmosphere, acquire a singular virulence; and that in that state being applied to the bodies of men, become the cause of a fever, which is highly contagious. The existence of such a cause is fully proved by the later observations on jail and hospital fevers; and that the same virulent matter may be produced in many other places must be sufficiently obvious.[25]

[23] *Ibid.*, p. 17.

[24] See J. Thomson, *An Account of the Life, Lectures and Writings of William Cullen*, 2 vols. (Edinburgh, 1832–59). Lettsom also attended the lectures given at the University by the anatomist Alexander Monro (secundus), (1733–1817), the botanist John Hope (1725–86), founder of the new Edinburgh Botanical Gardens in 1776 (friend of Linnaeus and Regius Professor of Botany and Medicine), and Francis Home (1719–1813), Professor of Materia Medica.

[25] W. Cullen, *First Lines of the Practice of Physic*, ed. J. C. Gregory (Edinburgh, 1829), pp. 55–6.

Cullen's view of contagion as a cause of fever is echoed in Lettsom's own book, *Reflections on the General Treatment and Cure of Fevers* (1775) where he says that

There is a matter constantly exhaling from the human body, whether in health, or under disease, which when diffused, or mixed with the air, seldom proves injurious to the individual from whom it proceeds, or to those who may be exposed to it in that diluted state; but the same effluvia, when accumulated in confined places, and for a considerable time retained about the body, acquires a virulence which often proves fatal to persons who receive the same, especially when these effluvia arise from people labouring under fevers, with symptoms of putrefaction. It is hence that the jail and hospital fevers are so alarming in their effects, which evidently prove what a degree of activity and virulence the effluvia from the human body and putrid animal matter may acquire, and the necessity of ventilation, change of clothes, and other circumstances conducive to cleanliness as preventatives.[26]

We do not yet know *why* this view of contagion was held in common by Cullen, Lettsom and Howard at this time but we can say with certainty that it influenced their perceptions of how and where to study and treat fevers. Lettsom's interest as a Quaker philanthropist to seek out and become familiar with the living conditions of the labouring poor in London – particularly institutions which reduced their independence and liberty through confinement – was complemented by his understanding of contagion as the cause of fevers. Lettsom may be placed within a larger group of physicians, philanthropists and reformers who shared the perception that contagion was made more virulent in closed or inadequately ventilated spaces, that it was preventable, and that jails, prisons, hospitals and other institutions of confinement did more harm than good. From what we know of Lettsom's efforts to extend the availability of medical care more widely to the labouring poor in London it makes sense that he would reject the hospital model as a means to this end. What he would need to do is to create a new kind of institution to fulfil his purposes and in 1770 he did just that: the General Dispensary was a solution to his particular problem.

Lettsom's belief that medicine cannot be improved by the practice of hospitals is seen in *Reflections on the General Treatment and Cure of Fevers* where he writes that

It might have been expected, that the hospitals established in this city, would have contributed more generally to extend the knowledge of medicine; but the public have been mistaken; and the cause will evidently appear from a candid review of their oeconomy and management. Many of the hospitals in London contain four hundred patients; half of which number are usually divided amongst three physicians, who visit them thrice a week, each time requiring about two hours' attendance: hence it appears, that one patient with another, two minutes at most are allotted to each, in order for the

[26] J. C. Lettsom, *Reflections on the General Treatment and Cure of Fevers* (London, 1775), p. 14.

> physicians to hear their complaints, to understand their different symptoms, and to prescribe proper remedies. Does any physician think, that two hours are sufficient to allow him to visit upwards of sixty patients conscientiously? Does any man of reflection expect, that the medical art will improve by the practice of the hospitals? Or is the great end of humanity answered in such receptacles of distress?[27]

For Lettsom, the answer to these questions was emphatically no. As a Quaker physician-philanthropist he put forward his case for the founding and support of dispensaries in four books: *Hints Designed to Promote the Establishment of a Dispensary for Extending Medical Relief to the Poor* (1770); *Reflections on the General Treatment and Cure of Fevers* (1772); *On the Improvement of Medicine in London on the Basis of the Public Good* (1773); and *Medical Memoirs of the General Dispensary in London, for Part of the Years 1773–1774* (1774). From these works we are able to see how the plan, organisation and aims of the General Dispensary addressed Lettsom's concern to bring about the improvement of medicine and the living conditions of the labouring poor while serving the interests of the philanthropists who supported it.

Typically for a Quaker at this time, in *Medical Memoirs* Lettsom makes it clear that there was a mutual obligation between the rich and the poor and that the

> poor are a large, as well as a useful part of the community; They supply the necessary and ornamental articles of life; and they have, therefore a just claim to the protection of the rich, whose interests must direct them to encourage the industrious in their employments, to frame laws for the maintenance of their rights, and to succor them in the misfortunes to which they are unavoidably incident.[28]

In other words, Lettsom would like to see the whole community and the relations between the rich and the poor guided by the ethics of the Society of Friends. As Lettsom points out to his readership, it is in the interest of the rich to encourage the *industrious* poor in their employment. Who were these rich people and industrious poor? We must remember that by 1770 the economic life of Britain was rapidly being transformed and that new classes of industrial employers (many of whom were Quakers) and skilled labourers were coming into being. The objects of charity at the General Dispensary were not the sick poor in general but a specific class of people upon whom the industrial capitalists depended for their wealth. Lettsom refers to these groups and the relationships between them. We read that there is a

> mutual obligation between the rich and poor, neither of whom could long subsist without the aid of the other . . . Artizans have always depended upon the affluent for

[27] *Ibid.*, preface. [28] Lettsom, *Medical Memoirs* (London, 1774), p. v.

employment. The success of the artizan being always necessary to the ease and convenience of the affluent.[29]

Presumably Lettsom felt that many rich people in London were failing to fulfil this obligation and that they should recognise the worth of artisans to themselves and the economy of the nation. Thus:

In a country where many people are enriched by commerce, and where all people are possessed of civil liberty, and the unrestrained exercise of their faculties, the ornamental and necessary arts must unavoidably flourish; but, whenever many persons are employed, labour must be cheap; the earnings therefore of the artizan will seldom exceed his expenses; and as many of these arts depend upon circumstances, changable in their nature, multitudes must thereby be liable to suffer temporary poverty.[30]

Thus the problem for the artisan is that 'whilst health continues, the resources which daily open to the industrious in a trading country, afford also a temporary subsistence to the families: but a long continuance of health, is the lot of few.'[31] Why is this so? Because

the poor, from the occasional want of employment and wholesome food, from exposure to all changes in the weather, and from various other causes, are often visited with sickness, as well as poverty; one, indeed, is consequent upon the other; and thereby they become the immediate objects of assistance; it is then peculiarly necessary that the hand of pity should be extended, to soften the pangs of a sick bed, and to restore health and ease to the poor in affliction.[32]

Lettsom establishes a link between poverty and illness and argues that one can lead to the other. Economic circumstances beyond the control of an artisan can leave him unemployed and thus unable to provide the necessary food and clothing to keep him and his family healthy and able to work to support themselves and the national economy. The health of sick artisans 'which is so necessary to their subsistence, will be sooner restored; famine and prison avoided; the nation enriched by industry, and a hardy race of useful members preserved to the community.'[33] And Lettsom argues that the design of the General Dispensary will fulfil these aims by administering

advice and medicines to the poor, not only at the Dispensary, but also in their own habitations; which later circumstance is an advantage peculiar to this plan. And notwithstanding the many excellent charities, already subscribing for relief of the sick, in and about this great metropolis, yet, when it is considered how many poor, from the nature of their circumstances and disorders, are still necessarily confined to their

[29] *Ibid.*, p. vi. [30] *Ibid.*, p. vi. [31] *Ibid.*, p. xii. [32] *Ibid.* p. iv.

[33] *Ibid.*, p. xii. The dispensary was very successful: in the first year of operation, Lettsom saw many sick poor people; he 'attended nearly seventeen hundred poor persons, into whose habitations I entered, and have been conversant with their sufferings, and their resignation under them', *Medical Memoirs*, p. x.

wretched dwellings, and perish through want of proper assistance, the utility of this institution becomes obvious.[34]

And the institution of the dispensary – not the hospital – could deal effectively with the immediate *cause* of illness as identified by Lettsom which was *poverty*.

Lettsom put forward the case that poverty caused illness, which in turn might lead to further impoverishment and eventual death. The loss of a skilled artisan through lack of assistance contributed immediately to the destitution of entire families and through this situation, an increase in immoral behaviour such as prostitution. When multiplied by thousands of skilled individuals and their families the larger effect, argued Lettsom, would be a diminution of the health of the economy of the nation. Only by providing assistance to the labouring poor through dispensaries could the dignity and independence of the artisan be maintained according to Quaker thinking, and for Lettsom founding and working in a dispensary was an example of 'living in the Light': by providing conditions suitable to fostering a healthy and independent class of labourers, the wealth of the nation would be increased.

In complete contrast to the situation found at the voluntary-subscription hospitals where the governors were repaid for their charity by the prayers and deference shown by the sick poor coming to them, the governors of the General Dispensary were rewarded in a practical and useful way:

A spontaneous gratitude will arise in the poor towards their benefactors, to repay by their industry those obligations which their unavoidable sickness had incurred; they not only meet their families with pleasure, but they are animated to follow their daily labour with redoubled chearfulness [*sic*].[35]

Through industriousness, perhaps the most highly valued Quaker quality, the artisan would be able to meet his part of what Lettsom saw

[34] *Ibid*., p. xix. A physician attended every day at 11 o'clock except Sunday to give advice to the recommended out-patients and to visit invalid patients in their homes (restricted to those living in the City). Out-patients who attended the dispensary were 'relieved without any restriction as to the place of residence', *Medical Memoirs*, p. xxiv. There was a restrictive admissions policy which favoured medical cases. Lettsom says that 'as there are *medical cases*, wherein *chirurgical assistance* is requisite, a surgeon attends on such occasions. However, *Chirurgical*, venereal, and lunatic cases are not admitted, being the peculiar objects of other charities', *Medical Memoirs*, p. xxiv. The first physician was Dr Nathaniel Hulme (1732–1807), formerly a naval surgeon who in 1774 had been appointed physician to Charterhouse in place of James Grieve (who had instructed Lettsom at St. Thomas's Hospital). Lettsom was appointed second physician to the dispensary in 1773 and Dr James Sims became the third serving physician in 1774. All three received an annual honorarium of £100. Mr George Vaux was the first surgeon to the dispensary and there was a resident apothecary.

[35] *Ibid*., p. xx.

as a social pact between the rich and poor: through dispensary-based philanthropy the mutual obligations of the poor labourer and the rich capitalist would work in harmony to contribute to the health of the economy and the wealth of the nation.

Between 1770 and 1800 there were thirteen dispensaries founded in London and no general hospitals. By looking at some surviving records of various London dispensaries and checking every entry in *Munk's Roll of the Royal College of Physicians* for this period we find that these institutions offered new careers to many Licentiates of the College of Physicians (LRCP), most of whom were Dissenters. I have not yet found any evidence that any Fellows of the College were involved in the establishment and running of the dispensaries in London, yet the dispensaries provided many Dissenting physicians with a means of improving medicine according to their own political interests. With the growing number of dispensaries scattered all across London and separated by great distances, many of these men felt the need for a forum where they could meet to share their experiences, read papers, discuss aspects of practice and generally act together to identify and further their common concerns and interests. For this purpose, Lettsom and others founded the Medical Society of London in 1773, yet another one of the many projects in his programme for social reform, and it was not a coincidence that most of its original members were Dissenters, Scottish-trained Licentiates and dispensary physicians. With a common experience of being excluded from the centre of power at the College of Physicians, the Medical Society offered them (through combination) an alternative venue for the advancement of their professional and political aspirations. The Medical Society was created for and by a new kind of physician, and, as we have seen, the hospital was *not* perceived by some of them as the obvious place for medical teaching, practice and research. By 1780 many London physicians had actually turned their backs on the hospitals and were engaged in an exciting and dynamic dispensary-based system for medical improvement.

On 28 February 1775 Lettsom gave the presidential address to the assembled members of the Medical Society and made it clear to them that he was going to use it as a forum for medical improvement and dispensary-medicine. Meeting together freely and on terms of equality was, argued Lettsom, a means in itself for physicians, surgeons and apothecaries to advance medicine by sharing information. He says that:

To me, I assure you, the happiness is not little, I experience from the ardor of our fellow members, in supporting the honor and welfare of our infant Society by every method which their relaxation from business will admit. Be assured, gentlemen, I shall always be ready to co-operate with you in every attempt to promote medical information. From my appointment in a public situation (Physician to the General Dispensary) I have an opportunity of observing the epidemics in this city, as well as many anomalous symptoms, which I shall at least once a month hope to lay before you. And as our members are gentlemen of extensive practice, may an unanimous zeal be exerted to promote those laudable views, for which the Society was instituted, and for which its members are so well qualified.[36]

Lettsom's dispensary-based research activities became well-known to practitioners in London through the weekly meetings of the Medical Society and via the publication of papers in *Memoirs of the Medical Society of London* which was first issued in 1787.[37] The divisions existing between the Fellows and Licentiates at the College of Physicians were not duplicated in the Medical Society and the sharing and cooperation of which Quakers were so fond constituted the basis of professional relationships in it. Moreover, it was only through the pursuit of *shared* interests and concerns that physicians, surgeons and apothecaries by finding common ground would be able to advance medicine. The role of societies in this quest for improvement was set out and clearly stated in the preface to the first volume of *Memoirs*:

Nothing has contributed more to the advancement of science, than the establishment of literary societies: these excite a generous ardour in liberal minds, and raise even envy into useful emulation.[38]

The corpus of knowledge comprising the 'science' of medicine has as its aim 'the preservation and restoration of health'. It is by the coming together as a society that contemporary problems are seen as being capable of being confronted and overcome and it is clear in Lettsom's mind that tradition and authority cannot be turned to for solutions: improvement is brought about by making personal observations and reporting them to colleagues. Thus

the principal part of our knowledge must be ever derived from comparing our own observations with those of others. In this view the utility of societies, which afford an

[36] Abraham remarks that Lettsom devoted most of his time to the Society and practically all the investigations he carried out, and the papers he wrote were presented before it. The first meeting of the Medical Society was on 19 May 1773 with 15 members which initially met at two public houses – the Queen's Arms, Newgate Street and the Sun Tavern. In August 1774 the Society acquired premises in Crane Court off Fleet Street where they met fortnightly. In 1788 Lettsom presented another building, no. 3 Bolt Court, to the Society as a permanent home under the care of a trust. T. Hunt (ed.), *The Medical Society of London 1773–1973* (London, 1972).

[37] The *Memoirs of the Medical Society of London* were published in six volumes between 1787 and 1805. [38] *Memoirs of the Medical Society of London* vol. 1 (1787), p. iii.

opportunity for the mutual communication of our thoughts, must be sufficiently apparent. Deceased authors cannot solve our difficulties, nor will the observations made in other ages and climates, hold always true in our own.[39]

Lettsom was aware that the members of the Medical Society were engaged on an exciting discovery of new knowledge with the aim of practical utility.

There are some circumstances peculiarly favourable to a rising society; each member thinking the honour of the association in some measure dependent upon himself, is stimulated to the highest exertion of his powers: unawed by the same, and fearless of being eclipsed by the lustre of his predecessors, no damp is cast upon the vigour of that genius, which alone can produce great discoveries.[40]

It is the image of a new society arising that strikes the reader most forcefully: that its members are actively rejecting what they consider to be outdated ways of thinking and moving towards a better future. While the dispensary as an institution brought physicians into contact with the sick poor on terms of greater equality (partners in the effort to defeat disease and unhealthy living conditions) the Medical Society redefined professional relationships in ways which saw cooperation as the first step towards improvement.

The aim of the Society was to build and support professional ties and friendships for mutual benefit and in the interest of the public good. We read that the

institution of this Society is to give practitioners in the healing art frequent opportunities of meeting together, and conferring with each other, concerning any difficult or uncommon cases which have occurred; or communicating any new discoveries in medicine which have been made, either at home or abroad.[41]

The Society actually created new opportunities for physicians, surgeons and apothecaries to work together and it fostered the ethic that research was an on-going and cooperative enterprise. New discoveries in 'science' and medicine were not to be used for private gain or kept

[39] *Ibid.*, pp. ii–iv. Quakers were eager to share their knowledge and experiences as Pettigrew (1817) shows: 'The Ministry among Friends (Quakers) is voluntary and gratuitous; nevertheless they exert themselves with great zeal, and frequently under great inconveniences. They travel from considerable distances to visit meetings, to inculcate their sentiments publically, as well as to convey private advice' (p. 6).

[40] *Ibid.*, pp. ii–iv. Lettsom was probably following on from the precedent set by Fothergill in London who had earlier established the Society of Physicians in 1752 (possibly based on the Royal Medical Society of Edinburgh of which Fothergill had been a member). The London society met on alternate Mondays at the Mitre Tavern in Fleet Street.

[41] *Ibid.*, pp. iv–v. Pettigrew (p. 3) says that 'the universality of his acquaintances, his extensive practice as a physician, his unbounded philanthropy, and his connexion with public institutions, for the promotion of Medical, Philosophical, Literary and Benevolent pursuits, introduced him to the knowledge of all classes of Society, and obtained for him universal esteem and admiration'.

secret, but to be brought forward for public debate and practical application. The Medical Society did not seek to keep the knowledge of its members to itself – it was not a cartel of men seeking to dominate and control an aspect of medical practice. What characterised them was their zeal and enthusiasm to spread their knowledge and experience as widely as possible.

The publication of *Memoirs* served this purpose and as its editors said,

> many useful facts are lost from the want of a proper opportunity of conveying them to the world; and though, when considered separately, they may not be of sufficient importance to claim the attention of the public, yet when a number of them are collected together, they may become highly deserving of notice: to such facts when properly authenticated, the Society will always be particularly attentive.[42]

And for Quakers 'living in the Light', the Medical Society was a practical expression of their concern to diffuse and disseminate practical knowledge to a wide audience. Their metaphorical description of this process was an apt one:

> In order to excite practitioners to bring those talents to light, which would otherwise lie buried, and useless to the community, the Society, on its first institution, proposed to hold forth honorary rewards to those who should improve the medical art.[43]

The talent, skills and knowledge inherent in each individual was to be brought *to light* and made useful in the service of the community. To spur members to this end, Lettsom gave a sum of money to the Society to support an annual gold medal of the value of ten guineas known as the Fothergillian Medal in honour of his patron and friend. A topic or question was posed to the Society each year and from these we are able to see that problems connected with the experiences of dispensary practitioners were uppermost in their minds.

The membership of the Society in its early years was comprised largely of dispensary practitioners and the topics dealt with by the annual Fothergillian Medal reflected their interests and concerns: the effect of air on the human body; how to prevent infection; contagion and how it is carried; diseases of great towns; and the various poisons that affect human beings in the community. Their theme was the diseases associated with life in the crowded and often dirty conditions of large towns such as London. This medal or award was seen by these men as an *honour* for bringing forth and sharing new knowledge of these problems with their professional colleagues and, through the

[42] *Ibid.*, pp. v–vi. [43] *Ibid.*, p. vi.

Memoirs, with the public. It was not payment for competitive and selfishly guarded information used for private benefit, but:

In order farther to promote the improvement of the healing art, in all its branches so intimately interwoven with the interest of the community, the Society continue to offer Medals, annually, as excitements to genius and abilities, that mankind in general may receive advantage from their exertions, and useful knowledge be diffused from the fountains of reason and experience.[44]

It was by exciting genius and ability, promoting medical improvement, diffusing new knowledge, and extending medical treatment to the sick poor that mankind in general and the interests of the community were served. The founding and support of dispensaries, the establishment of a Society which bridged the gaps between the 'branches' of the art, and the publication of papers based on personal observation and experience of contemporary conditions in the towns, was itself evidence of improvement.

The Medical Society not only allowed these physicians, surgeons and apothecaries to pursue 'medical improvement' but it also enabled them to be *seen* to be doing so. Evidently the first two volumes of *Memoirs* were so popular and well received by correspondents outside London that the editors had to apologise in the third volume for being unable to publish all worthy contributions. That the Society had attracted public attention is seen in the preface to volume three where we read that:

We should think ourselves defective in gratitude to the Public, if the favourable reception of our former Memoirs had not stimulated us to a farther exercise of attention, in order to render the present volume equally deserving of general approbation. We are truly sensible of the importance of various communications already received, and the utility of their early production, but we must necessarily lament that many of them are obliged, for want of room, to be postponed until our next publication, the manuscripts for the forming of which will be immediately committed to the press, and the volume completed with as much expedition as the nature of the work will admit of. This we have considered ourselves under an obligation to make known to our Correspondents, that they might not have the least reason to suppose us capable of disrespect, or of being inattentive to the importance of the medical information on several subjects with which they have favoured the Society. For the experience of every day not only evinces how beneficial to our fellow-creatures are the discoveries made in the Medical Art, but how that benefit is often enhanced by expeditious promulgation.[45]

[44] *Memoirs*, vol. 3 (1802), pp. vii–viii. Some of the annual questions for the Fothergillian Medal were as follows: (1788) 'How is the human body in health and in a diseased state, affected by different kinds of air?'; (1789) 'What circumstances accelerate, retard, or prevent the progress of INFECTION?'; (1791) 'What are the principal diseases of great Towns, and what are the best methods of preventing or curing the same?'; (1793) 'What are the effects of MINERAL POISONS upon living Animals, and more particularly upon MANKIND, when taken internally, or applied externally; and what are the most efficacious means of countering these effects?'; (1794) Vegetable poisons; (1795) Animal poisons; (1796) Aerial poisons.

[45] *Ibid.*, pp. ii–iv.

This apology to the correspondents shows a forthrightness and sincerity of intent which was part of the Quaker ethic. Lettsom and the other editors see an obligation between themselves and the contributors to their journal and, as in every other aspect of the relations between the members of the Medical Society, the editors of *Memoirs* believe that medical improvement will come about through a partnership of various practitioners based on honesty, mutual respect and a harmony of interests. Impediments to the free exchange and communication of information are never allowed to create conditions of division within the Society and through the 'expedious promulgation' of knowledge between medical practitioners in London and the provinces a community of like-minded professionals was sustained. Through the *Memoirs* the Medical Society had become a national forum for dispensary medicine which linked together practitioners from growing towns all over the country and by 1780 the Medical Society had ceased to be a parochial and small-scale London-based meeting-place and had been transformed into an active and dynamic focus of public interest throughout the kingdom.

The members of the society were aware that their activities were without precedent in the country and 'although *nothing similar has been hitherto attempted in this Kingdom*, yet, they hope that the example may appear not altogether unworthy of imitation'[46] Moreover the editors of *Memoirs* highlighted their concern that the relative distinctions of status between physicians, surgeons and apothecaries be abandoned in the interests of equality. Thus 'the members of this Society have extended its foundation as much as possible: wishing to rise superior to all low distinctions, they have endeavoured to render every person useful in that branch of the science to which he properly belongs.'[47] The message is clear to all and sundry: 'The Society consists of Physicians, Surgeons, and Apothecaries, divided into Fellows, Corresponding Members, and Candidates.[48] This invitation to all qualified practitioners of the three branches of medicine underlines the belief of the members of the Society that the breaking down of professional divisions was itself a form of medical improvement and fostered the awareness that many physicians, surgeons and apothe-

[46] *Memoirs*, vol. 1 (1787), pp. vii–viii. [47] *Ibid.*, p. ix.

[48] *Ibid.*, p. ix. In stark contrast to the College of Physicians where Licentiates and Fellows were segregated, the Medical Society sought 'to give the practitioners in the healing art, frequent opportunities of meeting together, and conferring with each other, concerning any difficult or uncommon cases which may have occurred; or communicating any new discoveries in medicine which have been made, either at home or abroad', *Memoirs*, vol. 1, pp. iv–v.

caries had a common experience of being excluded from direct representation at the College of Physicians, Company of Surgeons and Apothecaries' Hall. Power at the College of Physicians was vested entirely in the hands of a small group of Oxford- and Cambridge-educated Fellows, and at Surgeons' Hall, the twenty-one man Court of Assistants was comprised wholly of London hospital surgeons with life tenure and who were self-electing. The disenchantment felt by many members of these two corporate bodies was great and growing in the late eighteenth century. The exclusion of these men from power and influence in these corporations was the result of their position as Dissenters and the educational experiences which followed thereon.

The dissolution of professional divisions in the Medical Society gave formal expression to what many general practitioners already knew from their daily work: there was no rigid separation of medicine from surgery. Dispensary physicians and surgeons were particularly sensitive to this reality. While in London it may have been possible for some physicians and surgeons among the elite practitioners at the hospitals and in private practice to restrict themselves solely to physic and pure surgery, among general practitioners (especially in the provinces) this was often impossible and economically disadvantageous. For many men calling themselves 'physicians' in the late eighteenth century (and Lettsom is one example), their training as apprentices to surgeon-apothecaries or man-midwives blurred the distinction of one branch of the profession from another. Many surgeons prescribed and administered medicines to their patients, and physicians often performed minor surgery. We must admit that historians are not yet able to specify with precision the activities of men calling themselves physicians, surgeons and apothecaries in this period. This approach is probably fruitless in any case because there were so many different routes to a successful medical and surgical career in the eighteenth century, and there was little if any control over or policing of practice by the London medical corporations. However we can see how the Medical Society gave a voice and legitimacy to the belief that the hierarchical division of the profession served private interests (especially those of the elite London practitioners) and that only by ceasing to maintain such barriers could the public interest be served. The foundation of the Medical Society may be seen as a constructive and positive step by these men to create new situations and circumstances to suit themselves. Rather than seeking conflict and confrontation with the powerful but numerically small groups of elite physicians and surgeons in London, the members of the Medical Society simply sidestepped them and through peaceful cooperation implemented their programme for the reform of medicine.[49]

From what we know about the lives of some of the leading members of the Medical Society we are able to see why it was attractive to them and how it reflected their interests as dispensary-based practitioners and Dissenters. Although the Society had members drawn from all three branches of the profession, leadership was clearly provided by the physicians. By looking at who were the Presidents of the Medical Society between 1773 and 1825 a distinct pattern may be seen: they were *all* Licentiate physicians, most of whom had dispensary affiliations in London.[50] One of these men, Dr James Sims (1741–1820) held the office of President continuously for twenty-two years from 1786 to 1808 and he served at least four dispensaries as a physician: the General, Surrey, Middlesex and Dispensary for General Inoculation. He was a major supporter of the Royal Humane Society and a vice-president of the Philanthropic Society. From Sims's published work we are able to see that his interests were similar in many respects to Lettsom's and other philanthropist-physicians: *Observations on Epi-*

[49] The roots of the Medical Society probably lie in the earlier struggle for the reform of the College of Physicians in the 1760s which exploded in the 'Siege of Warwick Lane' in 1767 and culminated in Fothergill's failure to establish the rights of the Licentiates in the courts in 1770 to become eligible for the Fellowship. They were excluded by the indirect application of religious tests through the reservation of the Fellowship to Oxbridge graduates. By this time, the number of Licentiates had greatly outstripped the Fellows. The date of Fothergill's suspension of legal action against the College in 1770 and Lettsom's efforts to set up the General Dispensary in Aldersgate Street (a five-minute walk from Warwick Lane) less than a year later is no coincidence. Lettsom had earlier proposed to help frustrated licentiates by organizing a 'Scheme for Instituting a Society of Physicians in London, Instituted for the Improvement of Medical Knowledge and also for building a New College of Physicians'. Nothing came of this. See: L. G. Stevenson, 'The Siege of Warwick Lane, Together with a Brief History of the Society of Collegiate Physicians 1767–98', *Journal of the History of Medicine* 7 (1952), pp. 105–21; I. Waddington, 'The Struggle to Reform the Royal College of Physicians 1767–1771: A Sociological Analysis', *Medical History* 17 (1973), pp. 107–26. Nearly all the founding members of the Medical Society were Scottish-trained Licentiates, many of whom were (or would become) involved with London dispensaries. They were: John Coakley Lettsom; John Millar; John Hayes; James Sims; Thomas Bradley; James Wake; Edward Bancroft; Joseph Hart-Myers; William Woodville; Nathaniel Hulme; Sayer Walker; Robert Hooper; Edward Ford; John Haighton; Robert Thornton; John Shadwell; John Aiken; William Blair; William Babington; Charles Combe; John Relph and William Saunders. None of these men were Fellows of the College of Physicians and most were Dissenters of various descriptions.

[50] The Presidents of the Medical Society for 1773–1825 were: John Millar (1773); John Coakley Lettsom (1775); Nathaniel Hulme (1776); George Edwards (1779); Samuel Foart Simmons (1780); John Sims (1783); John Whitehead (1784); John Relph (1785); James Sims (1786–1808); Lettsom (1809); George Pinckard (1811); Lettsom (1813); Joseph Adams (1815); Thomas Walshman (1817); Henry Clutterbuck (1819); David Unwins (1821); William Shearman (1823); Clutterbuck (1825). I have looked at every entry in *Munk's Roll* and found that of the Physicians shown to have dispensary affiliations, *all* were Licentiates, mostly Scottish educated. No Oxbridge-educated Fellows held such appointments.

demic Disorders, With Remarks on Nervous and Malignant Fevers (1773); *A Discourse on the Best Methods of Prosecuting Medical Enquiries* (1774) – derived from the first oration given to the Medical Society by him in 1773; *Observations on the Scarlatina Anginosa, Commonly called the Ulcerated Sore Throat* (1776); and he completed and edited Edward Foster's *Principles and Practice of Midwifery* (1781). He contributed papers on the subject of fever to the Medical Society and actively supported it by giving his valuable library to the society in 1802.

The office of President was held between 1780 and 1783 by Samuel Foart Simmons,[51] author of the famous *Medical Register*, which first appeared in 1779, and which according to Bynum 'is a reminder both of eighteenth-century enterprise and of the visibility of medical men exactly seventy-five years before the Medical Act made the annual publication of a medical register a legal matter.'[52] But the *Medical Register* is less *evidence* of visibility, but rather a *cause* of greater visibility to the public of physicians, surgeons and apothecaries. This book is yet another example of the efforts of many Dissenting Licentiate physicians in this period to promulgate information to a wider audience about the medical profession, charities and the conditions of great towns. Through the *Medical Register* many medical charities and other philanthropic enterprises in London and the provinces became better known to people throughout the country, at a time when Britain was fast becoming a national economy through improved communication and trading links. This book was a further step towards the improvement of medicine and highlights the self-consciousness of many philanthropist-physicians outside London at this time.

The most characteristic feature of the Medical Society was that it was conceived as a venue for self-improvement, providing many medical men from a wide variety of educational backgrounds and professional experience with an opportunity to come together for the purpose of exchanging information, comparing observations, presenting research findings and building and cementing ties of friendship among professional colleagues. Through the *Memoirs* these men

[51] Samuel Foart Simmons (1750–1813) studied medicine at Edinburgh University and Leyden where he qualified (MD. 1776); he was an active member of numerous learned societies including the Royal Society (FRS 1779), Society of Antiquaries, Royal Society of Medicine at Paris, Medical Society of Edinburgh, and the Philosophical Society of Manchester.

[52] W. F. Bynum, 'Physicians, Hospitals and Career Structures in Eighteenth-Century London' in W. F. Bynum and Roy Porter (eds.), *William Hunter and the Eighteenth-Century Medical World* (Cambridge, 1985), p. 105.

created a new voice for the advocacy of their interests in medical philanthropy and improvement to a wider readership: it was in part a platform for dispensary medicine because they believed that this institution – and not hospitals – provided the solution to the problem of disease in the community, and particularly in the great towns. The writings of these men were not polemical attacks on hospital medicine and everything it represented, but rather an attempt to put forward their case in positive and alternative terms. In this sense, their approach to medical and social reform contained the best qualities of the Quaker ethic which so inspired Fothergill, Lettsom, Howard and other philanthropists. The Medical Society was not wholly dominated by Quakers, but many of its most active members were Quakers, and their influence within the larger community of philanthropist-physicians in London was great. The Medical Society served the interests of the Licentiate physicians and other practitioners with grievances against the professional medical corporations in London and it did so within the context of medical improvement of a particular kind: dispensary-based medicine in the service of the public. It was at the very worst a conspiracy of humane men, and at its best an attempt to circumvent the monopoly of practice enjoyed by the medical corporations in London, but one which in the long run was doomed to failure.

11

Measuring virtue
eudiometry, enlightenment and pneumatic medicine

SIMON SCHAFFER

To man the contemplation of the skies is permitted, but the practice of virtue is commanded . . . About ten years ago, my daily observations of the changes of the sky led me to consider whether, if I had the power of the seasons, I could confer greater plenty upon the inhabitants of the earth. This contemplation fastened on my mind, and I sat days and nights in imaginary dominion, pouring upon this country and that the showers of fertility, and seconding every fall of rain with a due proportion of sunshine. I had yet only the will to do good, and did not imagine that I should ever have the power.

Samuel Johnson, *The History of Rasselas*, 1759, chapter 42

PNEUMATICS AS AN ENLIGHTENMENT SCIENCE

A Swiftian pneumatic experiment at the Milan public baths – in February 1780 Pietro Verri, *philosophe*, journalist and editor of the organ of the Lombard Enlightenment, *Il Caffè*, wrote to his brother in Rome:

Last summer our two physico-chemists, Moscati and Landriani, were at the baths. It came into their heads to collect some flatus which rose through the water in a fine great bubble. They analyzed it; they found that it was inflammable; they cried: Discovery! Discovery! Now everyone knows that such an air comes from places where there is fermentation. It was considered whether an economical lamp could be made with such a substance. And why not consider lighting a city at night?[1]

[1] Pietro Verri to Alessandro Verri 26 February 1780, in Peter K. Knoefel, *Felice Fontana: Life and Works* (Trento, 1984), p. 142. Compare Squire Bramble's 'swoon' at the spa at Bath, envisaged by the physician and novelist Tobias Smollett in *Humphry Clinker* (1771): 'It was indeed a *compound of villainous smells* in which the most violent stinks, and the most powerful perfumes, contended for the mastery. Imagine to yourself a high exalted essence of mingled odours, arising from putrid gums, imposthumated lungs, sour flatulencies, rank armpits, sweating feet, running sores and issues, plasters, ointments and embrocations, hungary-water, spirit of lavender, assa foetida drops, musk, hartshorn, and sal volatile; besides a thousand frowsy steams which I could not analyse. Such is the fragrant aether we breath in the polite assemblies at Bath – such is the atmosphere I have exchanged for the pure, elastic, animating air of the Welsh mountains.' For spas and baths as sites of medical debate and culture see C. F. Mullett, 'Public Baths and Health in England', *Supplements to the Bulletin of the History of Medicine* 5 (1946), pp. 1–85, and, specifically, G. S. Rousseau, 'Matt Bramble and the Sulphur Controversy', *Journal of the History of Ideas* 28 (1967), pp. 577–89.

Throughout the late Enlightenment, and particularly in Habsburg Italy, the workings of the aerial economy repeatedly drew public attention. During the 1770s, following Italian translations of the pneumatic experiments of Joseph Priestley, a new technology developed to measure the 'virtue' (*bontà*) of airs and thus to provide a quantitative basis for the management of the medical environment. The technology was commonly known as 'eudiometry', a coinage of 1775 due to the Milan physics professor Marsilio Landriani.[2] Landriani transformed a test reported by Priestley into an instrument which would be accurate, portable and, he claimed, revolutionary. In this chapter I shall document the emergence and fate of this technology, and place it in the context of medical and managerial ambitions of physicians and natural philosophers of the late Enlightenment. In particular, I seek to connect varying interpretations of eudiometry's therapeutic meaning with changing schemes of political reform, including Priestley's rational Dissent, Italian *illuminismo* and Benthamite constitutionalism.

Priestley's work on airs began soon after his move from Warrington Academy to become minister of Mill Hill Chapel at Leeds in 1767. This followed a series of alliances forged between Priestley, physicians and reformers. In 1764, Priestley gained an LLD from Edinburgh University on the recommendation of the Manchester physician Thomas Percival. In 1766, on the nomination of the leading reformist physician Sir John Pringle, Priestley was elected to the Royal Society. In 1772, following demonstrations of his experiments on the impregnation of water with fixed air at the College of Physicians, Priestley composed a lengthy paper on pneumatic chemistry which won him the Royal Society's Copley Medal the following year. Priestley's publications in chemistry, natural philosophy and political theology soon drew warm attention from readers such as Jeremy Bentham, then a young Oxford lawyer, for whom the Dissenting philosopher's works struck with the force of a revelation. In 1773, Priestley moved from Leeds to the south, where he worked at Bowood and London as librarian for the leading Whig reformer Lord Shelburne.[3]

These connections gave pneumatic chemistry its reformist meaning. It provided a knowledge which reformers could use; a description of their social function; and an account of the strategies by which reform could be achieved. This knowledge included the understanding of matter and its powers developed in the laboratories. Such understand-

[2] R. Watermann, 'Eudiometrie', *Technikgeschichte* 35 (1968), pp. 292–319.

[3] Maurice Crosland, 'A Practical Perspective on Joseph Priestley as a Natural Philosopher', *British Journal for the History of Science* 16 (1983), pp. 223–38; Simon Schaffer, 'Priestley's Questions', *History of Science* 22 (1984), pp. 151–83.

ing involved a new practice of policy recommendations for the better management of the social economy and the human body. The atmosphere was taken to be a major site at which principles of health and disease were produced. Under Priestley's aegis, this practice was also used to revise the picture of body. The distinction between mind and body was erased by changing the definition of the attributes of matter. Since the mind now became just as accessible to material analysis, it also became just as accessible to management. So medical managers, using their knowledge of medical meteorology, could also be moral managers, using their knowledge of the powers of the mind. When medical management turned its attention to the discipline of minds, it produced a new story about the way interests and passions should be governed for the cause of social welfare. A revised account of pneumatology was therefore a necessary companion of the science of pneumatics.[4]

This science became an important component of late Enlightenment philosophy. The link between Priestley and jurists such as Bentham or physicians such as Pringle shows how this worked. Bentham and Priestley both became Shelburne's clients, and Bentham's writings of the 1770s and 1780s are eloquent testimony to his close encounter with Priestley's rational Dissent. Priestley's pneumatics and Bentham's panopticism were both versions of this model of mind and body. Bentham's Panopticon, a visionary scheme for the design and administration of factories, prisons and schools, first projected in the 1780s, was an exercise in the economy of powers, 'a marvellous machine' where the effects of power could be deployed in the setting of a laboratory: 'it could be used as a machine to carry out experiments on men'. Bentham explicitly considered the claim that the Panopticon made 'machines under the similitude of men'. It became an experimental machine for experiments upon machines. 'O chemists!', Bentham exclaimed, 'much have your crucibles shown us of dead matter – but our industry-house is a crucible for men!' If the Panopticon was an exercise in political anatomy and the mechanics of power, then Priestley's technology of airs provided a similar repertoire of strategies for the investigation of powers under a regime of observation, classification and experiment. His pneumatics investigated those powers on which life depended, and modelled an economy in which these powers were distributed.[5]

The preface to Bentham's celebrated *Fragment on Government*

[4] C. J. Lawrence, 'Priestley in Tahiti' in C. J. Lawrence and R. Anderson (eds.), *Science, Medicine and Dissent: Joseph Priestley* (London, 1987), pp. 1–10.

[5] Michel Foucault, *Discipline and Punish* (London, 1977), pp. 202–3; John Bowring (ed.), *The Works of Jeremy Bentham*, 11 vols. (Edinburgh, 1838–48), vol. 4, pp. 63–4.

(1776) provides evidence of his use of Priestley's pneumatics as the mark of progress. In 1767, in his *History of Electricity*, Priestley argued that the history of natural philosophy was the best way of capturing human interests, through the processes of association, for the cause of progress: no history 'can exhibit instances of so fine a rise and improvement in things, as we see in the progress of the human mind in philosophical investigations.'[6] David Hartley's associationist principles worked to good effect here: in Priestley's histories of electricity, optics and pneumatics, the sympathetic reader could recapitulate the course of actual experimental advance. This was a way of showing what was wrong with established authorities – in Bentham's case, with the conservative legal theorist William Blackstone. Bentham identified the Oxford lawyer as an enemy of progress because he stood opposed to the true principles learnt from the history of natural philosophy. 'Correspondent to *discovery* and *improvement* in the natural world, is *reformation* in the moral'. Blackstone resisted such a reformation. Yet the successes of the pneumatic chemists could and should be extended to the moral realm:

> If it be of importance and of use to us to know the principles of the element we breathe, surely it is not of much less importance nor of much less use to comprehend the principles, and endeavour at the improvement of those *laws*, by which alone we breathe it in security.[7]

The axiom of utility, the analogy between natural improvement and moral reformation, and the aim of the 'security' of respiration, were all aspects of the meteorological programme which both Bentham and Priestley pursued. In the 1770s Priestley and his colleagues aimed to show how a benevolent aerial economy functioned and to mark the processes which governed this economy. Human beings were an integral part of this system, and their welfare was a consequence of its actions.[8]

Natural philosophical understanding of the atmospheric powers was to become linked with civil policy. John Pringle was a typical practitioner in this field. His treatises in the 1750s on hospital and gaol fevers based themselves on the pneumatics of restored and corrupted

[6] Priestley, *History and Present State of Electricity*, 3rd edn (London, 1775), vol. 1. pp. ii–iv; J. G. McEvoy, 'Electricity, Knowledge and the Nature of Progress in Priestley's Thought', *British Journal for the History of Science* 12 (1979), pp. 1–30.

[7] Priestley, *Hartley's Theory of the Human Mind* (London, 1775), pp. xi–xx; Bentham, *Fragment on Government*, ed. F. C. Montague (Oxford, 1931), pp. 93–4. Compare Priestley, *Remarks on Some Paragraphs in the Fourth Volume of Dr Blackstone's Commentary on the Laws of England* (London, 1769).

[8] Simon Schaffer, 'Priestley and the Politics of Spirit' in Lawrence and Anderson, *Science, Medicine and Dissent*, pp. 39–54.

airs. As Christopher Lawrence has suggested, Pringle and his reformist colleagues, including Priestley, were instrumental in the construction of a specifically aerial analysis of slow epidemic fevers, locating their aetiology in noxious components of the atmosphere detectable by pneumatic chemistry.[9] Priestley defended Pringle's doctrine against Scottish critics in 1773, while successive volumes of *Experiments and Observations on Air* during the 1770s carried testimonies by physicians on the medicinal uses of airs and the aerial causation of fever. When Pringle presented Priestley with the Royal Society's Copley Medal in 1773, he placed Priestley's pneumatics in the context of the aerial system of fevers, and also linked it with the model of a benevolent economy which Priestley had begun to map: 'from these discoveries, we are assured that . . . every individual plant is serviceable to mankind, if not always distinguished by some private virtue, yet making a part of the whole which cleanses and purifies our atmosphere'. Storms and tempests would shake 'the waters and the air together to bury in the deep those putrid and pestilential effluvia which the vegetables upon the face of the Earth have been insufficient to consume.'[10] The pneumatic system proposed by Priestley and Pringle gave an account of the circulation of virtuous power in the world. It was deeply influential on the work of radicals in the 1790s, including Edinburgh-trained physicians such as Erasmus Darwin and Thomas Beddoes. Beddoes said that through pneumatic medicine 'Man may sometime come to rule over the causes of pain and pleasure with . . . absolute dominion.' The enterprise provided an image of the perfectly managed economy in human society, where medical administration and civil hygiene, the 'burial of pestilential effluvia,' were equally important.[11]

THE NITROUS AIR TEST AND PHLOGISTIC CHEMISTRY

Priestley's isolation of nitrous air in 1772 and dephlogisticated air in 1775 was part of this strategy of diagnosis and cure. He described a

[9] Lawrence, 'Priestley in Tahiti', pp. 5–6; D. W. Singer, 'Sir John Pringle and his Circle', *Annals of Science* 6 (1948–50), pp. 127–80 and 229–61.

[10] Douglas McKie, 'Joseph Priestley and the Copley Medal', *Ambix* 9 (1961), pp. 1–22; Priestley, 'On the Noxious Quality of the Effluvia of Putrid Marshes', *Philosophical Transactions* 64 (1774), pp. 90–5, pp. 90–1; Jan Ingenhousz, *Experiments upon Vegetables* (London, 1779), preface; Thomas Percival, 'Observations on the Medicinal Uses of Fixed Air', *Experiments and Observations on Different Kinds of Air*, 2nd edn (London, 1775), vol. 1, 288–324.

[11] Albert Goodwin, *The Friends of Liberty* (London, 1979), chapter 3; Dorothy Stansfield, *Thomas Beddoes: Chemist, Physician, Democrat* (Dordrecht, 1984), chapter 7; Maureen McNeil, *Under the Banner of Science: Erasmus Darwin and his Age* (Manchester, 1987), chapter 6. See Beddoes, *Notice of Some Observations Made at the Medical Pneumatic Institution* (Bristol, 1799), pp. 26–7.

series of processes which vitiated common air by phlogisticating it. Such processes included 'the amazing consumption of air by fires of all kinds, volcanoes, &c,' together with respiration and putrefaction. Respiration and putrefaction as medical terms were given meaning through phlogistic pneumatics. The air left above calces or remaining after animal respiration was revealed to be highly phlogisticated by a test comparison with nitrous air.

> It is not peculiar to nitrous air to be a test of the fitness of the air for respiration. Any other process by which air is diminished and made noxious answers to the same purpose but the application of them is not so easy or elegant and the effect is not so soon perceived. In fact, it is *phlogiston* that is the test.

Bad air supported neither respiration nor combustion, and did not diminish in volume when shaken with nitrous air. This gave the test its key place in his pneumatics.[12]

This was recognised by Pringle in his Copley Medal speech, and by Priestley himself in his paper at the Royal Society. Priestley and Pringle carefully traced the genealogy of 'nitrous air' to the well-established heroic achievements of two generations of British pneumatic chemists. The tradition involved a technology and a doctrine. The technology centred on the pneumatic trough. In his *Vegetable Staticks* (1727), Stephen Hales reported trials which extracted 'air' from various substances, vegetable, animal and mineral. He used the 'force of fire', as when he mixed Walton pyrites (our iron sulphide) with spirit of nitre (nitric acid). Hales's pedestal apparatus allowed him to collect the air emitted over water and so estimate its volume. For Hales, there was but one air, and it had one decisive property, elasticity. The water level measured its spring. But when he found that the water levels would change with time, he attributed this to loss of spring and so felt it necessary to wash the emitted air before collection, and thus developed a pneumatic trough.[13]

Only during the mid century, in Joseph Black's work in Edinburgh and that of spa physicians such as William Brownrigg, did the trough come to be seen as a means for collecting *different* kinds of air, in particular those forms which were 'fixed' in matter and useful for therapy, for analysis of mineral and spa waters and for the combat against sepsis. In this version it was a key tool in Priestley's pneumat-

[12] Priestley, 'Observations on Different Kinds of Air', *Philosophical Transactions* 62 (1772), pp. 147–264, p. 162; *Experiments and Observations*, second edition (London, 1775), vol. 1, pp. xx and 111; *Experiments and Observations on Different Kinds of Air and Other Branches of Natural Philosophy*, 3 vols. (Birmingham, 1790), vol. 1, p. 359.

[13] Stephen Hales, *Vegetable Staticks* (London, 1727), pp. 183–84.

ics.[14] Priestley's earliest pneumatic experiments used the trough to collect airs and test their electrical conductivity and spring.[15] In spring 1772 Priestley went to London to meet Henry Cavendish, who had isolated 'inflammable air' (our hydrogen gas) six years earlier. They discussed Hales's experiments, including that of the production of nitrous air from pyrites and nitric acid. Hales found the reaction generated a great volume of red fumes and then condensed to something less than its original volume. Cavendish made the crucial suggestion that the air was a specific substance fixed in the spirit of nitre alone, and that any kind of pyrites would serve to release it. In June Priestley used his trough to collect colourless samples of nitrous air, and swiftly determined that this air would absorb and diminish the volume of common air when mixed with it.

This was the basis of the nitrous air test. In its primitive form Priestley mixed one volume of nitrous air with two volumes of common air. At the end of effervescence the two volumes would diminish by about one-ninth; after two days standing over water, about 1.8 volumes of gas would remain. This became the standard of goodness, for Priestley soon found that 'this effervescence or diminution . . . is at least very nearly, if not exactly, in proportion to its fitness for the purpose' of respiration, and that 'the degree of diminution being from nothing at all to more than one fourth of the whole of any quantity of air, we are, by this means, in possession of a prodigiously large *scale*, by which we may distinguish very small degrees of difference in the goodness of air'. The test was troubled in at least two respects. First, Priestley immediately interpreted respirability as goodness. A scale of absorption by nitrous air became a scale of *virtue*. Second, the residual volume was hard to fix. It diminished if left standing, and varied whether over water or mercury. Priestley worked hard to make the test secure, and successfully sought aid from Cavendish to get the final volume stabilised.[16]

When Priestley published his results in autumn 1772, he emphasised that a measure of virtue was now available and it gave good, fixed values. Traditional techniques, such as the use of mice, could be

14 William Brownrigg, 'An Experimental Enquiry into the Mineral Elastic Spirit of Air Contained in Spa Water', *Philosophical Transactions* 55 (1765), pp. 218–48; John Parascandola and Aaron Ihde, 'History of the Pneumatic Trough', *Isis* 60 (1969), pp. 351–60; N. Coley, 'Physicians and the Chemical Analysis of Mineral Waters in Eighteenth Century England', *Medical History* 26 (1982), pp. 123–44.

15 Priestley, *History of Electricity* (London, 1767), p. 598.

16 Priestley, *Experiments and Observations* (Birmingham, 1790), vol. 1, pp. 354–64; Aaron Ihde, 'Priestley and Lavoisier' in Lester Kieft and Bennett Willeford (eds.) *Joseph Priestley* (Lewisburg and London, 1980), pp. 62–91, pp. 66–8.

avoided; above all, pneumatic chemistry now became a potentially quantitative technology which could assess the goodness of the aerial environment. 'Virtue' gained its meaning in a cosmology which Priestley derived from received assumptions of civic humanism. It was a moral quality contrasted to 'corruption'. Its social and pneumatic meanings were closely associated.[17] Priestley argued that the aerial economy must act to preserve the virtue of airs. There must be processes which restored vitiated air and rendered it virtuous and respirable. 'It becomes a great object of philosophical inquiry, to ascertain what change is made in the constitution of the air by flame, and to discover what provision there is in nature for remedying the injury which the atmosphere receives by this means.' Evidence of restorative processes was produced in the long series of pneumatic trials Priestley made at Bowood between 1774 and 1779 using the 'noble apparatus' Shelburne provided him. These processes included atmospheric purification by shaking over water and the beneficient action of green vegetable matter on air under the influence of light. His isolation of dephlogisticated air and his production of evidence for the restoration of air by vegetable life were easily fitted into the scheme of a well-judged economy which balanced vitiation with restoration.[18]

These researches were closely linked with human welfare through the scheme of medical meteorology – restoration of respirable air and its variation in quality governed the physiological fate of the human and the social frame. The standard of the atmosphere was a mark of its fitness for human existence. Respirability elided into dephlogistication, dephlogistication into health, health into virtue.[19] This was how John Pringle immediately interpreted the reports of 1772:

> A phial of air having been sent [Priestley] from the neighbourhood of a large town, it appeared upon a comparative trial to be inferior in quality to that taken up near Leeds, where he then resided. It was upon such a prospect of obtaining a criterion for distinguishing good air from bad, that Lord BACON almost in a rapture breaks out:

[17] J. G. A. Pocock, 'Virtue and Commerce in the Eighteenth Century', *Journal of Interdisciplinary History* 3 (1972), pp. 119–34; J. G. McEvoy and J. E. McGuire, 'God and Nature: Priestley's Way of Rational Dissent', *Historical Studies in Physical Science* 6 (1975), pp. 325–404; H. Laboucheix, 'Chemistry, Materialism and Theology in the Work of Joseph Priestley', *Price–Priestley Newsletter* 1 (1977), pp. 31–48.

[18] Priestley, 'Observations on Different Kinds of Air', p. 162; compare Priestley, *Experiments and Observations on Different Kinds of Air*, first edition (London, 1774), vol. 1, p. 53. See J. G. McEvoy, 'Joseph Priestley, Aerial Philosopher: Metaphysics and Methodology in Priestley's Chemical Thought, 1772–1781', *Ambix* 25 (1978), pp. 1–55, 93–116, 153–75 and 26 (1979), pp. 16–38 on pp. 96–101, 158–64.

[19] For vitiation, corruption and fixed air see Priestley, *Experiments and Observations*, second edition (London, 1776), vol. 2, pp. 115–19; for vitiation, corruption and nervous electricity see Priestley, *Experiments and Observations*, second edition (London, 1775), vol. 1, pp. 274–9.

[20] McKie, 'Copley Medal', p. 9.

'These are noble experiments that can make this discovery; for they serve for a natural divination of seasons!' and again, 'they teach men to choose their dwelling for their better health.'[20]

The morality of this scale of virtue initially suggested to Priestley that while atmospheric air was no doubt a compound of variously virtuous sections, nevertheless it must now be the best possible air for human respiration. 'I had no idea of procuring air purer than the best common air.' Yet his work of 1774–5 did yield such an air, dephlogisticated air. It was only after eighteen months that Priestley managed to position his new 'luxury' air as the ultimate in his scale of virtue and, consequently, the perfect commodity. Between summer 1774 and spring 1775, before and after his decisive journey to Paris in the autumn, Priestley was working on an air extracted from heating mercury *calcinatus per se*. A series of tests, particularly the nitrous air test, finally convinced Priestley that he had found his new virtuous air diminished more than any other in the test. His war against French chemists was therefore launched as a consequence of the technology which adequately embodied his phlogistic cosmology.[21]

The response of Lavoisier to the test and the claims Priestley based upon it show the theoretical system which made sense of the test. It only made sense for experimenters committed to the reality of phlogiston and to the measure of virtue as a determination of an air's character. Transmission of skill with the test was the vector for the transmission of Priestley's theoretical language and phlogistic cosmology. During the winter of 1773–4 and most of the following year, Lavoisier found the nitrous air test very useful. Details of the test were communicated to Paris by Priestley's colleague in London, Jean Magellan. The test provided a means for separating respirable and non-respirable airs, a key point for the Frenchman's emerging theory of the function of respiration: respired air was phlogisticated, and would diminish less in the test. At the end of February 1775, Lavoisier made some notes about why this diminution took place. His view at this point was that nitrous air was combined with phlogiston. When mixed with common air the phlogiston left the nitrous air and combined with common air. Dephlogisticated nitrous air became liquid nitrous acid. Phlogisticated common air became fixed air. That was what was left at the end of the reaction. All this was good Priestleyan doctrine. Lavoisier noted: 'all of this agrees very much with the system of Priestley.'[22]

[21] Priestley, *Experiments and Observations*, first edition (London, 1775), vol. 2, pp. 39–40; *Experiments and Observations* (Birmingham, 1790), vol. 2, pp. 102–19.

[22] F. L. Holmes, *Lavoisier and the Chemistry of Life* (Madison, 1985), p. 33.

One month after this memorandum, at the end of March 1775, Lavoisier performed the nitrous air test on the air extracted from mercury calx, just as Priestley had done the previous summer and as Priestley may have told Lavoisier in autumn of that year.[23] Whatever the source, Lavoisier treated the nitrous air test as decisive. Even though the new air supported combustion much better than common air, Lavoisier found that the reduction of the air by nitrous air was the same as that for common air (about one-fifth), so it was only as good as common air. When he reported these experiments to the Paris Academy in April 1775, therefore, Lavoisier announced that this was 'not only common air' but 'the air itself entire.' While more respirable, it was only as good as common air in the crucial test. During the next year Lavoisier set out to improve his command of Priestley's techniques. By mid March 1775, Priestley had already announced 'dephlogisticated air' at the Society. News reached Paris in December. Experiments by Lavoisier in spring 1776 and a memoir of April *still* mentioned that 'the air was found to be the dephlogisticated air of Priestley,' and at last managed to show that its diminution was greater than that for common air. Only with a different range of experiments on the synthesis of atmospheric air of spring 1776 performed at his new laboratory at the Arsenal could Lavoisier start to disengage from the technology which he had painfully learnt to use. Lavoisier continued to use Priestley's terminology, notably that of 'vitiation', even in his respiration theory. Until at least 1777, Lavoisier wrote and rewrote a series of memoirs designed to show that in respiration dephlogisticated air was fixed in the blood. This became a central dogma of his chemical theory, but it needed some sensitive reconstruction of his past involvement in the technology of the nitrous air test for phlogistication. By then, Priestley's nitrous air test was already embodied in a series of instruments built by his allies in Britain and Italy. Eudiometry, as this technology was to be called, was an accompaniment and constituent of the fate of phlogistic chemistry. Lavoisier needed to learn and undermine this technology to build a new theory of air, respiration and life.[24]

To use the nitrous air test as a tool of medical meteorology was to become committed to a more complex account of the cosmos and the social order. Priestley planned a collection of airs from different sites. In 1779 he asked his friend and patron, the Birmingham manufacturer Matthew Boulton, for 'air as it is actually breathed by the different

[23] C. E. Perrin, 'Prelude to Lavoisier's Theory of Calcination', *Ambix* 16 (1969). pp. 140–51.
[24] Holmes, *Lavoisier*, pp. 48–62.

manufacturers in this kingdom' to be gathered from different workshops in the Midlands. He also sampled the air left in rooms at Shelburne's house after gatherings there. Vials of air were sent round the kingdom; the test began to engross the social world. In the early 1780s Priestley collaborated with the reforming farming journalist Arthur Young on a general survey of the eudiometric characteristics of waters in different agricultural regions. They concluded that phlogisticated waters aided crop production and sought to win the Board of Agriculture to this pneumatic theory. For economic and political reformers in the critical period of radical Dissent, careful calculation and marketing were crucial tools. Potential allies were also customers. Physicians bought Priestley's electrical machines (one was sold to Leeds Infirmary, for example); manufacturers such as Boulton and Wedgwood helped him market new glassware and chemicals. From 1777 eudiometers were on sale at a fashionable cut-glass factory in London's West End. Making a market for pneumatics aided the spread of pneumatic doctrine and gave meaning to its utilitarian vocabulary. For example, Priestley's new 'pure air' might be 'peculiarly salutary to the lungs in certain morbid cases', and 'pure dephlogisticated air might be very useful as a medicine', even if too powerful in common measure: 'a moralist may say that the air which nature has provided for us is as good as we deserve.'[25]

This mixture of utility, technology and pneumatics won adherents. Magellan told Priestley that the nitrous air test, 'the happy discovery you have made for the benefit of mankind, and perhaps of almost the whole animal creation of this globe', was of an importance 'infinitely superior to that of the numerous trifling novelties which so often spread with prodigious rapidity through remote provinces of the Earth'. Similarly, Bentham began work on eudiometry when he contacted Priestley in 1774–5. He told Priestley that 'in using nitrous air as a test of the comparative purity of the atmosphere in different places, it is of importance to be certain of its being utterly free from all previous admixture with Common air'. To use such a test in this way was to

[25] Priestley, *Experiments and Observations*, second edition (London, 1776), vol. 2, pp. 40–9, 100–3; Priestley to Boulton, ?1777, in R. E. Schofield (ed.), *Scientific Autobiography of Joseph Priestley* (Cambridge, MA, 1967), pp. 161–2; Priestley and Richard Price, 'On the Noxious Quality of the Effluvia of Putrid Marshes'. For farming and eudiometry see Priestley, *Experiments and Observations* (Birmingham, 1790), vol. 3, p. 305; M. Betham-Edwards, *Autobiography of Arthur Young* (London, 1898), pp. 99 and 150–3; McNeil, *Under the Banner of Science*, pp. 180–3. For the market, see J. H. de Magellan, *Description of a Glass Apparatus*, third edition (London, 1783), p. iv and compare J. V. Golinski, 'Utility and Audience in Eighteenth-Century Chemistry', *British Journal for the History of Science* 21 (1988), pp. 1–32, pp. 17–23.

declare allegiance to the principles of pneumatics. Throughout the 1770s Bentham was concerned with the development of this programme: his 'Athanor' was one contribution to it, anticipating 'eudiometers' made by Cavendish and the Tuscan natural philosopher Felice Fontana in the 1780s. He talked to Fontana about publications on the improvement of the virtue of airs and better ways of making artificial airs. He also became involved in Priestley's disputes with chemists such as Scheele, who denied that vegetation purified airs.[26] As Bentham's case suggests, commitment to eudiometry often involved both discipleship and disputes. It was with Italian colleagues that Priestley and Bentham most strenuously debated the possibilities for a new medical meteorology. The context of the work in enlightened Italian culture gave 'eudiometry' its new political meaning.

EUDIOMETRY AND ENLIGHTENED DESPOTISM

The protagonists of the eudiometric campaigns were three officials of Habsburg regimes in Austria and Italy who later became sympathetic to radical reform. They were Marsilio Landriani, appointed through the influence of Joseph II's secretary for Italian affairs to the physics chair at the Brera Gymnasium in Milan in 1776; Felice Fontana, court physicist to Peter Leopold II in Florence and, from 1771, director of the Grand Ducal Museum of Physics and Natural History; and Jan Ingenhousz, graduate of Louvain and Leyden, encouraged by Pringle to lead inoculation campaigns in Britain and Austria, and, from 1768, court physician to Maria Theresa. All were skilful publicists, committed to medical meteorology and to Priestley's pneumatic chemistry. The three were also distinguished *philosophes*, studious readers of anticlerical and reformist French publications. Fontana was strongly identified with Leopold's medical and anticurial programmes, and was purged by anti-Jacobins in 1799 before enjoying a brief return to power as President of the Napoleonic Academy in Florence in 1801.[27] Landriani was a contributor to *Il Caffè*, founder of the improving Milanese Patriotic Society in 1778, and a close colleague of the Professor of Medico-Surgery at the Ospedale Maggiore, Pietro Moscati, who later became a leader of the Cisalpine Republic under French occupation in 1796–7.[28] Ingenhousz was an intimate of Priestley, Pringle and

[26] Priestley, *Experiments and Observations* (London, 1777), vol. 3, pp. 379–80; Magellan, *Description*, pp. 29–30; Correspondence of Bentham, vol. 1, pp. 210–16, 225–6, 314–15, 344; Schofield, *Scientific Autobiography of Priestley*, 182–6.

[27] Knoefel, *Felice Fontana*, part 1.

[28] For Landriani see P. Moscati, *Dei vantaggi della educazione filosofica nello studio della chemica* (1784), ed. L. Belloni (Milan, 1961), pp. 70–86.

Benjamin Franklin, whom he met in London in 1766. He later became a client of Shelburne, residing at Bowood for the last two decades of his life, whence he led campaigns for reformist physic and against what he perceived as the ignorant errors of the new stories of vaccination peddled by Edward Jenner and his establishment friends.[29] These features suggest a set of interests in reform and social management which became actual in their eudiometric work. Each display a representative pattern of research interests: Franklinian electricity, including arguments for lightning rods; work on the influence of light on vegetable growth; concern for public health, particularly slow fevers and epidemics; hostility to Lavoisier's chemistry. This work was to be characterised by a mixture of good marketing, complex pneumatic doctrine and energetic propaganda.[30]

Landriani began his enquiries into pneumatic medicine in collaboration with Moscati at the Milan Hospital from 1772. The vocabulary of Italian work on environmental medicine drew its sense from Bernadino Ramazzini's work at Modena in the 1690s and from that of Giovanni Lancisi at Rome in 1717. The very laxity of the tenets of environmentalism was a licence for the new Milanese work of the 1770s. Resources drawn from the earlier work included a warm admiration of British experimental philosophy, so that Priestley could easily be seen as the heir of Robert Boyle and Stephen Hales; a faith in the accumulation of *quantitative* meteorological data; and a strict attention to what seemed to be obviously mephitic sites, such as marshes, sewers and graveyards.[31] Such, for example, were the views on air and health publicised in *Il Caffè* in 1756 by another Brera professor, Giuseppe Parini. Most important, perhaps, was the causal nexus which figures such as Ramazzini and Lancisi documented. The air was at once a source of disease and of cure. Environmentalism, insofar as it indicated air-borne pathology, did not rule out contagion, for the sick released pathogenic vapours too. The key resource of this rich set of variables was the combination of measurement and pneumatics. A powerful weapon seemed at hand for use in efforts to win authority from the State and over civil society.

State patronage accompanied contests with what these men perceived as the ignorance of the plebs and the prejudice of priestcraft.[32]

[29] H. Reed, 'Jan Ingenhousz: Plant Physiologist', *Chronica Botanica* 11 (1949), pp. 285–396, pp. 291–4. For Ingenhousz against vaccination, see P. Van der Pas, 'The Ingenhousz–Jenner Correspondence', *Janus* 51 (1964), pp. 202–20. For the campaign for inoculation and Pringle's role, see A. S. Emch-Dériaz, 'L'inoculation justifiée – or was it ?', *Eighteenth Century Life* 7 (1982), pp. 65–72. [30] Antonio Pace, *Franklin and Italy* (Philadelphia, 1958), chapter 2.

[31] James Riley, *The Eighteenth Century Campaign to Avoid Disease* (London, 1987), chapter 2.

[32] F. Venturi, *Utopia and Reform in the Enlightenment* (Cambridge, 1971), pp. 100 and 135.

Leopold's notes on his accession to power in 1765 diagnosed the ills of Tuscan society: 'the difficulties for merchants, the estates of the Church, the excessive numbers of monks and nuns, the tolls'. The cure proposed involved careful mixtures of free trade, agricultural planning and anticlericalism.[33] Riots against new church reforms spread through Tuscany and elsewhere in the 1780s following ecclesiastical attacks on the aims of Joseph II in the Empire itself.[34] Meanwhile, both in Milan and Tuscany a new class of professional administrators was to be recruited to displace landed patrician dominance. Men like Landriani and Fontana plied their trade under a 'new discipline of office-holders'. Landriani's Patriotic Society, patronised by Joseph II and his ministers, was a chief target for suspicion from clerics and journalists alike. The great Milanese legal reformer Cesare Beccaria, co-founder of *Il Caffè*, wrote to the encyclopedist André Morellet in 1766 that 'the Milanese do not forgive those who wish to make them live in the eighteenth century'. Pietro Verri's scepticism of the despotic Habsburg regime helps explain his satires against Landriani's pneumatics, which was obviously linked to the physicist's rise to authority in Milan. In the same way, clerical hostility to Leopold was widely held to be at the root of the series of controversies which bedevilled Fontana's medical chemistry: an alliance of patricians and priests rallied against his natural philosophy in the 1780s. In contrast, Leopold detailed Fontana's valuable instruction of his son Francis in physics when seeking to guarantee Francis's succession to the Imperial throne.[35]

These intellectuals in public service needed techniques of management which would help sustain this discipline against its critics. As we shall see, a suitable case for treatment with these methods was the disastrous grain crisis which afflicted central Italy in the mid 1760s. The new government responded by deregulating the grain trade (in contrast to traditional protectionism) and replacing magistrates' control over provision with a supervisory statistical office.[36] The Habsburg government was making demands on a complex of quantitative and environmental skills which it expected its officers to provide.

[33] R. Burr Litchfield, *Emergence of a Bureaucracy: The Florentine Patricians 1530–1790* (Princeton, 1986), chapter 14.

[34] G. Turi, *Viva Maria: la Reazione alle Riforme Leopoldine* (Florence, 1969), p. 139.

[35] F. Venturi (ed.), *Illuministi Italiani*, vol. 3: *Riformatori Lombardi, Piemontesi e Toscani* (Milan and Naples, 1958), p. 207; D. Carpanetto and G. Ricuperati, *Italy in the Age of Reason* (London, 1987), pp. 210 and 225–9; Knoefel, *Felice Fontana*, pp. 85 and 184.

[36] Franco Venturi, 'Quatro anni di carestia in Toscana 1764–1767', *Rivista Storica Italiana* 88 (1976), pp. 649–707 and 'Scienza e riforma nella Toscana del settecento', *Rivista Storica Italiana* 89 (1977), pp. 211–105.

Management of airs would aid grain production and land reclamation; it would also sustain hospital reform and public hygiene. And these reforms brought the new managers into direct conflict with established medical elites. 'In Tuscany', a visitor reported, 'the hospitals are apparently the grand duke's palaces.'[37] The technology was also to be extended to the mad, notably after 1780 in alliance with the proposals of the *philosophe* and physician Vincenzo Chiarugi. Chiarugi adopted the pneumatic and environmental interpretation of mental derangement, and so made ventilation and respiration key sites for his bold therapy, licensed after a new law on the insane of January 1774.[38] The link between pneumatics and economical reform became explicit during the 1770s, especially in government schemes to drain the poisonous Maremma marshes and to reclaim new farmland there: the fight against *mal aria* (bad air) was led by a combination of agriculturalists and naturalists from the Tuscan capital backed with dictatorial State powers.[39] So even before Priestley's paper on nitrous air was translated into Italian at Milan in 1774, it already seemed plausible that a machine which measured respirability would *ipso facto* be a device for the manufacture of numbers which would allow the mapping and control of public health and the social body.

Landriani and Moscati began their work on the nitrous air test soon after reading Priestley's paper in spring 1775, carnival time in the city. After some weeks spent preparing good samples of the air and designing a portable version of the trial, the two toured celebrated Milanese sites of what they felt were obvious public dangers. The term 'eudiometry' was coined to describe this technology: literally, the measurement of good weather. The results were gratifying for the eudiometrists, and offered as condemnations of Milanese public order: 'the air of the pit at the Theatre during the last days of Carnival was found to be as infected as that of tombs'. Such statements drew immediate comment in Milan and elsewhere, including derision from members of the old governing classes. Landriani reported the public

[37] Eric Cochrane, *Florence in the Forgotten Centuries* (Chicago, 1973), p. 433; A. Corsini, 'La medicina alla corte di Pietro Leopoldo', *Rivista CIBA* 46 (1945), pp. 1,510–40.

[38] George Mora, 'Vincenzo Chiarugi and his Psychiatric Reform', *Journal of the History of Medicine* 14 (1959), pp. 424–33.

[39] Carpanetto and Ricuperati, *Italy in the Age of Reason*, p. 213; Eric Cochrane, *Tradition and Enlightenment in the Tuscan Academies* (Rome, 1961), pp. 151–6. In this effort the Tuscans shared the views of Beccaria, whose lectures on 'political agriculture' (1769–70) argued that priestcraft and peasant prejudice were principal obstacles to the use of medical science in rural improvement: Cesare Beccaria, 'Elementi di economia pubblica', p. 172 in F. Venturi, *Illuministi Italiani*, vol. 3. They were also helped by publication of past texts on pneumatics and drainage, including Sallustio Bandini's *Discorso sopra la Maremma di Siena* (1737, pb. 1775): see Venturi, *Illuministi*, pp. 883–941. See above, note 25.

fascination for pneumatics. His colleagues sought the basis of these judgements of virtue. Landriani responded with a theoretical gloss: the volume remaining at the end of the reaction was proportional to the fixed air and phlogiston contents of the sample. This gloss, in contrast with that of Priestley, pointed to eudiometry's ability to determine both the health of towns and of individuals, since respired air was widely held to be both phlogisticated and fixed. Landriani also varied Priestley's method in a number of ways, including the use of mercury and water together and the treatment of each volume of test air successively. This was a technique tooled to allow the estimate of the virtue of a wide range of combustible substances, including the air left over oils and waxes and in closed chambers.[40] Landriani also received criticism and satire: the latter from Pietro Verri, who castigated his 'chemical and literary charlatanism' and baptised him 'mister fixed air', the former from the young Como natural philosopher Alessandro Volta. In June 1775 Volta and Moscati received a copy of a treatise by Fontana sent from Florence, in which a similar range of instruments using Priestley's technology was outlined. Volta alleged that Fontana was trying to steal a march on the Milan physicist; Landriani temporised and then published an account of his own work, dedicated to the Austrian minister in Milan and including a major appeal for eudiometry's relevance to the State. He argued that the new technology was

> surely more useful and important than all meteorological observations, since it is not limited to the dry curiosity of the number of lines or inches by which the barometer or thermometer change from one day to the next, but instead shows the greater or less respirability of the air, the wind, the healthiness of a season, etc., all objects of the greatest importance and which if thoroughly studied could help us guard against infinite abuses, and thence also prognosticate and prevent the most terrible epidemics.[41]

Landriani's book (see plates 7, 8 and 9) presented eudiometry as a moment of radical discontinuity in the history of environmental medicine. But this discontinuity had to be carefully managed. Eudiometers took their place as one of a battery of meteorological devices which Moscati and Landriani developed for their experiments in Lombardy, including those designed to detect atmospheric electricity and elasticity. Landriani's career was seen as depending on these techniques: when he got the Brera job from the government in summer 1776, Pietro

[40] Luigi Belloni, 'L'eudiometro del Landriani', *Actes du symposium international d'histoire des sciences*, Florence-Vinci, 8–10 October 1960, ed. M. Righini Bonelli (Florence, 1962), pp. 130–51.

[41] Landriani, *Ricerche fisiche intorno alla salubrità dell'aria* (Milan, 1775), p. xi.

RICERCHE FISICHE
intorno
alla salubrità dell' aria

*Occulta res est salubritas presertim perfecti
:or aeris et potius experimentis quam dis
:cursu et conjectura elicitur* Bacon. Hist. vit. et mortis

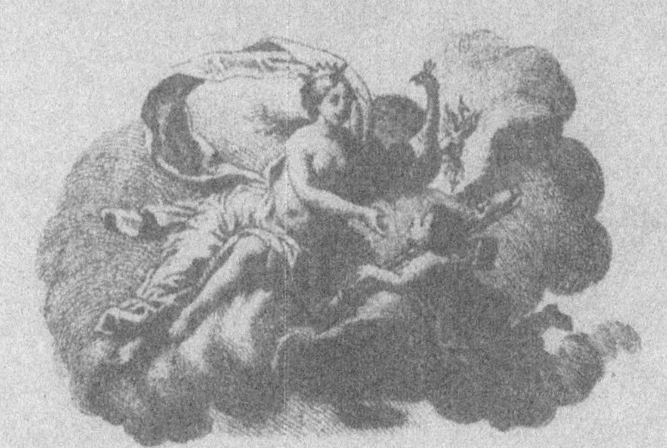

MILANO

M. DCCLXXV

7 Title-page of M. Landriani, *Ricerche fisiche intorno alla salubrità dell'aria* (Milan, 1775)

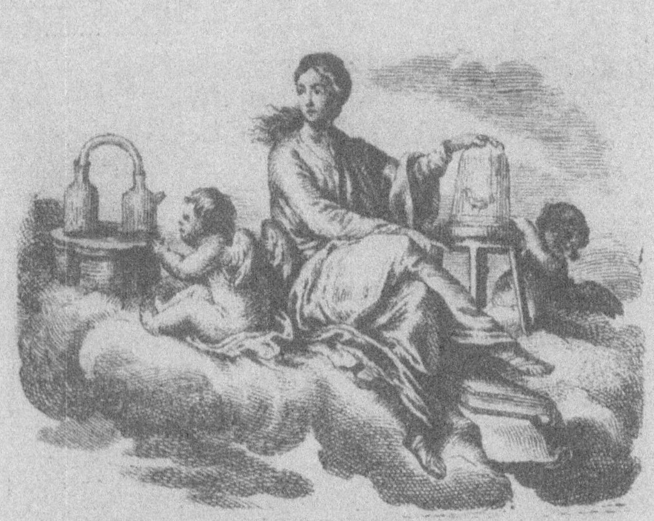

RICERCHE FISICHE

INTORNO

ALLA SALUBRITÀ DELL' ARIA.

SIno dall' anno 1727. il Dottore Stefano Hales (*) avea oſſervato che il vapor elaſtico, che ſvolgeſi dalla diſſoluzione delle ſpiriti di Walton nello ſpirito di nitro, oltre aver uno ſpiacevoliſſimo odore avvicinanteſi d' aſſai

(*) *Vegetable Staticks ch. 6. exp. 96.*

A

8 First page of M. Landriani, *Ricerche fisiche intorno alla salubrità dell'aria* (Milan, 1775)

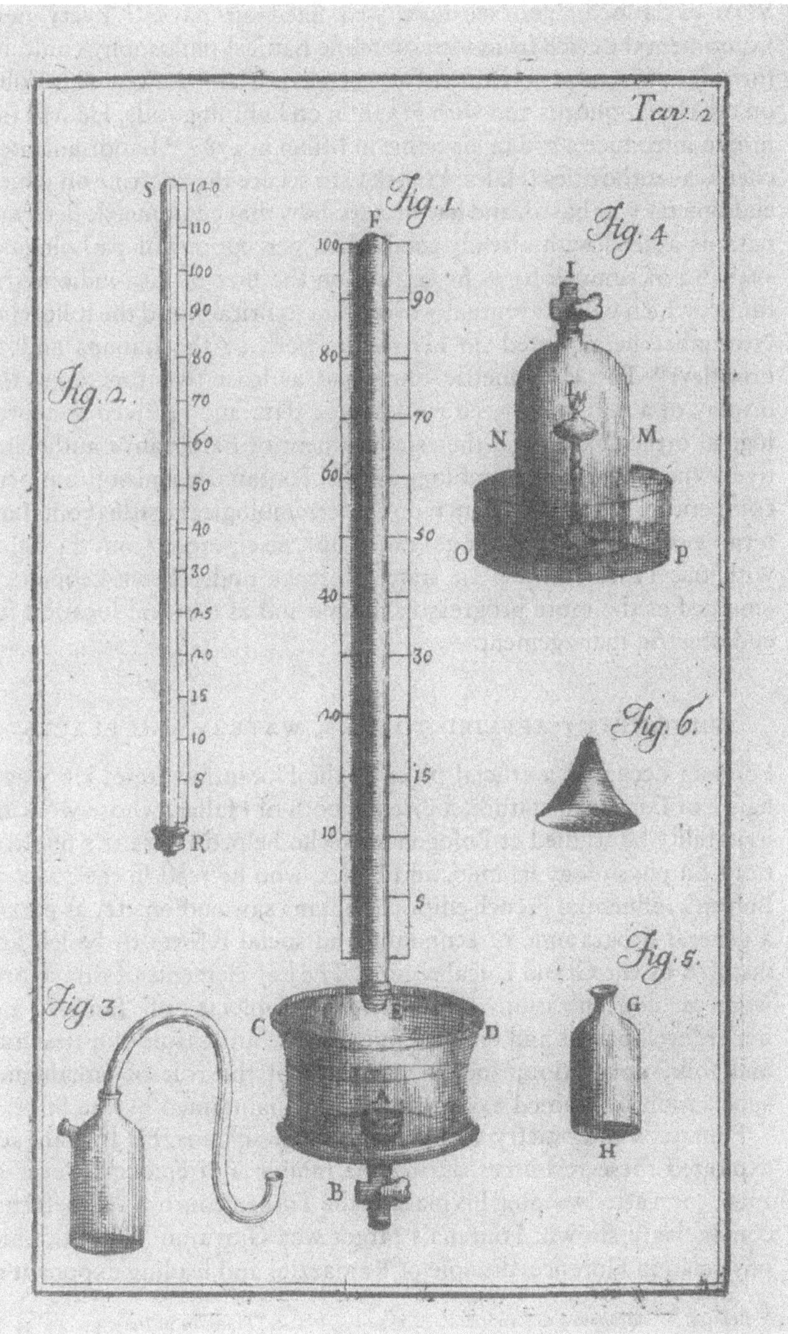

9 Table 2 from M. Landriani, *Ricerche fisiche intorno alla salubrità dell'aria* (Milan, 1775)

Verri exclaimed: 'you see how well fixed air pays.'[42] Every new experimental device from ultramontane natural philosophy could be turned to this end, as became clear when Landriani worked with Volta on the electrophorus and with Franklin on lightning rods. He was the first to introduce a rod in his home in Milan in 1781.[43] Landriani cited chemical authorities (Hales, Priestley) to secure the doctrine on which eudiometry was based, and had also to show that eudiometric determinations agreed with already established perceptions of pathological sites. So in summer 1776 he set out on the first of his 'eudiometric tours', which would eventually bring him to Britain, and the following November he reported on his results both to the Italians and to Priestley.[44] The eudiometric tours had at least two functions: the display of a match between eudiometric data and received meteorological orthodoxies; and the establishment of Landriani's authoritative ownership of the technology against Fontana, his most prominent competitor. While Landriani won the terminological battle (Fontana's term 'evaerometer' did not get taken up), he emerged from the fights with the Tuscan in a poor state. Florence under Peter Leopold II emerged as the more progressive regime and as an ideal location for eudiometric management.

EUDIOMETRY APPLIED TO AIRS, WATERS AND PLACES

Fontana occupied a crucial place in the Florentine State. He was a figure of European stature, a disciple both of Haller, whose work on irritability he studied at Bologna and who helped Fontana's publications on physiology in 1760, and Hales, who he read in the 1760s in Buffon's influential French edition. Fontana saw eudiometry as part of a general programme of economic and social reform to be led and inspired by the Grand Ducal regime. The key elements of this reform were a concentration on endemic problems of famine and underdevelopment and on epidemic disease; an assault on priestcraft and folk superstition; and an advocacy of the role of enlightened supervision by trained expert naturalists maintained by the State.

Fontana's eudiometry was made to fit these aims. He had already exploited these resources during the famine and epidemic fever of 1766, soon after winning his place at the Tuscan court. As Knoefel has convincingly shown, Fontana's target was Giovanni Tozzetti, chief physician in Florence, disciple of Ramazzini and leading exponent of

[42] Belloni, 'L'eudiometro di Landriani', p. 133. [43] Pace, *Franklin in Italy*, pp. 26, 39–40.
[44] Priestley, *Experiments and Observations* (London, 1777), vol. 3, pp. 380–1.

meteorological medicine in Tuscany. Tozzetti published a text on weather and famine which catalogued ancient and modern authorities on famine and epidemic, and announced the identification of microscopic organisms responsible for the disastrous wheat rust which frequently affected Tuscan grains. Fontana immediately gave Tozzetti's work a violently hostile review, condemning it above all for its devotion to ancient authority and its defence of what he saw as miracles and folk superstitions against moderns, iconoclasts and naturalists. Fontana followed up with his own work, published through the help of the Milanese *philosophes*, and argued that most popular remedies for rust were impotent and superstitious, while detailed microscopy and statistical comparison of different farms showed how to combat the disease. The satire worked: a comparison between early harvests of affected grains (Fontana's remedy), and the burning of ox horns (attributed to Tozzetti), gained Fontana respect at court and condemned Tozzetti to ridicule, albeit ephemeral. Fontana's integration of new pneumatics and government statistics won him influential patronage from the reformist agricultural managers in the Florentine Accademia dei Georgofili. More substantively, Fontana outlined the work on rust as part of a generalised strategy of supervision and investigation by elite savants: 'it does not suffice to say in general that such a practice may be useful; we must determine when and to what extent it may be of value. In order to accomplish this, the eye and hand of a sagacious observer are necessary'. 'Sagacity' now meant enlightened medical chemistry.[45]

Like Landriani, Fontana swiftly seized on Priestley's work when it reached Italy. In early 1775 he completed a paper on fixed air destined for the Royal Society in London, in which Priestley was both praised for experimental skill and yet attacked for the claim that this air was acidic. The paper did not appear in the *Philosophical Transactions* but it was widely distributed in French and Italian journals. So were the comments Fontana added to the paper announcing his invention of a number of devices based on the nitrous air test and the claim that such research should be of particular interest to governments and sovereigns.[46] It was this comment, and the substantial *Descrizione e usi di alcuni stromenti per misurare la salubrità dell' aria* of the same year which drew Landriani's and others' attention to Fontana's work. The

[45] Knoefel, 'Famine and Fever in Tuscany', *Physis* 21 (1979), pp. 7–35; Fontana, *Osservazioni sopra la ruggine del grano* (Lucca, 1767); English translation (Washington DC, 1932), p. 35.

[46] Fontana, 'Recherches physiques sur l'air fixe', *Observations sur la physique* 6 (1775), pp. 280–9.

Descrizione pictured eight eudiometers, all elaborately wrought and most rather clearly impracticable (see plate 10). Few protocols were provided, and in some cases Fontana's silence was remarkable, notably on the issue of the function of water, since he always used mercury as a means of measuring the residual volume of air. Just as Landriani, for one, doubted whether Fontana had built or could use any of these machines, so Fontana was equally sceptical about Landriani's device. Thus it is clear that both in Milan and in Florence a eudiometer was built, but that the public descriptions of these devices were published to establish the priority of the inventor and the social worth of the technology, and clearly not as instructions for other eudiometricians. In the event, for example, Fontana's working eudiometer only appeared in an account of 1779 by Ingenhousz, which pictures and describes a device very similar to Priestley's tubes. Eudiometry had an iconography appropriate to enlightened conventions of taste: it also maintained a problem of replication characteristic of experimental philosophy.[47]

Fontana and Ingenhousz created an iconography for eudiometry – they also developed a technique for representing its results. The technique depended on Fontana's aerial cosmology. He asserted it was possible to fix the minimum degree of salubrity of air quite easily, since this would be marked by a failure to react with nitrous air. The most salubrious air was harder to mark: Priestley had assumed common air was the most healthful, and if this could be fixed, Fontana argued, epidemics could be predicted and differences between regions assessed. The character of Fontana's scale also depended on his peculiar technique: unlike Priestley, who added volumes simultaneously, the so-called 'Fontanist' method involved the sequential addition of volumes, in an effort to get a fixed end-point. Most importantly, Fontana developed eudiometric representation only after discussions with Ingenhousz and his colleagues during his eudiometric tour of 1776–9. He left Florence for Paris soon after the publication of the *Descrizione* in autumn 1775, despatched by the government to purchase instruments for the new Museum with the aid of the young *illuministo* Giovanni Fabbroni. He was in Paris from early 1776 until autumn 1778, when he travelled to London. One decisive lesson Fontana learnt was the superiority of British over French and Italian instrument makers. Another was the enormous difficulty of replicating eudiometric results. Finally, he encountered the emerging controversies on air and phlogiston now raging in Paris and in Britain.

[47] Knoefel, *Fontana*, pp. 165–73; Ingenhousz, *Experiments*, pp. 152–81.

Tav. IIII.

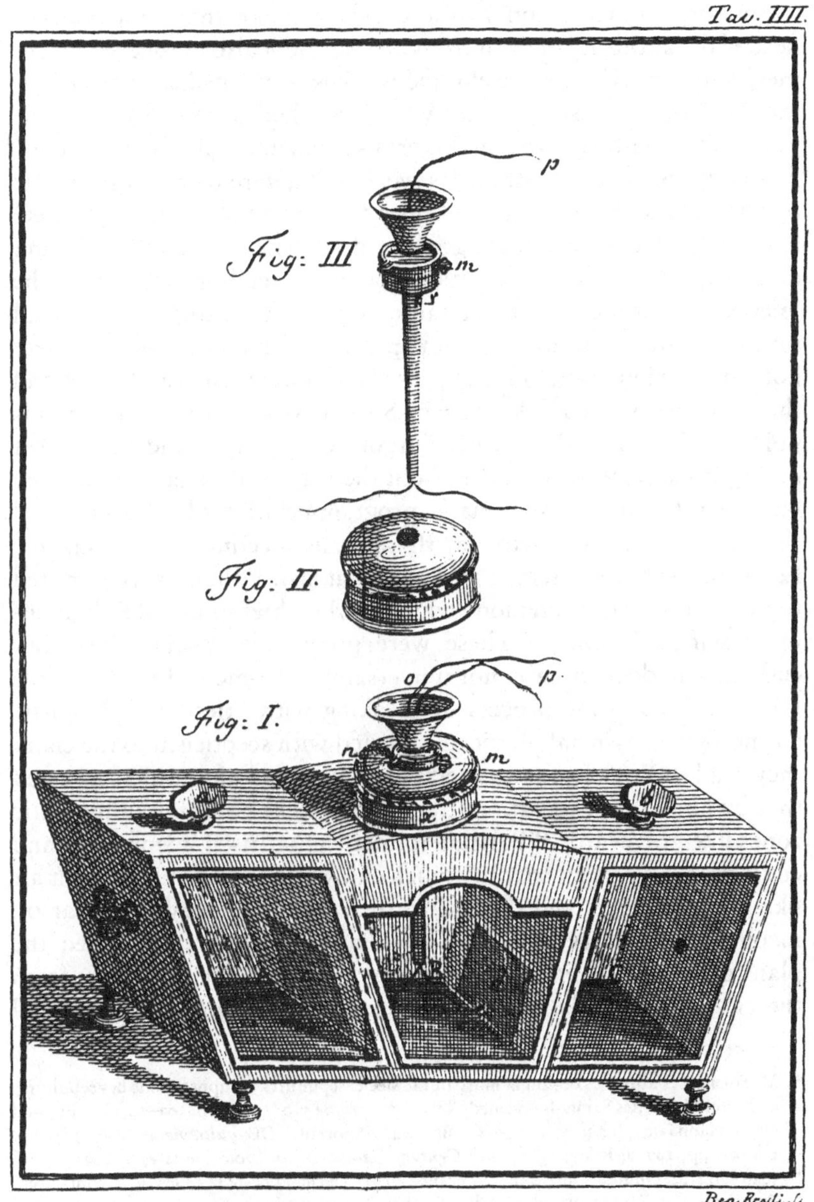

10 Table 4 from Felice Fontana, *Descrizione e usi di alcuni stromenti* (Florence, 1775)

Fontana's intervention in these debates, like that of Lavoisier, needed the authority of the nitrous air test and it also needed establishment support. His most celebrated work was pursued with the aid of the Paris pharmacist Cadet de Vaux, who had been ordered by the police to investigate the malodorous Cemetery of the Innocents. Evidently the French authorities were well aware of new pneumatic technology, and the Fontana–Cadet team soon showed the Société Royale de Médecine that the graveyard was eudiometrically foul and dangerous.[48] The confirmation between eudiometry and the 'mephitism' of the French capital took place in a fraught ideological setting. Traditional doctrines on epidemiology and oeconomy were hotly debated in France in the 1770s.[49] Physiocrats such as Turgot and the members of Vicq d'Azyr's new Société Royale were active in this polemic: Fontana talked with Turgot, Vicq d'Azyr and Condorcet during his stay, learning more about the ways eudiometry could now be integrated into a systematic programme of medical and social reform. Fontana was active at the famous meeting of the Masonic Lodge of the Nine Sisters in 1778 when, at last, Voltaire was admitted to their number in a ceremony which marks a high-point of Enlightenment self-celebration.[50] These were potentially crucial allies, but eudiometric doctrine was not universally welcome in France. While Lavoisier was in the process of breaking with Priestley's phlogistic cosmology, provincial physicians reacted with scepticism to the claim they read in Priestley that vegetable life purified air. Some suggested that by hindering circulation, trees would raise pollution in mephitic zones like graveyards.[51] Parisian journalists satirised 'mephitism' and eudiometry: 'Parisian frivolity much enjoys seeing chemists decant air like thimbleriggers and then bring their olfactory nerves to bear on mephitized lavatory seats.'[52] The clergy strenuously contested the plans prompted by Fontanist eudiometry to ship buried corpses from the city's graveyards. Enlightened management violated traditional

[48] M. Foisil, 'Les attitudes devant la mort au 18è siècle: sépultures et suppressions des sépultures dans le cimitière des Saints-Innocents', *Revue Historique* 510 (1974), pp. 303–30; Caroline and Owen Hannaway, 'La fermeture du Cimitière des Innocents', *Dix-huitième siècle* 9 (1977), pp. 181–91, pp. 187–8; Riley, *Eighteenth Century Campaign to Avoid Disease*, p. 109.

[49] Jean Ehrard, 'Opinions médicales en France au 18è siècle: la peste et l'idée de la contagion', *Annales* ESC 12 (1957), pp. 46–59; Alain Corbin, *The Foul and the Fragrant* (Leamington and New York, 1986), chapter 1.

[50] C. Hannaway, 'The Société Royale de Médecine and Epidemics in the Ancien Régime', *Bulletin of the History of Medicine* 46 (1972), pp. 257–73; Venturi, *Illuministi Italiani*, vol. 3, p. 1,085.

[51] Hannaway and Hannaway, 'Cimitière des Innocents', p. 186; compare Ingenhousz, *Experiments upon Vegetables*, conclusion, on nocturnal pollution by vegetation.

[52] L. S. Mercier, cited in Corbin, *The Foul and the Fragrant*, p. 59.

structures of kinship and collective feeling: one influential abbé complained in 1788 that 'if we gain in respect of the purity of the atmosphere, it is to be feared that we lose much so far as morality is concerned'. Significantly, just the same fights broke out over the Benthamite provisions of the Anatomy Act in Britain half a century later. Both cemetery closure and compulsory dissection involved appeals to the authority of pneumatics and medicine, and deprecation of traditional pneumatology.[53]

The Parisian milieu gave new meaning to eudiometry. In an essay published on his arrival in Paris, Fontana appealed to experiments performed the previous year in Florence. He now allowed, as he had not done in 1775, that nitrous air worked as a simple phlogiston donor and that the virtue of an air could be restored by shaking with water. By September 1776, Fontana had performed a series of trials aping those of Priestley on dephlogisticated air. His contacts in the cemetery survey drew him into the network of Paris apothecaries who supplied Lavoisier with his prized mercury calx and witnessed the celebrated trials of summer 1774 and spring 1775, in which the nitrous air test was used to assay the air left after the reduction of this precipitate.[54] In an effort to confront French chemistry, the Florentine argued that when metals were calcined the consequent weight gain was not due to fixed air but to the replacement of the metals' phlogiston by a substance which became common air through the loss of its natural phlogiston content.[55] Reports of these trials were sent to the Paris Academy – they remained unpublished. In spring 1777 Lavoisier read the Academy a paper on respiration held over from the previous autumn and now much altered in form. This address at last decisively rejected Priestley's claim that respiration and phlogistication were equivalent processes. The fight was to show that measures of phlogistication could still be taken as measures of vitiation and hence of insalubrity. In 1783, Lavoisier and Laplace helped themselves to Fontanist eudiometric techniques in their decisive work on animal respiration: crucially, this work led the Frenchmen to reject Fontana's claims about the dephlogistication of air during respiration.[56] While Priestley later treated Fontana's trials as support for his doctrine, Fontana himself worked hard with his new collaborator, Ingenhousz, on the eudiometry of Paris. This collaboration and its aftermath soon led to a dramatic crisis for Italian eudiometry.

53 John McManners, *Death and the Enlightenment* (Oxford, 1985), p. 314; Ruth Richardson, *Death, Dissection and the Destitute* (London, 1987), chapter 1.

54 A. Berman, 'The Cadet Circle', *Bulletin of the History of Medicine* 40 (1966), pp. 101–11.

55 Fontana, *Recherches physiques sur la nature de l'air nitreux et de l'air déphlogistiqué* (Paris, 1776), pp. 128 and 155.

56 Holmes, *Lavoisier*, pp. 82–9, 170 and 201.

INFLAMMABLE AIR AND NITROUS AIR: THE TRANSFORMATION OF EUDIOMETRY

Fontana first met Ingenhousz in Florence in 1769 when the Dutch physician was engaged in inoculating members of the ruling house, including Leopold himself. Elected FRS in 1771, and subsequently a physician and experimenter of distinction in both the British and French capitals, Ingenhousz was a key figure in eudiometry's fate and in the development of pneumatic chemistry in general, publishing a series of important papers in the journals and his great book, *Experiments upon Vegetables* of 1779. In November 1775, while working for the Habsburg court at Vienna, he received a copy of Fontana's *Descrizione*, and soon saw many of the defects of Fontana's methods. The trouble upon which Ingenhousz concentrated was that of ascertaining whether 'the nitrous air had dislodged all the common air out of it, or had dislodged always the same quantity of common air'. This was a genuine trouble, since the constancy of added volumes of nitrous air dictated the fixed outcome of evaluations of samples of common air. Ingenhousz devised a rubber bottle to force the air mixture together. By calibrating his machine with a mercury manometer, Ingenhousz sought to show that this novel technique was an improvement on Fontanist eudiometry. His account was sent to John Pringle in London and published there in spring 1776.[57]

This paper from Ingenhousz prompted fresh experiments with Fontana in Paris in 1776–7. They worked on the ways in which Cavendish's inflammable air could be used instead of or as a supplement for nitrous air. The polemical context was an attack by Scheele upon Priestley: Scheele had claimed, against the English chemist, that inflammable air was non-toxic and respirable, even if it showed up as bad on the nitrous air test. Both Bentham and Fontana defended Priestley against the Swede.[58] Fontana explained away Scheele's results by pointing out that the lungs kept residual air which would mix with any inflammable air inhaled, and by claiming once again considerable authority for his eudiometer, which showed the pathological effects of the inflammable air. Medical eudiometry hinged on maintaining this connection between diminution, respirability and virtue. To reaffirm this technique, Fontana described a new version of the machine, with

[57] Ingenhousz, 'Easy Methods of Measuring the Diminution of Bulk, Taking Place Upon the Mixture of Common Air and Nitrous Air', *Philosophical Transactions* 66 (1776), pp. 257–67.

[58] Schofield, *Scientific Autobiography*, pp. 161–62; *Correspondence of Bentham*, vol. 1, pp. 314–15 and 344.

water and mercury, and a new way of representing its results. The paper also included dramatic reports of the effects of breathing inflammable air: Fontana aimed to show that the air could be breathed safely but that this did not invalidate the nitrous air test. 'I never felt a like sensation even when I breathed the purest dephlogisticated air.'[59] It drew considerable public attention, including both a supporting paper by Ingenhousz in the *Philosophical Transactions*, in which Fontanist eudiometry was endorsed, and a spectacular show by the appealing popular lecturer on natural philosophy, Pilâtre de Rozier.[60]

The significance of the issues in the inflammable air controversy was dramatised by Ingenhousz and Pilâtre. Soon after the appearance of his own paper on inflammable air in 1779, Ingenhousz published his book on the effect of light on vegetable life, incorporating his work with Fontana and specifications of the new eudiometer design developed in Paris. On the one hand, Ingenhousz and Fontana reported that the variation in eudiometric assays was now reduced to less than 1/500, 'which accuracy in exploring the degree of goodness of respirable air surpasses the exactness of judging the degree of heat and cold by the thermometer of Réaumur', a bold claim. On the other, Ingenhousz testified to a new method Fontana had developed for medical therapy: using the fact that fixed air easily dissolved in lime water, the Tuscan designed a respirator in which exhaled air would be passed through limewater to deprive it of fixed air and restore its dephlogisticated character. Ingenhousz touted this as a cheap, safe method of aerial therapy.[61] Pilâtre, in contrast, had been trained as a pharmacist in 1776–77 and was beginning courses in dramatic experimental philosophy at his new Musée in Paris. He was a disciple of Lavoisier, deeply hostile to eudiometric technology, premised as it was on the claim that the constitution of common air varied and that there was a link between phlogistication, respirability and health. When Fontana claimed that inflammable air was respirable because it was mixed with dephlogisticated air from the lungs, Pilâtre tried breathing a mixture of inflammable and dephlogisticated air, and found, according to Chaptal's later report, that 'there resulted such a terrible explosion that it was feared his teeth had been carried away'. Five years later in

[59] Fontana, 'Experiments and Observations on the Inflammable Air Breathed by Animals', *Philosophical Transactions* 69 (1779), pp. 337–61.

[60] Ingenhousz, 'Account of a New Kind of Inflammable Air', *Philosophical Transactions* 69 (1779), pp. 376–418.

[61] Ingenhousz, *Experiments upon Vegetables*, pp. 129 and 152; compare Ingenhousz, 'Observations sur la construction et l'usage de l'eudiomètre de M. Fontana', *Journal Philosophique* 26 (1785), pp. 339–59.

June 1785, Pilâtre was killed in an exploding balloon at Boulogne, travelling on an expedition to which he had been recommended on Lavoisier's authority.[62]

Fontana's response to Pilâtre's heroic trial, and his subsequent eudiometric tours, show the crisis which eudiometry now faced. In brief extracts published in Paris from a much longer manuscript despatched to the influential Duc de Chaulnes, Fontana maintained Priestleyan orthodoxy with some new, important qualifications. First, he condemned the modish notion that the air contained some vital principle as but an occultist revival of an ancient superstition.[63] Next, he asserted that respiration dephlogisticated the blood. But, last, he conceded that there were differences between airs such as inflammable air and phlogisticated air, non-respirable but non-noxious, and fixed air, both non-respirable and noxious. Yet these airs showed up as similar in the nitrous air test. The problem this implied for eudiometry was not yet fully faced. Furthermore, in seeking to replicate Pilâtre's showmanship in London, Fontana almost asphyxiated inhaling inflammable air, needing to be revived by his countryman Tiberio Cavallo.[64]

Similar troubles emerged in trials on the eudiometry of Paris and its environs conducted by Ingenhousz and Fontana during 1777 and 1778, and continued by them in London with Cavallo when Fontana went there at the end of 1778. The results of these trials were sent by Fontana to Priestley in spring 1779 and later printed in the *Philosophical Transactions*. The trials included a long series on common water, distilled water, water from the Seine and water from the spring at Arceuil. Each water was tested eudiometrically for the air trapped in it. The results were partially satisfactory. Seine water was not as healthy as Arceuil spring water, but the air trapped in distilled water was the best. This showed, as pneumatic chemists agreed, and as Lavoisier and his collaborators were beginning to question, that shaking over water dephlogisticated air. Fontana insisted this 'must certainly be one of the

[62] C. Duval, 'Pilâtre de Rozier: Chemist and First Aeronaut', *Chymia* 12 (1967), pp. 99–117; C. C. Gillispie, *The Montgolfier Brothers and the Invention of Aviation* (Princeton, 1983). For the future role of the Musée and the Paris Athénée in hygiene, see William Coleman, *Death is a Social Disease* (Madison, 1982), p. 18; B. Haines, 'The Athénée de Paris and the Bourbon Restoration', *History and Technology* 5 (1988), p. 249–72 on pp. 251 and 262.

[63] On 'ancient chemistry' compare Lavoisier, 'Mémoire sur l'existence de l'air dans l'acide nitreux' in *Receuil de mémoires sur la formation et la fabrication du salpêtre* (Paris, 1776), pp. 601–17, p. 617; Pierre Macquer, *Dictionnaire de chimie*, second edition (Paris, 1778), vol. 2, p. 352, cited in Wilda Anderson, *Between the Library and the Laboratory* (Baltimore, 1984), p. 74.

[64] Fontana, 'Lettre à M. le Duc de Chaulnes', *Observations sur la physique* 23 (1783), pp. 262–9; T. Cavallo, *Treatise on the Nature and Properties of Air* (London, 1781), pp. 344–59.

methods by which nature keeps the atmosphere in a state constantly fit to support animal life, it being certain, that the water in various circumstances must lose either a part or the whole of that air which it hath absorbed from the atmosphere'. However, severe qualifications were now issued about the basis of medical eudiometry. Fontana published a series of worries: some applied to the cosmology of which eudiometry was a part, others to the protocols of his fellow experimenters. These were condemned: no other eudiometer worked well or gave consistent results. Moreover, differences between the airs of different places, as Paris and Mont Valérien or London and Islington, were far less than differences in airs taken from the same place at different times.

Nature is not so partial as we commonly believe. She has not only given us an air almost equally good every where and at every time, but has allowed us a certain latitude or a power of living and being in health in qualities of air which differ to a certain degree.

This was a decisive abandonment of a premise of eudiometry. Fontana argued that the air did carry steams and vapours which were pathogens: vapours like 'particles of arsenic', or health-giving balms from vegetables. The truth of environmentalism remained, but medical eudiometry was abandoned: 'this state of the air cannot be known by the test of nitrous air'. There might be a time when the test would work but that time had not yet come:

This curious enquiry, together with the method, &c., are the production of this eighteenth century, and our descendants must have some gratitude for the philosophers who found out, as well as for those who improved it. If our ancestors had known and transmitted it to us, we should perhaps, at present be able to judge of one of the greatest changes of our globe, of a change which very nearly interests human life.[65]

The response to Fontana's dramatic statement was mixed. Ingenhousz had already signalled its import in his paper on inflammable air, where the preservation of aerial medicine had also been outlined. Whatever the fate of eudiometry, he wrote, the ministration of dephlogisticated air would continue to be of service to physic. During autumn 1779, Ingenhousz commissioned a good new portable eudiometric set from Benjamin Martin, one of London's best makers, and set sail from London to Ostend on a eudiometric voyage. The voyage prompted a letter to Pringle published in London in spring 1780. Ingenhousz used

[65] Fontana, 'Account of the Airs Extracted From Different Kinds of Waters', *Philosophical Transactions* 69 (1779), pp. 432–53. For French interest in tests of water see P. Cosma-Muller, 'Entre science et commerce: les eaux minérales en France à la fin de l'Ancien Régime' in J. P. Goubert (ed.), *La médicalisation de la société française 1770–1830* (Waterloo, 1982), pp. 249–62.

eudiometric determinations to argue for a wide range of medical claims: sea air was better and consumptives should take seaside holidays; trials near his lodging in Carlton House showed that trees improved aerial health; warm, summer air was unhealthy; finally, there were, *contra* Fontana, genuine variations of place, so that islands or peninsulas such as Malta or Gibraltar were noticeably healthier. The evidence for these claims was as anecdotal as technical: once again the means for propagating eudiometry was to show its correspondence to popular belief. An excellent example occurred during early December 1779 when Ingenhousz was at The Hague. His determination was that mixing one volume of Hague air and one of nitrous air gave a resultant of 1.17 measures. This was to be compared with 0.94 on Ostend Beach.

> As I had never found the common air near so bad, I had some apprehension that my eudiometer was out of order, or that something was the matter with the nitrous air. I made therefore fresh nitrous air, and repeated the experiment many times, but the result was nearly the same. In the mean time, I had the following accidental meeting. The father of the landlady of the house having been informed by the servant, that I was about some extraordinary pursuit, of which he could have no conception, was led to come and see what I did. He had scarce been a minute with me but I perceived he laboured under a severe asthma. He explained his case to me, knowing me to be a physician, and told me, *that he had passed these two days very uncomfortably, finding the air so uncommonly heavy that he could scarce draw his breath*: which convinced me, that the element was in reality become of an inferior quality.[66]

Ingenhousz worked hard, and continued to do so for the rest of his career, to establish this relationship between eudiometric determination and medical reasoning. He used the same strategy in his polemics for inoculation and against vaccination. He enlisted the eminent physician William Heberden in the cause of assessing the eudiometric effects of trees. He encouraged Martin to manufacture portable telescopic eudiometers. But others were less sanguine, and with the work of Priestley, Cavendish and Volta we witness the disassociation, though not the disappearance, of the eudiometric regime.

The authority of eudiometry depended on a set of plausible but weak inferences sustained by phlogistic cosmology and environmen-

[66] Ingenhousz, 'On the Degree of the Salubrity of the Common Air at Sea', *Philosophical Transactions* 70 (1780), pp. 354–77. For a similar case of reconciliation with popular medical belief, see *Experiments on Vegetables*, conclusion, where Ingenhousz refers to the evil effects of trees which blocked light: 'I remember to have heard people say, that it was unwholesome to sit under a walnut tree and that they found themselves affected by its shade. But I looked upon such an apprehension as one of those popular or vulgar errors which are propagated from father to son. I should now be inclined to think, that an apprehension of some mischief might not be entirely ill-grounded, when such a tree stands, as is often the case, in a narrow yard confined by the surrounding buildings.'

talist vocabulary. Pneumatic chemists now began to separate means by which phlogiston content could be assessed from the consequent inference to *virtue*. Magellan conceded that eudiometry did not reveal 'all the bad qualities of the atmosphere, only its phlogistication'. Volta had been an early advocate of this split. In August 1775, he told his friend Landriani that eudiometry was not an adequate means of assessing salubrity, even if it measured respirability.

> Imagine that you use it to examine the air of some closed room, in which someone has been sleeping or several lamps have been burning, and you then compare the night air of some open place: doubtless the eudiometer would decide in favour of the latter. Yet who does not know that the risk of contracting disease is much greater sleeping in the open air than in that of a closed room, corrupted as it would be by respiration and the lamps? I am persuaded that all the respect and devotion I have for your eudiometer, dear Marsiglio, would not tempt me to sleep with the windows open; and, further, that I would be bold enough to sleep some time not merely in closed air but in the suffocating pit of your Milan Theatre, even if the air of that place has already been found by your eudiometer no less bad than that of tombs![67]

During 1776, Volta extended this thought through a detailed investigation of the reports of Ingenhousz, Fontana and Priestley on inflammable air. By 1777, following the development of a pistol fired by the explosion of inflammable air with dephlogisticated air, Volta proposed the inflammable air eudiometer. In July 1777 he told Landriani that the explosion of any air with inflammable air measured its phlogistication, since during the process inflammable air would phlogisticate the test air. The conventional, nitrous, test he baptised 'dark combustion'; his new explosive method, which he claimed to be more accurate, he named 'luminous effervescence'. From autumn 1777 until late 1779, principally in correspondence with Priestley and with Senebier, Volta reported more crafted explosive techniques, and pushed his proposal that with this accurate eudiometry a technology now existed for the investigation of combustion, the key problem of what he saw as pneumatic chemistry.[68]

Volta's concentration on combustion and phlogistication was interpreted as a challenge to medical pneumatics, notably by Ingenhousz and Fontana. The British experimenters were more sanguine. Volta became a conspicuous beneficiary of Habsburg patronage, winning the physics chair at the reformed University of Pavia in 1778 and

[67] Belloni, 'Landriani', p. 146–8; Magellan, *Description*, third edition (1783), p. 48.

[68] W. A. Osman, 'Alessandro Volta and the Inflammable Air Eudiometer', *Annals of Science* 15 (1959), pp. 215–42. Compare Magellan's comment (1777) that Volta's early work on inflammable air should be used to help eudiometrists survey miasmic sites 'before any building is erected or country seat fixed upon' (Magellan, *Description*, pp. 30–1).

negotiating with the State for huge endowments of the laboratory, cabinet and library. He was well known to Priestley and Ingenhousz as a disciple of Boscovichean matter theory and the inventor, in summer 1775, of the dramatic 'electrophore', a device for purveying electricity which obsessed Franklinist and anti-Franklinist electricians from the late 1770s.[69] Priestley published Volta's paper on inflammable air as an appendix to his *Experiments and Observations* in 1777. In 1779 and 1780 Priestley was preoccupied with his fight with Ingenhousz over the vegetable character of the green matter he produced in experiments on the influence of light, and his correspondence with the Italians such as Volta, Landriani and Fabbroni, carried requests for their support. The nitrous air test mattered here because it was with this test that Priestley showed that the air emitted from the green matter was very good, certainly as good as dephlogisticated air. When he read in Ingenhousz's book that Fontana now claimed that eudiometric tests could not discriminate aerial differences, he was furious, seeing this as one aspect of the contest over photosynthesis and vital matter. In March 1780 he told Shelburne's secretary, Benjamin Vaughan, that:

> I have been busy with some *experiments* and among other things have satisfied myself that it is altogether without reason that the Abbé Fontana (in Dr Ingenhousz) pretends that the measure of *good* and *bad* nitrous air comes to the same thing in his method of applying the test. I am astonished, and provoked, at the little care with which some persons make experiments and the confidence with which they report them.[70]

This criticism was amplified in a thorough paper given to the Royal Society by Cavendish in 1783, reporting trials performed during 1781. Cavendish pointed out that eudiometric determination would be more accurate if a way could be devised to bubble the test air into the nitrous air rather than add it in bulk. Fontana had tried to avoid bubbles in his method. Since phlogiston, according to Priestley and Cavendish, absorbed dephlogisticated air continuously, bubbling was necessary to correct for this. Cavendish gave very detailed protocols for his new machine: nitrous air should only be prepared from copper; weight not volume measures should be employed; nitrous air must always be present in excess. Common air and phlogisticated air should be used as the fixed points of the eudiometric scale. Common air was conventionally taken as 1, phlogisticated air as zero, giving a reading of 4.8 for dephlogisticated air. The implication of these fresh designs was that

[69] Schofield, *Scientific Autobiography of Joseph Priestley*, p. 157; J. L. Heilbron, *Elements of Early Modern Physics* (Berkeley, 1982), p. 210; Ingenhousz, 'Improvements in Electricity', *Philosophical Transactions* 69 (1779), pp. 661–73.

[70] Schofield, *Scientific Autobiography of Joseph Priestley*, p. 181.

the machine was no longer a eudiometer as the Fontanists understood it. It could not detect really phlogisticated air, but was now to be used to determine the type of air in question, not its degree of phlogistication. The composition of any air was uniform, so that aerial structure was a question of quantitative chemistry. 'Our sense of smelling can, in many cases, perceive infinitely smaller variations in the purity of the air than can be perceived by the nitrous test', Cavendish concluded.[71]

Cavendish's paper accompanied a violent controversy between Magellan, Priestley's long-time ally and correspondent, and Cavallo, representative of the 'Fontanists'. This fight centred on the right way of making eudiometric trials, but it also touched on all the social and intellectual troubles of pneumatics. There were suggestions that the conservative President of the Royal Society, Joseph Banks, was hostile to Priestley and Magellan and so helped aid Cavallo's medical campaign. Cavallo and Magellan were noted designers of pneumatic machines and fought for market leadership. Cavallo emphasised the need for 'regular management' of such instruments as the key to their successful use by physicians.[72] The abandonment of medical eudiometry by Priestley and Cavendish, and their acceptance of Volta's methodology for investigating combustion, was amply demonstrated during the water controversy with Lavoisier in 1783–4, for in this exchange the British started using explosive eudiometry to demonstrate that elementary water lost its phlogiston. Thomas Day, fellow member of the Lunar Society, argued in 1784 that eudiometry could not be relied upon as a means of managing polluted airs either in medicine or agriculture.[73]

The division between therapeutics and experimental natural philosophy seemed to be the division between the trained nose of the physician and the precision instrumentation of the philosopher. This split was decisive, and most environmentalists soon abandoned the technology completely by the end of the 1780s. Typical was the work of

[71] Cavendish, 'An Account of a New Eudiometer', *Philosophical Transactions* 73 (1783), pp. 106 ff.

[72] Priestley, *Experiments and Observations* (London, 1777), vol. 3, p. 379; Magellan, *Description*, third edition (1783), p. 67; Cavallo, *Treatise*, pp. 326–33. For Banks's hostility to Cavallo, see *Autobiography of Arthur Young*, p. 151.

[73] Thomas Day, *Considerations on Different Ways of Removing Confined or Infectious Air* (Maidstone, 1784), pp. 28–9. For the water controversy, see Cavendish, 'Experiments on Air', *Philosophical Transactions* 74 (1784), pp. 119–53; J. B. Meusnier and A. L. Lavoisier, 'Mémoire où l'on prouve par la décomposition de l'eau, que ce fluide n'est point une substance simple', *Mémoires de l'Académie Royale des Sciences* (1781; pb. 1784), pp. 269–83; J. R. Partington, *History of Chemistry*, vol. 3 (London, 1962), pp. 325–38; Holmes, *Lavoisier*, chapter 7.

the Swiss naturalist Jean Senebier, who argued against the nitrous air test in his own crucial work on the exchange between fixed and vital air in plant respiration.[74] The enterprises of environmental medicine did not depend on eudiometry's truth, but the meanings given to terms such as 'virtue' and 'goodness' did derive explicitly from that vocabulary. Different audiences became customers for different techniques of quantifying virtue and health. The importance of these audiences for the varieties of eudiometry was hilariously dramatised in the Florentine response to the water controversy. In 1784 Fontana read reports of Lavoisier's alleged 'decomposition' of water into inflammable air in a heated iron pipe.[75] Fontana replicated the trials but supported Priestley in denying that they showed the decomposition of water. A local physician, Francesco Giorgi, claimed that water did decompose, but into respirable rather than inflammable air. The dispute between Fontana and Giorgi, used by many as a Galilean allegory for the crisis wracking church–state relations in Tuscany, reached the law courts in 1785 amidst wild public enthusiasm.[76] This was an apt conclusion of the efforts to make Fontanist eudiometry a State-backed technology of reform; it had become a source of dangerous ridicule.

CONCLUSION: THE ATMOSPHERE OF REFORM

What of eudiometry's fate? Medical eudiometry is commonly seen as a noble failure situated at the meeting-point of two highly successful enterprises: analytic chemistry and public hygiene. Historians of chemistry note that the original eudiometers were designed to assay moral and medical welfare, but point out that eventually 'correct' views prevailed, leaving the eudiometric machines as excellent means of determining the oxygen content of gas samples, usually by firing or exploding the gas in the way that Volta developed.[77] Similarly, histori-

[74] J. Senebier, *Recherches sur l'influence de la lumière solaire* (Geneva, 1783), pp. 297–301. For the development of *chemical eudiometry* after the 1780s, including the use of assays with phosphorus, hydrogen and potassium sulphide, see Partington, *History of Chemistry*, vol. 3, p. 325; Watermann, 'Eudiometrie'.

[75] J. Meusnier and A. Lavoisier, 'Extrait d'un mémoire où l'on prouve par la decomposition de l'eau que ce fluide n'est point une substance simple', *Observations sur la Physique* 24 (1784), pp. 368–80; Fontana, 'Extrait d'expériences sur la decomposition de l'eau', *Observations sur la physique* 27 (1785), pp. 228–9.

[76] Knoefel, *Felice Fontana*, p. 84; Cochrane, *Florence*, p. 430.

[77] Compare George Wilson, *Life of Henry Cavendish* (London, 1851), pp. 230–31: 'We are still as much in need of an eudiometer, properly so called, as the contemporaries of Priestley and Cavendish were . . . Medicine, as well as meteorology and chemistry, have the deepest interest in such inquiries, and we may anticipate the period when a laboratory will form an essential part of our meteorological observatories.'

ans of public health and hygiene reform note that for a brief moment chemists believed that a quantitative scale of healthy air could be established, a faith abandoned when 'the failure of this device' bred pessimism about 'the environment–disease association.'[78] In both stories, eudiometry appears as a pause on the path to disinterested rational understanding of the environment. These stories neglect the range of interests, political, commercial and moral, which furthered eudiometry's career. The different forms of pneumatic medicine failed or succeeded with the political movements which sustained them. Leopold's reformism was fatally undermined in the violent priest-and-peasant riot in Florence in June 1790; Priestley's rational Dissent was challenged in the church-and-king riot in Birmingham in July 1791. Under Revolutionary and Napoleonic administrations, there is considerable evidence of the survival of respectable medical eudiometry. Italian naturalists and members of the Société Royale de Médecine kept on searching for assessment techniques to determine the quality of noxious airs given off by human bodies. Volta's students sewed young beggars into water-soaked sacks to gather their fumes before testing.[79] Distinguished chemists such as Gay-Lussac, Dumas and Leblanc continued the search for quantitative methods of matching gas level to health in air samples. After the Restoration, and especially under the July monarchy, this campaign gained important allies amongst the new Paris statisticians, political economists and hygienists such as Louis-René Villermé, and was sustained until at least the 1840s.[80]

The complex of medical management and aerial chemistry which was used to make this authority won new power and fresh constituencies. Corbin rightly stresses the intriguing contrast between the search for physico-chemical measures and the triumph of the physicians' sense of smell as a means of divining disease. 'Miasma remained elusive.'[81] Did medical eudiometry fail because the expert technicians could not match physicians' intuitions about stench? This would be a convincing story only if chemists had as their sole aim the scientific rationalisation of common-sense experience of foul air. But much more was at stake. An ensemble of juridical and ideological themes helped sustain the eudiometric tours: alliance with enlightened despotism; integration with cameralist management of the public body; the

[78] Riley, *Eighteenth century campaign*, p. 51.

[79] Louis Jurine, 'Mémoire sur les avantages que la médecine peut retirer des eudiomètres', *Mémoires de la Société Royale de Médecine* 10 (1789), pp. 19–100.

[80] Corbin, *The Foul and the Fragrant*, pp. 42–3 and 113. For hygiene after the Restoration see William Coleman, *Death is a Social Disease* (Madison, 1982), pp. 14–24.

[81] Corbin, *The Foul and the Fragrant*, p. 55.

search for new markets for complicated glassware and techniques; the appeal to polite audiences of journalists, academics and civil servants. Once this ensemble is understood, then the appropriate accompaniments and successors of eudiometry become apparent: the tradition of military medicine developed in John Pringle's *Diseases of the Army* (6th edn, 1815), the contest between reformist inoculators and the novel techniques of Jennerian vaccination, and, decisively, Benthamite reform and Chadwick's 'sanitary idea.'[82] Here the early interest Bentham displayed in eudiometry takes on great significance.

In 1774, as we have shown, Bentham began corresponding with Priestley on medical and chemical philosophy and condemned Scheele for his 'metaphysical' inquiry as to whether 'fire be a real or fictitious entity'. He identified the close connection between the forms of chemical nomenclature and the flourishing of corrupt fantasy. 'In speaking of any *pneumatic* (or say *immaterial* or *spiritual*) object, no name has ever been employed, that had not first been employed as the name of some *material* (or say *corporeal*) one. Lamentable have been the confusion and darkness produced by taking the names of *fictions* for the names of *real* entities'. Utilitarianism expelled what Bentham called 'the pestilential breath of fiction' from society and legal discourse: pneumatic chemistry expelled it from nature and natural philosophy.[83] Hygiene became a key principle of Bentham's vision of civil order. In his mature survey of that order, the *Constitutional Code*, the 'Health Minister' was to discharge a range of eudiometric functions: the 'exemplificational-antimalarial function' involved the control of dangerous exhalations; other roles included registration of changes in the air and its relation with health. These were, perhaps, Hippocratic commonplaces: their management and the knowledge which sustained them were not. The utilitarian State was to be compared with the strategy of medical police fostered by the German cameralists, for example. Where authorities such as Justi, Sonnenfels and Frank argued during the period 1750–80 for a centralised State bureaucracy invigilating social and moral conduct in order to control welfare and population growth, Priestley and Bentham proffered an

[82] P. Mathias, 'Swords and Ploughshares: The Armed Forces, Medicine and Public Health in the Late Eighteenth Century' in *The Transformation of England* (London, 1979), chapter 14; M. Fitzpatrick, 'Science and Society in the Enlightenment', *Enlightenment and Dissent* 4 (1985), pp. 83–106; Van der Pas, 'Ingenhousz–Jenner Correspondence'. For pneumatic criticisms of Jenner, see Thomas Beddoes, *Contributions to Physical and Medical Knowledge* (Bristol, 1799), pp. 387–402.

[83] *Correspondence of Bentham*, vol. 1, pp. 214 and 216; vol. 2, p. 315; for pneumatic objects, see Bowring, *Bentham's Works*, vol. 8, pp. 119–20.

account of philosophical necessity and reasoned self-interest in civil society; the role of the State was as guarantor of that society, not as its despot. The progress of society was safely left in the hands of expert philosophers and medical managers whose legitimacy was derived from their understanding of the natural powers, not from their subservience to the civil powers.[84]

Bentham's campaign was to go further: the legislator could wisely extend the accomplishments of the medical manager. In the 1770s he argued that 'the art of legislation is but the art of healing practised upon a large scale. It is the common endeavour of both to relieve men from the miseries of life. But the physician relieves them one by one: the legislator by millions at a time.' The accumulation of numbers and the collective origin of social pathology were essential principles of reformist medical management. Bentham insisted that 'this is not a fanciful analogy': it was to be taken as a literal account of the managers' work.[85] 'Medicine, commonly so called . . . has for its basis the observations of the axioms of pathology, commonly so-called. Morals is the medicine of the soul. The science of legislation is the practical part of this medicine.' Hence, 'mental pathology' should provide the axioms for the science of legislation: 'God forbid that any disease in the constitution of a state should be without its remedy.'[86]

Medical eudiometry was an important example of this understand-

[84] For the Health Minister, see Bowring, *Bentham's Works*, vol. 9, pp. 439–45. For medical police and cameralism, see George Rosen, *From Medical Police to Social Medicine: Essays on the History of Health Care* (New York, 1974), pp. 120–41 and 189–90; Michel Foucault, 'The Politics of Health in the Eighteenth Century' in C. Gordon (ed.), *Power–Knowledge: Selected Interviews and Other Writings by Michel Foucault* (New York, 1980), pp. 166–82; Marc Raeff, *The Well Ordered Police State: Social and Institutional Change Through Law in the Germanies and Russia, 1600–1800* (New Haven, 1983), pp. 119–35. See Benjamin Spector, 'Jeremy Bentham: His Influence Upon Medical Thought and Legislation', *Bulletin of the History of Medicine* 37 (1963), pp. 25–42. In view of the eudiometric interests shared by Bentham and the *philosophes*, the question of Chadwick's 'debt' to Bentham or to French hygienists becomes otiose: see A. F. La Berge, 'Edwin Chadwick and the French Connection', *Bulletin of the History of Medicine* 62 (1988), pp. 23–41; S. E. Finer, 'The Transmission of Benthamite Ideas' in G. Sutherland (ed.), *Studies in the Growth of Nineteenth Century Government* (London, 1972), pp. 11–32.

[85] M. P. Mack, *Jeremy Bentham: An Odyssey of Ideas, 1748–92* (London, 1962), p. 264, citing Bentham MSS, University College, London, 27.13. This was just the sense of Southwood Smith's parliamentary evidence in 1840: the Government must relieve the poor of 'the sources of poison and disease', for otherwise 'the effect is the same as if twenty or thirty thousand of them were annually taken out of their wretched homes and put to death' (C. L. Lewes, *Southwood Smith: A Retrospect* (London, 1898), p. 104).

[86] For Bentham on the medical comparison, see Bowring, *Bentham's Works*, vol. 1, pp. 304–5, 367 and vol. 2, p. 204; R. Harrison, *Bentham* (London, 1983), p. 141, citing Bentham MSS, University College, London, 32.6; Mack, *Jeremy Bentham*, pp. 264–6. For 'mental pathology', see Bentham, *Introduction to the Principles of Morals and Legislation* (Oxford, 1876), p. vii; for the cure of disease in the state, see Bentham, *Fragment on Government*, p. 224. Compare Richardson, *Death, Dissection and the Destitute*, pp. 107–14.

ing. The Benthamite reforms of the 1830s testify eloquently to this fact. Edwin Chadwick was Bentham's amanuensis at the time when his master was composing the *Constitutional Code*. Chadwick's 1842 *Report on the Sanitary Condition of the Labouring Population* was a homage to the connections between management and medical meteorology which Bentham had discussed: 'bad ventilation or overcrowding, and the consequences on the moral habits' were demonstrably based on 'an original cause we have high scientific authority for stating to be easily and economically controllable.' As Roger Cooter has suggested, Bentham's loyal disciples among reforming physicians made the atmosphere the key site of medical management: Cooter cites the work of Southwood Smith, a convert from Calvinism to Priestley's Unitarianism and the personal physician to Bentham. Southwood Smith's anticontagionism refused to speak of disease-causing miasmas and refused to define the aerial principle which might be pathogenic. In his *Treatise on Fever* (1830), he argued that disease was spread via air because 'poverty in her hut . . . striving with all her might to keep out the pure air and to increase the heat, imitates Nature but too successfully.' As a result, 'penury and ignorance can create a mortal plague.' At the hands of the Benthamite anticontagionists, the air became the proper concern of expert managers and the way to moralise society. Using lessons their master had learnt from Enlightenment chemists in Wiltshire and Tuscany, these reformers reckoned that the human and the social body should be engrossed by pneumatics.[87]

[87] Edwin Chadwick, *Report on the Sanitary Condition of the Labouring Population of Great Britain* (1842), ed. M. W. Flinn (Edinburgh, 1965), pp. 29–43 and 167; Thomas Southwood Smith, *Treatise on Fever* (London, 1830), p. 324; Roger Cooter, 'Anticontagionism: History's Medical Record', in P. Wright and A. Treacher (eds.), *The Problem of Medical Knowledge: Examining the Social Construction of Medicine* (Edinburgh, 1982), pp. 87–108. Compare Southwood Smith, *Treatise*, p. 349: 'Vegetable and animal matter, during the process of putrefaction, give off a principle or give origin to a new compound, which, when applied to the human body, produces the phenomena constituting fever'. See F. N. L. Poynter, 'Thomas Southwood Smith – the Man', *Proceedings of the Royal Society of Medicine* 55 (1962), pp. 381–92.

Index

Abraham, J., 262n, 272n
Absolutism, 67, 87, 89, 90
Adam, 119
Adams, J., 278n
Addington, A., 145 and n, 146 and n, 147, 151
Aikin, Dr J., 218, 220, 225, 227, 228, 230, 234, 237, 245, 247, 253, 264n, 278n
Aikin, Mr J., 234
air, inflammable, 306–14; nitrous, 306–14; and eudiometry, 300–6
Aiton, E., 71n
Alberti, M., 84
Alexander, G., 187n
Allan, D., 174n, 184n
Altmann, E., 80n
Akenside, M., 142
America, North, 194–216
Ammerman, D., 212n
Amsterdam, 42
Amyand, C., 30
Anderson, J., 33n
Anderson, R., 58n, 64n, 283n, 284n
Anderson, W., 308n
Andrew, J., 144 and n
Anglicanism, 21, 166, 167n
animism, 103–10
animists, 90, 101, 103, 104, 106–7, 110
Anne, Queen, 21, 23, 167
Apothecaries' Hall, 277
Aquinas, St Thomas, 45, 107
Arbuthnot, J., 9, 29, 30, 131, 177
Aretaeus, 49, 55
Aristotle, 45, 107, 110, 117, 119
Armet, H., 60n
Armstrong, G., 255, 256
Armstrong, J., 255n
Arndt, J., 89, 91
Arnold, G., 73, 74, 79 and n
Aronson, K., 159n
Ashcroft, M., 142n
Ashplant, T., 5n
Astruc, J., 103, 104, and n
atomists, 79
Atterbury, Bishop, F., 32
Augustine, St, 107
Austen, J., 84
Aveling, J., 35n
Ayers, M., 167n
Aylett, G., 154, 155 and n, 160
Ayn, G., 84n

Babington, W., 278n
Bacon, F., 49, 99, 100, 112, 114, 116 and n, 117, 118, 124, 137, 191n, 221, 288
Baddeley, J., 254
Baglivi, G., 112, 114, 115–18, 120–6, 129, 136
Bajollet, J., 104n, 105
Baldick, R., 142n
Bancroft, E., 278n
Bandini, S., 295n
Banks, Sir J., 313 and n
Baptists, 228
Barber-Surgeons' Company, 196, and *see* Surgeon's, Company of
Barclay, D., 225
Barclay, family of, 260, 263n
Barfoot, M., 165n
Baron, J., 248n, 249n
Barrie, J. M., 41
Barry, J., 171n
Bartholin, T., 47
Bartram, J., 214n, 215
Basker, G., 150n
Baxby, D., 24n, 236n
Baylies, W., 149, 150 and n, 151 and n, 155
Beccaria, C., 294, 295n
Bechler, R., 38n
Beddoes, T., 285 and n, 316n

Bell, W., 204n, 206
Bellers, J., 16, 18
Bellini, L., 129
Belloni, L., 292n, 296n, 300n, 311n
Benjamin, B., 232n, 233n
Bentham, J., 282, 283 and n, 284 and n, 291, 292, 306, 316, 317 and n, 318
Bentley, R., 185n
Benwell, J., 155n
Benz, E., 80n
Berg, A. La, 317n
Berg, F., 127
Berkeley, Bishop, 165–93
Berkeley, D., 214n
Berkely, E., 214n
Berlin, 68, 73, 83
Berman, A., 305n
Berman, D., 166n, 167n, 192 and n, 193n
Bernouilli, D., 102, 129
Betham-Edwards, M., 291n
Bickerstaff, J., 41n
Bickley, A., 261n
Bigg, T., 146 and n, 147
Black, J., 286
Blackmore, Sir R., 29, 30
Blackstone, W., 284 and n
Blair, W., 278n
Blake, J., 197, 198n, 205n, 209n, 210n
Blandy, M., 147 and n
Blanton, W., 203n, 205n
Bligh, Revd R., 159n
Bloch, M., 33n
Blondin, T., 70n
Blundell, N., 161
Boerhaave, H., 40–66, 75, 83, 98 and n, 101, 105, 121, 129, 164, 175, 176 and n, 182, 190, 191
Boerhaavians, 108
Böhme, J., 74n, 79 and n, 89
Bolingbroke, Viscount H., 22
Bond, T., 200, 206
Bonelli, M., 296n
Bonham, T., 141 and n
Borelli, G., 102, 105
Bornkham, H., 72n, 78n
Bossy, J., 140n
Bostock, J., 227, 234
Boulton, M., 158, 290, 291
Boulton, R., 157 and n
Bowles, G., 171n
Bowring, J., 283n, 316n, 317n
Boyle, Hon. R., 48, 49, 51 and n, 54, 55, 94, 96, 185 and n, 293
Boylston, Z., 209
Bracken, Harry, 192n
Bracken, Henry, 30n, 140n, 148 and n, 155 and n, 161–4
Braddyll, R., 163
Brady, Dr S., 30, 31
Bradley, L., 29n
Bradley, T., 278n
Bramble, Squire, 281n
Brandenburg–Prussia, 73, 83, 84, 90
Breithaupt, J., 89
Brennan, T., 160
Brigden, T., 21n
Brock, C., 199n, 200n
Brock, W., 200n
Brockliss, L., 112n
Bromfield, W., 154 and n, 155 and n, 156, 160
Brooke, R., 214
Brooks, C., 16n
Brown, A., 49n, 113n, 140n
Brown, J., 265n
Brown, P., 231n
Brown, T., 113n, 130n, 173n
Brownrigg, W., 286, 287n
Bryan, R., 208
Buchan, W., 177n, 201, 215
Buddeus, J., 83 and n
Buer, M., 236n
Buffon, 300
Burke, E., 247
Burke, P., 160n
Burnby, J., 37n
Burton, J., 144 and n
Burton, W., 43n, 44n, 48n, 49n, 56 and n
Bury St Edmunds, 151, 153
Butler, S., 157n, 222n, 224n, 242n
Butterfield, H., 4n
Butterfield, T., 161, 162
Bynum, W., 36n, 49n, 75n, 142n, 199n, 221n, 279 and n
Byrom, Dr J., 30, 31, 32

Cadbury, family of, 263n
Cajori, F., 131n, 132
Cambray, N., 105n
Campbell, R., 57n
Cant, R., 57n
Cantor, G., 105n, 165n, 171n, 186 and n
Cappel, Dr, 245
Carl, J., 79n, 80, 82 and n
Carlisle, G., 161, 162
Carolina, South, 194
Caroline, Princess, 179
Carpanetto, D., 294n, 295n
Carroll, C., 199
Carstares, W., 60, 61, 62, 64
Carter, E., 179
Carter, L., 202n
Cartesians, 51, 114, 129, 130, 133, and *see* Descartes
Cash, A., 144n
Cash, P., 202n

Cassedy, J., 231n
Catherine the Great, 1
Catherine II, Empress, 236
Catholic church, 79
Cavallo, T., 308, 313 and n
Cavendish, H., 287, 292, 296, 310, 312, 313 and n, 314n
Chadwick, E., 316, 318 and n
Chamberlen, family, 35
Chambers, E., 30
Chandos, Duke of, 34
Chapman, E., 30n
Charitable Society, of Westminster, 15–21, 23, 24, 38
Charles II, 42n
Chartism, 7
Chaulnes, Duc de, 308 and n
Chaytor, M., 5n
Chesterfield, Earl of, 149
Chester Smallpox Society, 218, 227, 240, 241–3
Cheyne, G., 102, 107, 131, 171n, 173
Chiarugi, V., 295
Chicoyneau, F., 103, 113, 114, 115, 120, 136; father and son, 104
childbirth, 2, 34–9
Chirac, P., 113, 114 and n, 115, 120, 125, 136
Chitnis, A., 57n
Choulant, L., 86, 92n
Christianson, E., 196n, 197n, 199n, 202n, 204n
Christopherson, P. 161, 162
Cicero, 50
Clark, A., 5
Clark, Mr G., 156n
Clark, James, 245
Clark, Jonathan, 5n
Clark, Sir G., 138, 145, 178n, 260n
Clarke, S., 30, 167, 168, 187n
Clark-Kennedy, A., 14n
Clayton, Revd J., 214
Cleland, A., 138 and n, 148, 149 and n, 151
Clement of Rome, 45
Clutterbuck, H., 278n
Cochrane, E., 295n, 314n
Cockburn, Revd P., 17, 21n, 22
Cockburn, W., 208n
Cohen, I. B., 185n
Colbatch, Dr J., 17, 18
Colden, C., 186, 200, 210 and n
Coleman, W., 308, 315n
Coley, N., 287n
Collegium Medicum, 83
Colley, L, 21n
Collins, A., 167 and n, 168
Colquhoun, P., 5, 6, 254n
Combe, C., 278n
Condillac, 1
Condorcet, 304
Cook, J., 174
Cooke, H., 138, 141n
Cooter, R., 318 and n
Cope, Sir Z., 255n
Corbin, A., 304n, 315 and n
Cork, 146
Corresponding Society, 7
Corsini, A., 295n
Cosma-Muller, P., 309
Cotes, R., 130n, 132n
Covenanters, 59
Cowper, W., 130n, 173
Crawford, J., 60
Crosland, M., 282n
Cullen, W., 57n, 65, 166, 218, 220–3, 225, 227, 230–3, 237, 239, 240, 241, 243, 245, 252, 257, 266 and n, 267
Cunningham, A., 62n, 88n, 113n, 122n, 140n
Currie, J., 218, 220, 225, 228, 229 and n, 230, 241, 245, 247, 248, 253, 257

Darby, family of, 260, 263 and n
Darlington, W., 214n
Dartmouth, Lord, 225
Darwin, E., 158, 159n, 285
Darwin, R., 158, 159 and n
Daston, L., 33n
Dawson, J., 219, 220, 225, 230, 244, 245
Day, E., 20n
Day, T., 313 and n
Deacon, T., 144
De Gorter, D., 100
De Gorter, J., 99 and n, 100, 101n, 102 and n, 106, 110
Deidier, A., 103, 104 and n, 105, 113 and n, 114, 136
Delarbre, L., 105n
Democritus, 50, 55
Denman, T., 35
Derham, W., 94
Desaguliers, J., 175 and n
Descartes, 45, 49, 54, 77, 88, 95, 129, 133, and *see* Cartesians
Deventer, H. van, 35, 36, 38
Deventerians, 36, 37
Dickinson, H., 168n, 170n
Diderot, 1
Dimsdale, T., 236
Dippel, J., 73 and n, 79n, 80n, 82 and n
dispensaries, 254–80
Dissent, 3, 217–53; Dissenting Academy at Warrington, 225, 234
Dissenters, 144, 157, 257, 258, 259, 263, 271, 278 and n, 279, 282
Dixon, H., 265n
Dobson, M., 220, 227, 229n, 232, 234, 237, 241

Dod, Dr P., 30
Donnison, J., 14n, 34n, 35n, 148n
Donovan, A., 220n, 239n, 240n
Douglass, W., 198, 199
Dover, T., 177
Drélincourt, C., 46
Dreyhaupt, C. von, 73n
Drummond, G., 57n, 61, 62, 64, 65
Duffy, J., 205n, 209n, 210n
Dulieu, L. 112n, 113n, 127, 133n
Dumas, J.-B., 315
Duncombe, W.W., 179
Dunlop, I., 60n
Dunster, H., 197
Duval, C., 308n

Eckart, W., 62n
Edinburgh, 40–66; Philosophical Society of, 222
Edwards, G., 278n
Edwards, J., 186
Eggleston, E., 215n
Egmont, Lady, 179
Ehrard, J., 304n
Einem, J.J. von, 73n, 74n
eirenicism, 48, 50, 51, 55, 56, 58
Eklund, J., 183 and n
Elers, H., 74 and n, 79n
Eliot, J., 197
Elliot, J., 217n, 253n
Ellis, R., 116n
Enlightenment, 1, 2, 3, 78, 88, 110, 281–318; Enlightened despotism, 292–318; French, 136, 137; German, 67–87; Lombard, 281; Scottish, 57, 62, 65, 221; in Montpellier, 111–37
Epicurus, 54
Erasmus, 44, 45
Erb, C., 94n
Erfurt, 73, 74
Erlam, H., 64n, 65n
Estes, J., 202n
eudiometry, 281–318
Evans, A., 11n
Evanson, Revd E., 159n

Fabbroni, G., 302, 312
Falconer, Dr W., 220, 223, 224, 248
Falconer, T., 223, 227, 228n, 232, 237, 238
Fallopius, G., 47
Farr, A., 181n
Farrall, L., 230n
Faulkner, G., 179
Ferrall, S., 142n
Field, J., 265n
Fielding, H., 5, 6, 7, 8
Finer, E., 317n
Fitzgerald, Revd, 22
Fitzpatrick, M., 316n
Flage, D., 192n
Fletcher, J., 144n
Fleure, H., 225n
Flinn, M., 318n
Foisil, M., 304n
Fontana, F., 292 and n, 294 and n, 296, 300, 301 and n, 302, 303, 304, 305, 306, 307 and n, 309 and n, 310, 311, 312, 314 and n
Foot, J., 156 and n
Forbes, E., 11n, 172n
Forbes, T., 217n
Forbinger, S., 86 and n
Force, J., 168n
Ford, E., 278n
Foster, E., 279
Foster, J., 166n
Fothergill, A., 219
Fothergill, J., 139, 142, 204, 214, 218, 219, 225, 226 and n, 228–31, 236n, 237, 257–60 and n, 264, 273, 278n, 280
Fothergill, S., 259
Foucault, M., 11n, 74n, 283n, 317n
Fox, G., 261 and n
Fox, R., 225n, 226n, 227n, 229n, 236n
Francis II, Emperor, 294
Francke, A., 67, 73n, 79, 89, 90, 96n
Frank, H., 255n
Frank, J.-P., 316
Franklin, B., 225, 293, 300
Frederick III, of Prussia, 89
Frederick the Great, of Prussia, 1, 89
Frederick William I, of Prussia, 67, 68, 89, 96
Freind, J., 32, 113n, 114, 130n, 173n
Freke, J., 38n, 185
French, R., 11n, 33n, 50n, 97n, 102n, 103n, 105n, 122n, 171n
Frerichs, I., 71n, 77n
Frewen, T., 158
Frewin, R., 145, 146
Frowde, Mrs, 17
Fry, family of, 263n
Fulbrook, M., 89n, 93n

Galen, 2, 55, 98, 107, 109, 134
Galenists, 108, 129
Garrioch, D., 160
Gassendi, P., 50
Gaub, J., 98, 101, 102, 106
Gaustad, E., 169
Gay-Lussac, J.-L., 315
Geismar, M. von, 73n
Gelfand, T., 213n
George I, of England, 22, 24, 33, 38, 144

George III, of England, 242
George, D., 5, 6, 7, 8, 9, 10, 36
Germany, 72
Gerth, H., 144n
Geyer-Kordesch, J., 62n, 67n, 72n, 75n, 78n, 91n, 92n
Gibson, E., 265n
Gichtel, G. 73 and n, 79
Gillispie, C., 11n, 308n
Giorgi, F., 314
Gluckman, M., 140 and n
Goetz, J., 85 and n
Gohl, J., 84
Goldman, L., 141 and n
Golinski, J., 176n, 183n, 291n
Goodall, C., 157n
Goodwin, A., 285n
Gordon, C., 317n
Gotha-Eisenach, 73
Göttingen, 40
Goubert, J., 309n
Graeme (Graham), W., 57, 65n
Grafton, Duke of, 156
Granshaw, L., 24n
Grant, Sir A., 60n
Gray, S., 175
Gray, W. 21n
Grayling, A., 166n
Gregory, David, 171,
Gregory James, 221n
Green, J., 202n
Greene, D., 171n
Grew, N., 214
Grey, T., 179
Grieve, J., 270n
Griffenhagen, G., 202n
Grosvenor, Earl of, 223
Grosvenor, family of, 222, 223
Grotius, H., 96n
Grubb, I., 228n
Grünberg, P., 74n
Guerra, F., 208n
Guerrini, A. 102 and n, 171 and n

Hacking, I., 29n
Haigh, E., 111n
Haighton, J., 278n
Haines, B., 308n
Hales, Revd S., 102, 103n, 107, 131, 174 and n, 175, 183 and n, 184 and n, 286 and n, 287, 293, 300
Halle, 67, 73, 74, 78, 82, 83, 89, 90, 94, 97, 109, 110
Haller, A. von, 40, 71 and n, 83, 97n, 106n, 131n, 132n, 133n, 300
Halley, E., 186
Hamilton, B., 138n
Hannaway, C., 304n
Hannaway, O., 304n
Hansell, P., 18n
Hanway, J., 5, 6, 7, 8
Haresnape, S., 161, 163
Harris, B., 222n
Harley, D., 31, 140n
Harnak, A. 67
Harrison, J., 14
Harrison, R., 317n
Hartley, D., 149, 284
Hart-Myers, J., 278n
Hartston, W., 255n
Harvard, N., 159n
Harvey, W., 49, 55, 75
Hauksbee, F., 175
Hawes, J., 172n
Hawkins, Sir J., 139 and n, 142 and n, 155, 156
Haygarth, J., 25, 34, 217–53, 257, 258
Haygarth, J. (the younger), 230n
Hays, J., 278n
Hearne, T., 21n
Heath, D., 116n
Heberden, W., 226n, 242n, 310
Heilbron, J., 312n
Heimann, P., 172 and n, 190 and n
Hemingway, J., 223n
Henry, T., 225
Herder, J., 83
Hermann, P., 47
Herring, Archbishop, 179
Hicks, G., 192n
Highlanders, 61
Highmore, A., 254n
Higson, P., 226n
Hindesley, Bishop, 184
Hinrichs, H., 79n
Hippocrates, 46, 47, 48, 49, 50, 51, 54, 55, 56, 107, 109, 114, 134, 164
Hoadly, B., 143
Hoare, H., 17, 20, 21n, 22, 23
Hodge, J., 105n, 171n, 186n
Hoffmann, F., 75, 88–110
Hogarth, W., 7
Holbrooke, W., 148
Holmes, F., 289n, 290n, 305n, 313n
Holmes, G., 145n, 178n, 205n
Holmes, T., 163
Holt, R., 148, 228n
Hooper, R., 278n
Hope, J., 266n
Horace, 51n
Horwitz, H., 21n
hospitals, 2,
  Bath, 149, 150, 151
  Bristol, 156

hospitals, (*cont.*)
  Brownlow St., 13, 36
  Chelsea, 156
  Chester Infirmary, 25, 222, 223, 224, 229, 248
  Christ's, 145
  Cork Infirmary, 146
  Foundling, 6
  General, 14
  Greenwich, 156
  Guy's, 164
  Hôtel Dieu, 163
  Lock, 11
  London, 14, 164
  Lying-in, 11, 13
  Manchester, 222, 224n
  Middlesex, 36
  New York, 204
  Philadelphia, 195, 204
  Queen Charlotte's, 14n
  St Bartholomew's, 24 and n, 164
  St George's, 14, 15, 17, 259
  St Thomas's, 24 and n, 163, 270n
  Smallpox Inoculation, 11, 34, 236
  Westminster, 10–24
  Westminster Lying-in, 14
  Winchester, 11
Hospitals, voluntary, 10–24
Houston, J., 41 and n
Howard, John, 6, 25, 226 and n, 228, 229 and n, 264 and n, 265 and n, 266, 267, 280
Howard, Joseph, 208
Howard, L., 11n
Howell, J., 42 and n
Hoyme, L., 206n
Huguenots, 56, 73
Hulme, N., 270n, 278n
Humane Society, 219
Humble, J., 18n
Hume, D., 166n, 221
Hunt, T., 272
Hunter, W., 34, 35, 199 and n, 221n, 279n
Hutcheson, F., 109n, 68n
Hutchinson, J., 186
Hutton, Revd J., 21n, 22

Ideler, K., 69n, 82n, 87
Ihde, A., 287n
improvement, 4–39, esp. 4–10, 136
Ingenousz, J., 285n, 292, 293n, 302, 304n, 305–9, 310 and n, 311, 312 and n, 316n
Ingram, D., 155 and n, 156
Innes, J., 65
Innes, Revd A., 22
inoculation, 24–34
Irvine, W., 220, 245

Jackson, J., 142n
Jacob, J., 48, 167n
Jacob, M., 33n, 167n
Jacobites, 7, 31, 32, 33, 59, 61, 62, 144, 168, 170
Jacobs, J., 42n
James II, of England (and VII of Scotland) 24, 42, 58, 59, 60
James, R., 177
Jarcho, S., 206n, 210n
Jena, 67, 73, 74, 76
Jenner, E., 27, 218, 219, 236n, 248, 249, 252, 253, 293 and n, 316n
Jessop, T., 165n, 169n
Jewson, N.D., 15n, 42n, 178n
Johnson, Dr S., 139n, 142n, 281
Johnston, N., 143
Johnstone, E., 158
Jones, C., 112n
Jones, M., 19n, 61
Jordan, D., 212n
Joseph II, Emperor, 292, 294
Josselyn, J., 214, 215
Juncker, J., 108
Jurin, J., 30, 32, 130n, 131, 173, and n, 178, 180 and n, 181, 182
Jurine, L., 315n

Kamman, M., 203n
Kant, 1, 83
Kegel-Brinkgreve, E., 40n, 48n, 50n, 54n, 101n
Keill, James, 105, 112, 114, 129, 130, 131, 171, 173
Keill, John, 173, 175
Kenyon, J., 168n
Kett, J., 177n
Kieft, L., 287n
Kilpatrick, R., 11n
King, L., 111n, 135n
King-Hele, D., 159n
King's College, New York, 195
Knight, T., 179
Knoefel, P., 281n, 292n, 294n, 300, 301n, 302n, 314n
Kramer, G., 73n
Krüger, J., 84
Kuhn, A., 185, 186n
Kundmann, J., 86 and n

Labadie, J. de, 73
Laboucheix, H., 288n
Labroquère, F., 106 and n
Lamb, G., 179n
La Motte, G. M. de, 36
Lancisi, G., 293
Landriani, M., 281, 282, 292 and n, 293, 294,

295, 296 and n, 297–9, 300, 301, 302, 311 and n, 312
Langdon-Davies, J., 18n
Langen, A., 79n
Laplace, P., 305
Latitudinarians, 33, 167, 168, 172, 173, 176, 181, 186, 189
Lavoisier, A., 289 and n, 290, 293, 304, 305, 307, 308 and n, 313 and n, 314 and n
Law, W., 185
Lawrence, C., 65n, 177n, 221n, 283n, 284n, 285 and n
Leade, J., 73
Leake, J., 14n
Leblanc, N., 315
Lee, S. 156 and n
Le Fanu, W., 9, 10
Leibezeit, G., 84
Leibniz, 71 and n, 83, 84, 95, 130, 133, 168, 173, 187 and n
Leiden, 40, 42, 43, 44, 45, 58, 64, 65
Leigh, C., 157
Leipzig, 73, 74
Lenman, B., 170n
Lettsom, J., 142, 218, 220, 225, 228 and n, 229, 233, 255–62 and n, 264–74, 276, 277, 278 and n, 280
Levellers, 72
Levin, J., 32n
Levine, J., 142n
Lewes, C., 317n
Lewis, J., 5n
Lewis, W., 146, 147 and n
Lewis, W. S., 179n
Lindberg, D., 186n
Lindeboom, G., 40n, 43n, 44n, 47n, 50n, 54n, 56n
Linnaeus, C., 100 and n, 111, 127, 266n
Lister, M., 132
Litchfield, R., 294n
Lloyd, family of, 260, 263n
Lobo, F., 257, 258n
Locke, J, 1, 119 and n, 166n, 191
London, 4–49
Loss, F., 143n
Loudon, I, 35n, 139n, 148n, 156n, 177n, 255 and n
Lower, R., 143n
Lucas, C., 149, 150 and n, 154, 179n
Luce, A., 165n, 185n
Lunar Society, 158, 224, 225, 227, 313
Luther, 73
Lutheranism, 73
Luyendijk-Elshout, A., 40n, 48n, 50n, 54n, 101n
Macdonald, M., 171n
Macdonogh, F., 14
McEvoy, G., 284n, 288n
McGuire, J., 172n, 288n
Mack, M., 317n
McKie, D., 285n, 288n
McLachlan, H., 228n
McManners, J., 305n
McNeil, M., 285n, 291n
Macquer, P., 308n
Maddox, R., 148n
Magellan, J., 289, 291 and n, 292n, 311 and n, 313 and n
Magnol, P., 113
Maitland, C., 27, 28, 31
Malebranche, N., 185n
Malinowski, B., 140
Maloney, W., 255n
Malpighi, M., 115n
Mann, Sir H., 179 and n
Mansfield, Lord, 262n
Maria Theresa, Empress, 292
Marshall, H., 214n
Martin, B., 309, 310
Martin, G., 57, 65
Martin, R. R. J., 4n, 32n, 100, 113n, 173n
Massey, Revd E., 30, 31 and n
Mather, C., 208, 209, 213, 214
Mathias, P., 316n
Matthias, C., 44
Mead, R., 30, 32, 130n, 143n, 146, 173n
Meara, E. de, 143n
mechanism, 2, 82–5, 95, 96, 129
mechanists, 79, 90, 91, 99, 102, 103, 104, 110, 133
Medical Society of London, 258, 260, 271–80
Medical Society of Philadelphia, 203, 204
Medical Society of South Carolina, 194
Mercier, L., 304n
Methodism, 21
Methodists, 107, 108, 228
Meusnier, J., 313n, 314n
Middleton, P., 200
Milanese Patriotic Society, 292, 294
Millar, J., 278n
Miller, G., 24n, 32n, 181n, 182n, 195 and n
Miller, H., 178n
Millingen, J., 142n
Mills, C., 144n
Minard, R., 210n
Mitchison, R., 61n
Mittelstrass, J., 71n
Monardes, N., 213
Monro, A. (Primus), 57, 64 and n, 65 and n, 166
Monro, A., (Secundus), 266n
Monro, J., 64, and n

Monsey, M., 153
Montague, F., 284n
Montpellier, 111–37
Moogk, P., 140n
Mora, G., 295n
morality, 165–93
Moravians, 79
Morellet, A., 294
Morgan, J., 200, 203, 204n
Morrell, J., 58n
Moscati, P., 281, 292 and n, 293, 295, 296
Mullett, C., 281n
Murdoch, A., 61n
Murrell, P., 153n
Myer, G., 38n

Nader, L., 140 and n
Natural Law, 1, 2, 88, 96, 108, 109, 110
Natural Religion, 109, 110
Natural Theology, 110
nature, 78–82
Natzmer, General G.D. von, 68, 83
Neal, Revd D., 30
Nenter, G., 108
Nettleton, Dr T., 30
Newman, Sir G., 261n
Newport, Sir J., 226n
Newton, Sir I., 1, 45, 49, 50, 51n, 62n, 88, 113, and n, 115, 129–34, 136, 137, 165, 167, 168, 171, 172, 174, 175, 176, 184–90, 192
Newtonian natural philosophy, 128–31; Newtonians, 168, 169, 171, 173, 182, 185
Nicander, 49
Nicholl, H., 167n
Nicolai, E., 84
Nicolson, Malcolm, 15n, 42n
Nicolson, Marjorie, 178 and n, 180n
nitrous air, 285–92
Noble, V., 261n
nosology, 103–10, 134–7
Nuck, A., 47
Numbers, R., 196n, 213n
Nutton, V., 49n, 67n, 75n

Odier, Dr, 245, 249
Oldenburg, H., 185 and n
Oldmixon, J., 23n
Oliver, W., 149, 150 and n, 151, 155
Orange, House of, 58, 62
Osman, W., 311n
Otto, M., 96n
Owen, D., 11n
Owen, J., 144n

Pace, A., 293n, 300n
Packard, F., 203n
Padua, 41
Paltz, E., 79n
Paracelsus, 49
Paramore, T., 215n
Parascandola, J., 287
Parham, Lord Willoughby de, 226 and n
Parini, G., 293
Paris, 5
Partington, J., 313n, 314n
pathology, 88–110, 98, 99
Pattison, F., 142n
Pawpaw, J., 215
Payne, J., 260n
Peachey, G., 14n, 15
Peck, J., 159n
Peel, Sir R., 226n
Pelling, M., 199n
Pemberton, H., 130 and n, 173 and n
Penn, T., 203
Penn, W., 261 and n
Percival, T., 25, 157 and n, 170, 218, 220 and n, 224, 225 and n, 226, 227, 230, 231n, 232 and n, 233 and n, 234 and n, 235, 236, 237, 242, 245, 248n, 249, 257, 282, 285n
Perrin, C., 29
Peter Leopold II, Grand Duke of Tuscany, 292, 294, 300, 306, 315
Peterson, J., 73
Pettigrew, T., 262n, 273
Petty, W., 18n
Philadelphia, College of, 195
Philanthropic Society, 278
Philanthropy, 2, 254–80
Phillipson, N., 61n
Phlogistic chemistry, 285–92
Pickstone, J., 157n, 222n, 224n, 242n
Pietism, 67–87, 89–95
Pigott, F., 147 and n
Pillonière, F. de la, 144n
Pinckard, G. 278n
Pinson, K., 89n
Piquer, A., 159n
Pitcairne, A., 49n, 102, 112, 113n, 114, 115, 129, 131, 133, 136, 140n, 171, 173
Pitcairne, O., 155n
Pitt, W., the Younger, 247, 248
Place, F., 5, 7
Plato, 45, 191
Platonists, 191
Plumb, J., 32n, 170n
Plummer, A., 57, 65
Plumtree, Dr, 163
pneumatic medicine, 281–318
pneumatology, 2, 109 and n
Pocock, J., 288n
Port, M., 23n
Porter, R., 24n, 36n, 112n, 133n, 160n, 171n,

177 and n, 181n, 199n, 221n, 260 and n, 279n
Porterfield, G., 166
Porteus, Bishop, 229 and n
Posner, E., 159n
Power, E., 5
Poynter, N., 255n, 318n
Presbyterians, 60
Price, R., 226, 228, 230, 231 and n, 243, 244, 247, 253, 291n
Priestley, J., 224, 226, 228, 229, 282–93, 295, 296, 300 and n, 302, 304, 305, 308, 310–16, 318
Pringle, Sir J., 282, 283, 284, 285 and n, 286, 288, 292, 293n, 306, 309, 316
Prior, T., 170, 171n, 178n, 179 and n, 180 and n, 181 and n, 191n, 192 and n
professional disputes, 138–64
progress, 2
Protestants, 3; Enthusiastic, 77, 79, 81, 82, 83, 89, 91, 93, 110; radical, 68, 71, 72, 73, 74, 80, 81, 82, 83, 87, 91
Prussian Royal Society, 67
psychology, 2
Puffendorf, S., 96n
Puritans, 196
Pythagoreans, 191

Quaker, Quakers, 18, 219, 222, 225, 226, 228, 229, 236, 257, 259–68, 270, 272, 273, 274, 276, 280
Quedlinburg, 73, 74, 75
Quinn, A., 175n

Rack H., 171n
Radcliffe, J., 9
Raeff, M., 317n
Raistrick, A., 261 and n, 262, 263n
Ramazzini, B., 293, 300
Ramsay, D., 194, 195
Ranby, J., 155 and n, 156
Rand, B., 169n
Rannie, W., 21n
Ranters, 72
Rather, L. 71n, 77n
Ratte, H. de, 112
Ray, J., 94, 118, 119 and n
Razzell, P., 24n, 235n
Réamur, 307
Reason, 1, 2
Redwood, J., 168n
Reed, H., 293n
Reeve, T., 179n
Reformation, 90
Reich, J., 83, 86 and n
Relph, J., 278n
Rendall, J., 57n
Restoration, 75
Revelation, 1
Revolution, French, 2
Rhodes, P., 14n
Richardson, R., 305n, 317n
Richardson, S., 38n
Richetti, J., 166n
Richter, C., 78, 79n, 80 and n, 81 and n, 82, 86
Ricuperati, G., 294n, 295n
Riley, J., 293n, 304n, 315n
Risse, G., 213n
Ritterbush, P., 173
Roberts, H., 34n
Roberts, S., 141
Robinson, B., 174 and n, 185 and n, 188
Robinson, H., 166n
Rochford, Lord, 156
Rose, C., 21, 23, 24n
Rosen, G., 72n, 317n
Rosenberg, A., 255n
Rosetti, J., 101 and n, 102, 106
Rothstein, E., 178n
Rousseau, G., 177n, 178 and n, 180n, 281n
Rowntree, family of, 263n
Royal College of Physicians of London, 56, 113, 138, 139, 141 and n, 142, 144n, 145, 148, 152, 162, 173, 178, 179n, 196, 203, 243, 260, 271, 272, 276, 277, 278n, 282
Royal College of Physicians of Edinburgh, 63, 65
Royal Humane Society, 229, 278
Royal Medical Society of Edinburgh, 273n
Royal Society, 25, 27, 29, 32, 34, 38, 51n, 72, 113, 115n, 173, 175, 183, 195, 201, 214, 226, 233n, 282, 285, 286, 301, 312
Rozier, Pilâtre de, 307, 308 and n
Ruf, W., 87
Rule, G., 60
Rush, B., 214 and n
Russel, R., 145 and n, 146 and n, 147, 148
Russell, P., 226n
Russell, Revd R., 22
Rutherford, J., 57, 65
Rutman, A., 206n
Rutman, B., 206n

Sachsen-Weimar, 73
Sachsen-Weimar, Johann E. von, Duke, 68, 74, 75
St-Clair, A. (also Sinclair), 57, 65
Salusbury-Brereton, O., 226n
Samber, R., 35
Sasson, L, 56n
Saunders, W., 278n
Sauvages, F., 88–110; and nosology, 103–10, 111–37
Sayn-Wittgenstein, the Counts, 73

Schade, J., 93
Schaff, P., 48n
Schaffer, S., 38n, 48n, 130n, 175n, 282n, 284n
Scheele, K., 292, 306, 316
Schmidt, M., 79n
Schofield, R., 174n, 184n, 185n, 190n, 225n, 291n, 292n, 306n, 312n
Schreiner, O., 5
Schulz, M., 73n, 74, 75n
Schulze, J., 93n, 94n, 96n, 97
Scotland, 41, 57–66
Scotus, Duns, 45
Scull, A., 263, 264n
Sena, J., 72n
Senebier, J., 311, 314 and n
Seward, A., 227
Seward, W., 226n
Shadwell, J., 278n
Shapin, S., 48n, 166n, 167n
Sharpin, E., 152, 153n
Shaw, P., 176 and n, 182, 183 and n
Shearman, W., 278n
Sheils, W., 171n
Shelburne, Lord, 282, 283, 288, 291, 293, 312
Sheridan, A., 11n
Shippen, W., 200
Shuckburgh, Sir G., 226n
Siebenschuh, B., 182n
Siegel, S., 29n
Simbert, J., 192
Simmons, S., 278n, 279 and n
Simpson, A., 58n, 64n
Simpson, W., 143
Sims, James, 270n, 278 and n
Sims, John, 278n
Sinclair, see St-Clair
Singer, D., 285n
Skinner, A., 57n
Slayer, Dr, 184
Sleech, Archdeacon, 144n
Sloan, P., 119n
Sloane, Sir H., 27, 28, 29, 30, 34, 37
smallpox, 24–34, 217–53
Smellie, W., 35, 36
Smith, A., 220
Smith, G., 156n
Smith, J. R., 24n
Smith, J. S., 154n
Smith, S., 317n, 318 and n
Smith, V., 177n
Smith, W., 203 and n
Smith, W. H., 179n
Smollett, T., 36, 149 and n, 150n, 151, 281n
Snape, A., 132, 144n
Société Royale de Médecine, 304 and n, 315 and n
Société Royale des Sciences, 126
Society of Apothecaries, 196
Society of Friends, *see* Quakers
Society for the Promotion of Christian Knowledge, 19, 20, 21; Scottish, 61
Society for the Reformation of Manners, 61
Sosa, E., 166n
soul, 68–87, 88–110
South Sea Company, 169
Speck, W., 21n
Spector, B., 317n
Spedding, J., 116n
Spencer, H., 34n
Spencer, W., 18n
Spener, P., 74 and n, 78, 89, 93, 94 and n
Spinoza, 54, 95
Sprengel, K, 87
Sprögel, J., 73n, 74 and n, 75n
Stahl, G., 67–87, 88–110
Stahlians, 108
Stansfield, D., 285n
Starr, J., 140n
Steffan, T., 72n
Steigerthal, Dr J., 28, 30
Steiner, B., 198n
Steinmetz, A., 142n
Steinmetz, M., 73n
Stenhouse, A., 198
Stephens, J., 155
Sterne, L., 144n
Stevenson, J., 144n
Stevenson, L., 278n
Steward, T., 152 and n, 153 and n
Stewart, L., 29n, 32n, 34 and n, 167n, 181 and n
Stillingfleet, Bishop, 94
Stimson, D., 51n
Stoughton, J., 265n
Stuart, House of, 60
Stürzbecher, M., 68n
Sullivan, R., 167n
Surgeon-Apothecaries, Incorporation of, 63, 65
Surgeons, Company of, 154, 277
Sutcliff, A., 259
Sutherland, G., 317n
Sutton, family of, 25, 236
Swinton, A., 210n
Sydenham, T., 47, 49, 50 and n, 62n, 65, 75, 112, 113n, 122 and n, 129n

tar-water, 165–93
Tate, T., 212n
Tate, W., 33n
Tawney, R., 228n
Taylor, T., 265n
Tenon, J., 10, 11n

Terence, 44
Terry, family of, 263n
Thackray, A., 166n
Theophrastus, 119
Thomas, K., 33n
Thomasius, C., 83 and n, 84, 89
Thompson, E., 32n
Thompson, G., 144n
Thompson, R., 140n
Thomson, A., 202n
Thomson, J., 57n, 65n, 220n, 221n, 222 and n, 225n, 227n, 232n, 241n, 245n, 266n
Thornton, J., 22
Thornton, R., 278n
Thuringia, 75
Timonius, E., 208 and n, 214
Tindal, M., 167, 168, 171
Tipton, L., 180n, 191 and n
Toellner, R., 71n
Tofts, M., 155
Toland, J., 167 and n, 171
Tolles, F., 261n, 262 and n
Tonstall, G., 143 and n
Tory, Tories, 4n–39, 155, 157, 161, 166, 167, 170, 222, 223, 230
Tournefort, J., 100, 113, 118–20, 121, 122, 123, 126
Tozzetti, G., 300, 301
Treacher, A., 318n
Trebeck, Revd A., 21n, 22
Trevelyan, G., 7, 168
Trigland, J., 45
Trollope, W., 179
Tuke, family of, 263, 264
Turbayne, C., 191n
Turgot, A.-R.-J., 304
Turi, G., 294n

Unitarians, 224, 225, 228, 229
Unschuld, P. 140n
Unwins, D., 278n
Unzer, J., 84
Urrea, G. de, 142n

Van Helmont, 49
Van Swieten, G., 40
Vaughan, B., 312
Vaux, Cadet de, 304
Vaux, G., 270n
Venice, 42
Venturi, F., 294n, 293n, 295n, 304n
Verri, A., 281n, 296
Verri, P., 281 and n, 294, 300
Versluysen, M., 34n
Vesalius, A., 47
Vicq d'Azyr, F., 304
Vidal, A. 159n
Vienna, 40
Vieussens, R., 104
virtue, 281–318
Viseltear, A. 217n
vital motions, 131–4
Volta, A., 296, 300, 310, 311 and n, 312, 313, 314, 315
Voltaire, 1, 304
Vossius, G., 44

Waddington, I., 138, 144 and n, 157n, 278n
Wadsworth, Dr, 163
Wagstaffe, W., 27, 28, 30
Wake, J., 278n
Walker, S., 278n
Wall, M., 245
Wallis, P., 37n
Wallis, R., 37n
Walpole, Sir R., 32, 33, 168, 169, 170, 179
Walsh, L. 210n
Walshman, T., 278n
Ward, J., 177, 178n, 182, 184
Warder, J., 143, 144n
Wareing, J., 148
Warner, J., 217n
Waterhouse, B., 220, 226, 227, 245, 249 and n
Watermann, R., 282n, 314n
Watson, J., 261n
Watson, W., 226n
Watts, G., 158
Wear, A., 50n, 102n, 112n, 122n, 133n, 171n
Weaver, G., 217n, 219n
Webb, B., 6
Webb, S., 6
Weber, M., 144 and n
Webster, C., 11n, 18n, 39 and n, 157n
Wedgwood, J., 224, 229, 291
Weissbach, C., 83, 86
Wesley, J., 177 and n, 178, 186
Wesley, S., 20, 21 and n, 22
Weydenhain, C., 73n, 74
whig (whiggish) history, 4n
Whig, Whigs, 4 (note), 22–39, 58, 60, 151, 157, 161, 167, 168, 170, 172, 179, 181, 184, 223, 230, 282; Scottish, 61, 62
Whiston, W., 30, 168 and n, 171, 175
White, C., 161
White, T., 161, 163
Whitehead, J., 278n
Whytt, R., 97n, 98, 101, 102 and n, 103 and n, 105n, 106n, 166
Wilberforce, W., 229, 247
Wilde, C., 168 and n, 186n
Wildes, H., 261n
Wilhelm, J., 73
Wilkes, J., 7

Wilkinson, family of, 260, 263n
Wilkinson, K., 159n
Willeford, B., 287n
William III, of England, 24, 58, 60
Williamson, G., 72n
Williamson, R., 113n
Willis, B., 143n
Willis, T., 104, 143n
Wilson, A., 5n, 34n, 35n, 36n
Wilson, B., 219n
Wilson, G. 314n
Wilson, J., 248
Wisdom, T., 20, 22
Wise, F., 143n
Witham, R., 21n, 22
Withering, W., 158, 159n
Wittet, T., 37n
Wittie, R., 143 and n
Wogan, W., 17, 21n, 22
Wolff, C., 68, 69n, 71 and n, 82 and n, 83, 84, 89, 96 and n, 108, 109
Woodville, W., 278n
Woodward, John, 11n, 18n
Woodward, John (fl.1720), 27, 32n, 142 and n
Worthington, Revd, 248
Worthington, T., 161, 163
Wortley Montagu, Lady M., 27, 28, 30, 182 and n
Wright, P., 318n
Wright-St. Clair, R., 64n

York Retreat, 263, 264
Young, A. 291 and n

Zinzendorff, C., 79n
Zinzendorff, Count N., 73, 79n